Clinical Consult to

Psychiatric Mental Health Care

Jacqueline Rhoads, PhD, ACNP-BC, ANP-C, PMHNP, FAANP, is Professor and Director of Graduate Program of Nursing at University of Texas Medical Branch in Galveston, Professor at Louisiana State University Health Science Center School of Nursing, Adjunct Professor at Tulane University School of Public Health in New Orleans, and Adult Nurse Practitioner at Odyssey House Free Clinic in New Orleans and at the U.S. Army-Reserve Command in Washington, DC. Dr. Rhoads has taught in nurse practitioner programs since 1994. She has been awarded major research funding for a variety of research projects, including $1.5 million Tri-Service Dept of Defense Combat Readiness project, two HRSA grants ($1 million CRNA Specialization project and $600,000 CRNA and NP Distance Education Program), and a $150,000 Role Delineation Study: Acute Care Nurse Practitioner grant from ANCC. She has been Primary Investigator for research on behalf of March of Dimes, United Way, NONPF and the military. Dr. Rhoads earned her PhD from the University of Texas, Austin, and has earned post-master's degrees in Acute Care NP, Community Health Primary Care Adult NP, Gerontology NP, and Psychiatric Mental Health NP. She is a Fellow in the American Academy of NPs, and was awarded numerous commendations and medals for meritorious service in the U.S. Army Nurse Corps, including the Bronze Star, U.S. Army Meritorious Service Commendation, Army Commendation Medal (eleven times!), the Vietnam Service Medal, and numerous academic and teaching awards, including Outstanding Faculty Award (undergraduate and graduate), STT Care Award, Outstanding Demonstration of Research and Practice Award, ten Teaching Excellence Award nominations, Commander of Outstanding Reserve Unit Award, and, lastly, Reserve Nurse of the Year (American Association of Military Surgeons of the United States, 1997 and 1998). Dr. Rhoads has authored three books for major nursing publishers as well as numerous articles.

Clinical Consult to

Psychiatric Mental Health Care

Jacqueline Rhoads, PhD, ACNP-BC, ANP-C, PMHNP, FAANP

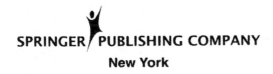
SPRINGER PUBLISHING COMPANY
New York

Springer Publishing Company, LLC
11 West 42nd Street
New York, NY 10036
www.springerpub.com

Acquisitions Editor: Margaret Zuccarini
Project Manager: Peter Rocheleau
Cover Design: David Levy
Composition: Aptara Inc.

ISBN: 978-0-8261-0501-1
E-book ISBN: 978-0-8261-0502-8

10 11 12 13 / 5 4 3 2 1

Library of Congress Cataloging-in-Publication Data

CIP data is available from the Library of Congress.

The author and the publisher of this Work have made every effort to use sources believed to be reliable to provide
information that is accurate and compatible with the standards generally accepted at the time of publication. Because
medical science is continually advancing, our knowledge base continues to expand. Therefore, as new information
becomes available, changes in procedures become necessary. We recommend that the reader always consult current
research and specific institutional policies before performing any clinical procedure. The author and publisher shall not
be liable for any special, consequential, or exemplary damages resulting, in whole or in part, from the readers' use of, or
reliance on, the information contained in this book.

The publisher has no responsibility for the persistence or accuracy of URLs for external or third-party Internet Web sites
referred to in this publication and does not guarantee that any content on such Web sites is, or will remain, accurate or
appropriate.

Special discounts on bulk quantities of our books are available to corporations, professional associations, pharmaceutical
companies, health care organizations, and other qualifying groups. If you are interested in a custom book, including
chapters from more than one of our titles, we can provide that service as well.

For details, please contact:
Special Sales Department, Springer Publishing Company, LLC
11 West 42nd Street, 15th Floor, New York, NY 10036-8002
Phone: 877-687-7476 or 212-431-4370; Fax: 212-941-7842
Email: sales@springerpub.com

Printed in the United States of America by Gasch Printing

To my husband Jim
who died before this book was completed.

Jim put up with me, taught me,
edited me, believed in me,
and encouraged me to believe I could be a writer...

After thirty years of shared laughter, love, and tears,
it's hard to let him go.

With deepest thanks.

I love you sweetheart.

Contents

II. Syndromes and Treatments in Adult Psychiatry

III. Syndromes and Treatments in Child and Adolescent Psychiatry

Reviewers

Marion Newton, PhD, PNP
Professor, Shendoah University, Winchester, Virginia

Meena Patel, ARNP, DNP (Candidate)
Overland Park, Kansas

Kristen Vandenberg, MSN, ARNP, FNP-BC
Instructor/Nursing, University of North Florida, Brooks College of Health

Alma I. Vega, EdD, MSN, ARNP-BC
Assistant Professor, University of Miami School of Nursing and Health
  Studies, Coral Gables, Florida

Lucinda Whitney, MSN, ARPN-BC
Marillac Home, Overland Park, Kansas

Contributors

Renee R. Azzouz, ARNP
Overland Park, Kansas

Athena J. Arthur, MS, LCDC
Doctoral Student, Fielding Graduate University, Santa Barbara, California

Sandra S. Bauman, PhD, ARNP, LMHC
Lecturer, School of Nursing and Health Studies, University of Miami School,
    Coral Gables, Florida

Virginia Brooke, RN, PhD
University of Texas Medical Branch Medical School, Galveston, Texas

Deonne J. Brown-Benedict, DNP, ARNP, FNP-BC
Assistant Professor and Family Nurse Practitioner Track Clinical Coordinator,
    College of Nursing, Seattle University, Seattle, Washington

Angela Chia-Chen Chen, PhD, RN
Assistant Professor, College of Nursing and Health Innovation, Arizona State
    University, Phoenix, Arizona

Lawrence S. Dilks, PhD
Clinical Neuropsychologist, Lake Charles, Louisiana

Susan O. Edionwe, MD
University of Texas Medical Branch Medical School, Galveston, Texas

Elizabeth Hite Erwin, PhD, APRN-BC
Assistant Professor, School of Nursing, University of Virginia,
    Charlottesville, Virginia

Deborah Gilbert-Palmer, EdD, FNP-BC
Associate Professor of Nursing and FNP Program Coordinator, Department of
    Nursing, Arkansas State University, State University, Arizona

Nnenna I. Igbo, MD
University of Texas Medical Branch Medical School, Galveston, Texas

Jose Levy, MA, BCBA, CBIST
Fielding Graduate University, Austin, Texas

Jo-Ann Summitt Marrs, EdD, FNP.BC
East Tennessee State University, Johnson City, Tennessee

Patrick J. M. Murphy, PhD
College of Nursing, Seattle University, Seattle, Washington

Meena Patel, ARNP, DNP (Candidate)
Overland Park, Kansas

Nancy Pierce, ARNP
Psychiatric and Counseling Associates, Leawood, Kansas

Theresa Raphael-Grimm, PhD, RN, CS
University of North Carolina, Chapel Hill, North Carolina

Judy Rice, BSN, MSN FNPCS
Johnson City, Tennessee

Victoria Soltis-Jarrett, PhD, PMHCNS/NP-BC
Clinical Associate Professor and Coordinator, University of North Carolina,
    Chapel Hill, North Carolina

Kimberly Swanson, PhD
Research Interventionalist, University of Washington School of Social Work,
    Seattle, Washington

Hisn-Yi (Jean) Tang, PhD, APRN
Assistant Professor, College of Nursing, Seattle University, Seattle, Washington

Kristen Vandenberg, MSN, ARNP, FNP-BC
University of North Florida, Jacksonville, Florida

Alma Vega, EdD, MSN, ARNP-BC
Assistant Professor, School of Nursing and Health Studies, University of
    Miami, Coral Gables, Florida

Lucinda Whitney, MSN, ARNP-BC
Overland Park, Kansas

Elizabeth Willford
University of Texas Medical Branch Medical School, Galveston, Texas

Preface

The devastation of the Gulf Coast after Hurricane Katrina has been imprinted in our memory, not only by the sensational news coverage but also by the personal experiences of many health care providers who volunteered countless hours in helping the people affected by this disaster. I was one of those providers who responded. From that experience came a realization of how many people were and are affected by mental illness, and how little I knew of the protocols that could be used to provide mental health care to those I served. I went back to school for my post-master's degree in psychiatric mental health and saw the lack of published information that would lend assistance to those caring for people with mental disorders.

I hope that this book gives readers a greater array of protocols that are helpful in offering optimal mental health care to those they serve. My goal is to integrate the latest pharmacologic and psychotherapeutic approaches to assist health care providers in treatment planning.

The concepts of mental health and mental disorder are vague and there is little agreement among mental health providers about how to define these concepts as well as how to diagnose and treat mental disorders. While the medical issues surrounding mental health and mental disorder are important, this book focuses on other key issues pertaining to mental health assessment and treatment. The overall goal of the book is to engage students, faculty, and mental health care providers. It is hoped that the book will be useful in providing evidence-based guidelines that could be considered in caring for those with a mental health disorder. The book also is designed to help those providers in the primary care specialties of family practice, internal medicine, pediatrics, and obstetrics/gynecology increase their "comfort zone" in working with the array of mental health issues in patients who present every week in a busy medical practice.

Although this book is written primarily for practicing primary care clinicians, I also hope to reach residents, medical and nursing students, and other providers who could benefit from guidelines about "what to do next" when working with and beginning the treatment of a patient with a mental health disorder. This book provides recommendations to help providers make treatment decisions for patients with psychiatric disorders. Because these decisions should be supported by the best available evidence derived from current research and expert consensus, these guidelines were developed by expert work groups, whose members reviewed available evidence using an explicit methodology. As a result, every guideline has been reviewed and approved for publication by consultants and a panel of experts. This process balances the conclusions of scientific research with the practical experience of professionals working in the field.

In addition to providing recommendations that may improve patient care, the guidelines can be used as a course textbook for advanced practice nursing students, physician assistant students, and medical students. They may also serve as a review book for psychiatric advanced practice nurses seeking certification or recertification, as well as other mental health professionals. Researchers may use the guidelines to identify important clinical questions for which further research could improve the treatment decision-making process.

This professional clinical reference is designed specifically to provide the information needed for the advanced practitioner to:

- Understand the clinical features and symptoms of a wide range of psychiatric disorders, both adult and pediatric.
- Make a confident differential diagnosis.
- Evaluate interventions commonly used to treat specific disorders.
- Select the appropriate site of service.
- Educate the patient and family.
- Assess the efficacy and risks of available medications.
- Develop an individualized treatment plan.

This book offers fast and efficient access to evidence-based diagnostic and therapeutic guidelines for managing psychiatric and mental health conditions, organized by *DSM-IV* disorder categories arranged into chapters. This design and organization enables the advanced practitioner to quickly access key information on disorders and syndromes that is presented using a the following standard format: definition of disorder, etiology, demograhics, risk factors, differential diagnosis, ICD codes, diagnostic workups and laboratory evaluations, initial assessment, clinical presentation, signs and symptoms, *DSM-IV* diagnosis, acute and chronic treatment, patient education points, and medical/legal pitfalls. Reference lists are provided at the end of each chapter.

In a few instances, such as the very complicated Disruptive Behavior Disorders, the content is presented in a format designed to help the reader compare and contrast the individual disorders that comprise the Disruptive Behavior "complex," including Conduct Disorder, Oppositional Defiant Disorder, and Attention Deficit Disorder. Because these disorders present somewhat differently in the very young child than in the school-age and adolescent person, the individual disorders are again presented in Chapter 19, "Disorders Usually Presenting in Middle Childhood or Adolescence."

Jacqueline Rhoads

I

General Psychiatry

The Psychiatric Interview

Introduction

- The psychiatric interview is the core of proper psychiatric evaluation. It plays an important role not only in clinical assessment but also in therapy. The interviewer should come to understand the patient's behaviors, emotions, experiences, and psychological, social, religious influences and motivations through verbal and nonverbal communication with the patient.
- The psychiatric interview can be divided into the following stages: building an alliance with the patient, psychiatric history, diagnostic evaluation, and treatment plan formulation.
- As with all interviews, the patient–provider relationship is very important. An intact relationship between the interviewer and the patient increases the patient's confidence and willingness to disclose the personal or sensitive information necessary for diagnosis and facilitates patient compliance.
- The psychiatric interview depends on more than verbal communication; it requires that the physician be observant and listens. Nonverbal communication can provide insight necessary for the patient's clinical assessment and diagnosis, especially in patients significantly impaired by psychiatric disease.
- The extent of psychiatric impairment may necessitate that the interviews occur in multiple sessions or depend on information from additional persons such as family members or friends.
- The interview should begin with an open-ended approach.
- A structured interview approach combines the psychiatric interview with diagnostic criteria in attempts to derive a thorough psychiatric history.

The Patient–Provider Relationship: Building an Alliance

- The patient–provider relationship is fundamental to providing excellent care, improving patient outcomes, and the healing process. It has special significance in psychiatry where the "stigma" of psychiatric treatment can make even seeking treatment difficult.
- A solid patient–clinician relationship requires optimization of the following seven principles
  - Communication
  - Office experience
  - Hospital experience
  - Patient education
  - Integration (information sharing among all members of the treatment team)
  - Shared decision making
  - Outcomes
- The patient–provider relationship involves a working or therapeutic alliance, which is an agreement between provider and patient, based on mutual rapport and trust, to undertake treatment together.
- The interviewer must be sensitive to the importance of empathy, respect, and trust to develop a good working alliance.
- Distrust is a common reason for noncompliance. In fact, most instances of noncompliance come from interruption to the provider–patient relationship.
- The interviewer should develop a rapport with the patient:
  - Remain attentive:
    - Maintain eye contact
    - Minimize distractions such as excessive note-taking or interrupting the patient while speaking
  - Be empathic:
    - Show the patient an understanding and appreciation for his or her situation.
    - Reinforce what the patient is feeling. One way to do this is by making statements such as, "I can see that was a very difficult time for you."
  - Listen! Listen! Listen!

The Interview: Nonverbal Communication

- Active observation of the patient should occur within the first minutes of the interview, before names have been exchanged and the "formal" interview has begun.
- Actively process the patient's nonverbal communication, such as:
  - How does the patient first greet the interviewer?
  - Does the patient make eye contact?
  - What items (books or pictures, etc.) are present?
  - What is the patient wearing and is his or her appearance disheveled or neat?
  - What (if any) unusual sounds or smells are in the room?
- Observation of the patient should continue throughout the interview. The interviewer should take note of the patient's body language and emotional expressions during responses to the questions.
- For example, a patient who becomes emotional when asked about a spouse may be depressed about a recent divorce or loss of a loved one.
- Certain kinds of nonverbal communication are included in diagnostic criteria and the interviewer should be cognizant of their presence.
- Active observation becomes increasingly important with increases in psychiatric impairments.

The Interview: Verbal Communication

- Open-ended questions
  - After formally introducing yourself and your role in the patient's care, start by asking open-ended questions.
  - Examples of open-ended questions:
    - Tell me what brings you here?
    - Tell me what kinds of problems you have had, lately?
  - Three reasons why an open-ended manner of interviewing is important:
    - It strengthens the patient–provider relationship by showing that the interviewer is interested in the concerns of the patient.
    - It provides insight into the patient's condition.
    - It allows the interviewer to understand what is most important to the patient rather than making assumptions.
  - The interviewer should engage in active listening as the patient responds to questions.
- Diagnosis-specific questions
  - As the history develops, specific questions such as, "Do you see things that others cannot see?" (hallucinations) or "Have you ever tried to harm yourself?" (suicidal ideations) become necessary.
  - These specific questions aim at gathering information necessary for diagnosis based on *DSM-IV* criteria.
  - The interviewer should be able to use transition from open-ended questions to more specific ones.
    - For example, "Now I would like to ask you about several psychological symptoms that patients might experience."

Structured Interviews

- A structured interview uses a series of questions that couple the interview method with the *DSM-IV* diagnostic criteria in attempts to explore the signs and symptoms necessary for diagnosis.
- Examples
  - The MINI-International Neuropsychiatric Interview (MINI[-Plus])
  - Structured Clinical Interview for *DSM-IV* disorders (SCID)
  - Composite International Diagnostic Interview (CIDI)
  - Schedules for Clinical Assessment in Neuropsychiatry (SCAN)

Psychiatric Interview ICD-9 Codes Volumes 1, 2, and 3 (2009)

- Interview, psychiatric NEC 94.19
- Interview, psychiatric NEC, follow-up 94.19
- Interview, psychiatric NEC, initial 94.19
- Interview, psychiatric NEC, precommitment 94.13

The Diagnostic Encounter

Phases of the Diagnostic Encounter

The diagnostic encounter is divided into three phases:
- Opening phase
- Body of the interview
- Closing phase

Opening Phase
- Initial 5–10 minutes
- Goals
  - Introductions
  - Preinterview preparation
    - For example, ease patient's fears or concerns about the necessity for the interview
  - Build a therapeutic alliance
  - Keep questions open-ended and allow the patient to speak uninterrupted for an appropriate amount of time

Body of the Interview
- Thirty to forty-five minutes
- Goals
  - Psychiatric history
  - Diagnosis-specific questions such as, "Does this patient meet *DSM-IV* criteria for diagnosis?"
  - Mental status exam (MSE)
  - Physical exam
  - Additional investigations

Closing Phase
- Five to ten minutes
- Goals
  - Review your assessment with the patient
  - Collaborate with the patient on a treatment and follow-up plan

Psychiatric History
- *Identifying data*: collecting basic details about the patient, such as name, sex, age, religion, educational status, occupation, relationship status, and contact details.
- *Chief complaint* (CC): the reason for the patient's presentation.
- *History of present illness* (HPI): the interviewer attempts to gain a clear understanding of the full history of the patient's problems, such as when they started, what they entail, worsening symptoms, or associated symptoms. The HPI allows the interviewer to formulate preliminary hypotheses as to a diagnosis.
- *Past medical history* (PMH): the interviewer should explore the PMH to look for surgical or medical diseases or medications that cause, contribute to, or mimic psychiatric disease.
- *Past psychiatric history*: explore previous diagnoses, treatments, and outcomes.
- *Family history* (FH): explore familial psychiatric disorders or medical conditions as a cause of or contributing factors to psychiatric disorders.
- *Social history* (SH): document the social circumstances of the patient, such as finances, housing, relationships, drug and alcohol use, and problems with the law, as these can contribute to the cause of psychiatric disease.
- *Development history*: past, present, family, social, and cultural.
- *Review of systems* (ROS): explore pertinent systems associated to the onset of psychiatric disease.

Mental Status Exam
- *Appearance*: physique, grooming, dress, habits, nutritional status, posture, nervousness, and eye contact.
- *Attitude/rapport*: attitude toward the examiner. For example, is the patient friendly, cooperative, bored, or defensive?
- *Mood*: the patient's emotions. Elicit by asking the patient questions such as, "How have you been feeling on most days?" List the mood in the patient's own words. Moods include being depressed, angry, anxious, stressed, or elevated.

- *Affect*: defined by the interviewer. Observable emotion: euthymic (normal), neutral, euphoric, dysphoric, or flat (no variation in emotion); the range: full, constricted, or blunted; appropriateness: appropriate or labile.
- *Speech*: quality, quantity, rate, and volume.
- *Thought process*: the organization of the patient's thoughts.
  - *Logical*: normal thought process
  - *Loose associations*: the patient slips off the track from one idea to an unrelated one
  - *Flight of ideas*: verbally skipping from one idea to another before the previous one has been concluded
  - *Tangentiality*: the responses never approach the point of the questions
  - *Thought blocking*: patient stops abruptly in the middle of a thought
  - *Circumstantiality*: delay in getting to the point because of unnecessary details and irrelevant remarks
  - *Neologism*: patient creates new words
- *Thought content*
  - *Suicidal ideation*: assess plan and previous attempts
  - *Homicidal ideation*: assess plan and previous attempts
  - Obsessions and compulsions
  - Phobias
  - Paranoia
- *Perceptual disturbances*
- *Hallucinations*: perception of a stimulus in the absence of a stimulus; auditory (hearing things), visual (seeing things), olfactory (smelling things), tactile (feeling things), and gustatory (tasting things)
- *Delusions*: grandiosity, religious delusion, persecution, jealousy, thought insertion (belief that someone is putting ideas or thoughts into his or her mind), ideas of reference (belief that irrelevant, unrelated phenomena in the world refer to him or her directly or have special personal significance)
- *Illusions*: erroneous interpretation of a present stimulus
- *Insight*: the patient's understanding of his or her illness
- *Judgment*: estimate the patient's judgment on the basis of the history or on an imaginary scenario. Ask the following question: "What would you do if you smelled smoke in a crowded theater?" (adequate response is, "Call 911" or "Get help"; poor response is, "Do nothing" or "Watch the smoke rise").
- *Impulsivity*: the degree of the patient's impulse control.
- *Reliability*: determine if the patient seems reliable, unreliable, or if it is difficult to determine.

Physical Exam

- Medical conditions (CNS malignancy, hypothyroidism, or pancreatic cancer) can mimic a psychiatric illness. A thorough physical exam (usually except genitourinary examination), including full neurological exam, should be documented.

Additional Investigations

- Lab investigations
- Additional information from accompanying friend or family members
- Other forms of pertinent information

Clinical Decision Making

- The decision-making process has been broken down into a systematic and individualized process involving
  - State-mandated criteria: clinical practice guidelines, *DSM-IV* criteria, etc.
  - Investigation of alternatives: for example, ruling out medical conditions that mimic psychiatric disease through lab investigations
  - Shared decision making: requires an adequate patient–clinician relationship
  - Intuitive reasoning and experiences such as years of experience or exposure to previous psychiatric disorders
  - Connection with the client, caution, and inability to control all contingencies
- Strategies of clinical reasoning and decision making include:
  - Tolerate uncertainty, avoid premature closure, and consider alternatives.
  - Separate cue from inference; be able to refer inferences to the salient cues from which they were derived.
  - Be aware of personal reactions to the patient.
- Be alert for fresh evidence, particularly evidence that demands a revision or deletion of a hypothesis or diagnosis.
- Value negative evidence above positive evidence.
- Be prepared to commit to a diagnosis when enough evidence has been gathered.
- Historically, decision making has shown variability among practitioners. As a result, efforts have been made to create practice guidelines, processes, and recommendations that will result in consistency in the diagnostic evaluation and, subsequently, in the treatment of psychiatric disease.
- Trend toward evidence-based clinical decision making:
  - For example, *DSM-IV-TR*, version of *DSM* modified to include evidence-based criteria
  - Goals
    - More clinical research independent of pharmaceutical companies
    - An efficient means of making evidence-based data easily accessible to clinicians

Diagnostic Formulation, Treatment Planning, and Modes of Treatment

Putting It All Together: Diagnostic Formulation

- Diagnostic formulation has been traditionally described as a summary of the relevant genetic, constitutional, and personality factors and their interaction with the etiological factors, taking into account the patient's life situation, together with a provisional diagnosis.
- Essentially, the full encounter, including psychiatric history, MSE, labs, referral information, additional information from family members/friends, and physical exam, is assessed to yield a diagnosis.
- Currently, a diagnostic formulation is best accomplished using the *DSM-IV* multiaxial system of assessment.

DSM-IV Multiaxial System of Assessment

- A systematic approach to the description of each patient's disorders.
  - *Axis I: Clinical Disorders; Other Conditions That May Be a Focus of Clinical Attention*
    - The major psychiatric and behavioral syndromes based on the *DSM-IV*
    - List the principal disorder or reason for the current visit first and follow with subsequent diagnoses
    - For example, major depressive disorder or adjustment disorder
  - *Axis II: Personality Disorders and Mental Retardation*
    - These disorders may coexist and complicate the diagnosis and management of Axis I problems
    - For example, borderline personality disorder
  - *Axis III: General Medical Conditions*
    - List general medical conditions
    - May be important in the understanding and management of the Axis I and II disorders

- *Axis IV: Psychosocial and Environmental Problems*
  - List problems in the psychosocial and surrounding physical environment of the patient. May influence the diagnosis, management, or prognosis of Axis I, II, and III problems.
  - For example, divorce or recent job loss.
- *Axis V: Global Assessment of Functioning*
  - The clinician's assessment of the patient's global level of function is recorded using the Global Assessment of Functioning Scale, a 0–100 scale descriptive of the degree of functioning and impairment as a consequence of the psychiatric (Axis I and II) disorders. The full scale is available in the *DSM-IV-TR*.

DSM-IV Disorders and ICD-9 Codes

- These disorders will be listed as Axis I or Axis II on the multiaxial system assessment
- Adjustment disorders
  - Adjustment Disorder Unspecified (309.9)
  - Adjustment Disorder with Anxiety (309.24)
  - Adjustment Disorder with Depressed Mood (309)
  - Adjustment Disorder with Disturbance of Conduct (309.3)
  - Adjustment Disorder with Mixed Anxiety and Depressed Mood (309.28)
  - Adjustment Disorder with Mixed Disturbance of Emotions and Conduct (309.4)
- Anxiety disorders
  - Acute Stress Disorder (308.3)
  - Agoraphobia (without a history of Panic Disorder) (300.22)
  - Generalized Anxiety Disorder (GAD; (300.02)
  - Obsessive-Compulsive Disorder (OCD; (300.3)
  - Panic Disorder—with Agoraphobia (300.21) or without Agoraphobia (300.01)

- Social Phobia (300.23)
- Posttraumatic Stress Disorder (PTSD; 309.81)
- Dissociative disorders
    - Dissociative Amnesia (300.12)
    - Dissociative Fugue (300.13)
    - Dissociative Identity (Multiple Personality) Disorder (300.14)
    - Depersonalization Disorder (300.6)
- Eating disorders
    - Anorexia Nervosa (307.1)
    - Bulimia Nervosa (307.51)
- Impulse control disorders
    - Intermittent Explosive Disorder (312.34)
    - Kleptomania (312.32)
    - Pathological Gambling (312.31)
    - Pyromania (312.33)
    - Trichotillomania (312.39)
- Mood disorders
    - Bipolar Disorder (296.8)
    - Cyclothymic Disorder (301.13)
    - Dysthymic Disorder (300.4)
    - Major Depressive Disorder (296.2)
- Sexual disorders
    - Exhibitionism (302.4)
    - Fetishism (302.81)
    - Frotteurism (302.89)
    - Pedophilia (302.2)
    - Sexual Masochism (302.83)
    - Sexual Sadism (302.84)
    - Transvestic Fetishism (302.3)
    - Voyeurism (302.82)
- Sleep disorders
    - Primary Insomnia (307.42)
    - Primary Hypersomnia (307.44)
    - Narcolepsy (347)
    - Nightmare Disorder (307.47)
    - Sleep Terror Disorder (307.46)
    - Sleepwalking Disorder (307.46)
- Psychotic disorders
    - Brief Psychotic Disorder (298.8)
    - Delusional Disorder (297.1)
    - Schizoaffective Disorder (295.7)
    - Schizophrenia
        - 295.2 Schizophrenia, Catatonic Type
        - 295.1 Schizophrenia, Disorganized Type
        - 295.3 Schizophrenia, Paranoid Type
        - 295.6 Schizophrenia, Residual Type
        - 295.9 Schizophrenia, Undifferentiated Type
    - Schizophreniform (295.4)
    - Shared Psychotic Disorder (297.3)
- Sexual dysfunctions
    - Dyspareunia (302.76)
    - Female Orgasmic Disorder (302.73)
    - Female Sexual Arousal Disorder (302.72)
    - Gender Identity Disorder (302.6)
    - Hypoactive Sexual Desire Disorder (302.71)
    - Male Erectile Disorder (302.72)
    - Male Orgasmic Disorder (302.74)
    - Premature Ejaculation (302.75)
    - Sexual Aversion Disorder (302.79)
    - Vaginismus (306.51)
- Somatoform disorders
    - Body Dysmorphic Disorder (300.7)
    - Conversion Disorder (300.11)
    - Hypochondriasis Disorder (300.7)
    - Pain Disorder (307.8)
    - Somatization Disorder (300.81)
- Substance disorders
    - Substance Abuse (305.9)
    - Substance Dependence (304.9)
- Personality disorders
    - Antisocial Personality Disorder (301.7)
    - Borderline Personality Disorder (301.83)
    - Narcissistic Personality Disorder (301.81)
    - Dependent Personality Disorder (301.6)
    - Histrionic Personality Disorder (301.5)
    - Paranoid Personality Disorder (301)

Treatment Planning

- Treatment planning is the next step after a diagnosis is evident.
- Selection of a therapeutic method depends on the mode, time, and setting of treatment.
- Patient involvement is necessary in formulating a treatment plan.
- Treatment plan goals
    - To clarify treatment focus
        - What the treatment is meant to accomplish and through what means.
    - To set realistic treatment expectations and goals
        - Treatment goals should have criteria for achievement, be achievable, and collaboratively developed and prioritized

- ◆ Expectations should adequately clarify to patients what they can realistically expect from a treatment course
  - ◆ Clarify patient and provider roles, setting ground rules for therapy and establishing realistic goals agreed on by the patient
- To establish a standard for measuring treatment progress
  - ◆ Include a plan for reevaluation or follow-up
- To facilitate communication among professionals
- For the purposes of managed health care, treatment plans also serve to support treatment authorization, to document quality assurance efforts, and to facilitate communication with external reviewers

Modes of Treatment

- Pharmacotherpy
  - *Antidepressants*: used to treat depression, panic attacks, OCDs, PTSD, social anxiety disorder, anxiety, premenstrual dysphoric disorder, nicotine withdrawal symptoms (buproprion [Wellbutrin])
  - *Mood stabilizers*: used to treat bipolar disorder, dementia (anticonvulsants), severe agitation, aggression, severe impulsive behavior, mania, and disinhibition
  - *Neuroleptics*: used to treat schizophrenia, mania, delusional disorder, symptoms of psychosis, Tourette's disease, Asperger's syndrome
  - *Anticholinergics*: used for anxiety and stress reactions
  - *Anxiolytics*: used to treat anxiety disorders
  - *Sedative hypnotics*: used to treat insomnia and sleep disorders
- Electroconvulsive therapy
  - Major depression with or without psychotic features
  - Bipolar illness (both depressed and manic phases)
  - Catatonic schizophrenia
  - Schizophrenia with strong affective components or schizophrenia highly resistant to treatment
- Behavior therapy and cognitive therapy
  - Used to help patients eliminate target behaviors; refer to additional texts for more information
- Group psychotherapy
  - Used to treat the following disorders in a group setting:
    - ◆ Most personality disorders
    - ◆ Most anxiety disorders
    - ◆ Somatoform disorders
    - ◆ Substance-related disorders
    - ◆ Schizophrenia and related psychotic disorders
    - ◆ Stable bipolar disorders
    - ◆ PTSD
    - ◆ Eating disorders
    - ◆ Medical illness
    - ◆ Depressive disorders
    - ◆ Adjustment disorders
  - Refer to additional texts for more information
- Family/marital therapy

The Diagnostic Evaluation

The Process of Diagnostic Evaluation

- A complete diagnostic evaluation involves obtaining a complete psychiatric history, including the presence of specific symptoms, course, and duration, in addition to the MSE, physical exam, pertinent labs, and other additional information. Diagnosis-specific questions for *DSM* criteria during the diagnostic encounter are the key.

Diagnosis-Specific Questions

- As the interviewer develops hypotheses for a diagnosis, diagnosis-specific questions are asked to elicit *DSM-IV* criteria for diagnosis
  - *How long have you felt depressed?*—the *DSM-IV* diagnosis for a major depressive disorder (MDD) requires at least 2 weeks of symptoms.
  - *Do you still derive pleasure from doing your favorite activities?*—the *DSM-IV* diagnosis for MDD must include the presence of lack of pleasure (anhedonia) or a depressed mood.
  - *Are you able to function during the day on little to no sleep?*—a decreased need for sleep is one of the possible criteria for a diagnosis of bipolar disorder.
  - *Do you have flashbacks or nightmares of the traumatic event?*—reexperiencing a trauma (via nightmares, flashbacks, obsessive thoughts) is part of the *DSM-IV* criteria of diagnosis for PTSD.
- The interview may refer to additional diagnosis-specific screening questionnaires such as:

- Mini-Cog—instrument to assess dementia
- Mini-mental state examination—screening tool for cognitive function and impairment
- Clock drawing test—screening tool to assess executive function
- Beck Depression Inventory
- Hamilton Depression Scale
- Prime MD instruments—screening tool for diagnosis of psychiatric disorders based on *DSM* criteria (intended for and sufficiently diagnostic in primary care settings)

The *Diagnostic and Statistical Manual of Mental Disorders (DSM)* Diagnostic Criteria

- Standard classification of mental disorders used by mental health professionals in the United States.
- Designed for use across settings, such as inpatient, outpatient, partial hospital, clinic, private practice, and primary care; with community populations; and by psychiatrists, psychologists, nurses, occupational and rehabilitation therapists, counselors, social workers, medical students, and other health and mental health professionals.
- Necessary tool for collecting and communicating accurate public health data.
- Three major components: the diagnostic classification, the diagnostic criteria sets, and the descriptive text.
- For each disorder in the *DSM*, a set of diagnostic criteria indicates inclusion criteria (symptoms and length of presence) and exclusion criteria to qualify for a particular diagnosis.

Psychological Testing in Psychiatry

What Is Psychological Testing?

Psychological testing offers objective data about mental functioning. It involves administration, scoring, and interpretation of specific tasks in a controlled fashion. Tests must be

- Normed on a representative population
- Administered in a controlled environment
- Administered in a standard fashion
- Reliable and valid
- Culturally fair
- Scored according to standardized procedures
- Interpreted according to acceptable professional practices

What Information Does Psychological Testing Provide, and for Whom Is It Appropriate?

Psychological testing has the ability to provide useful diagnostic information regarding level of intellectual functioning, identify and describe the nature of a mental disorder, and indicate underlying motivation, personality attributes and other variables.

- The patient must be able to participate in the assessment. Grossly confused or psychotic patients are not good candidates for psychological testing.
- Psychological testing is useful in treatment planning and outcome evaluation.
- Psychological testing is useful when objective data are required to establish a suspected diagnosis (sanity boards, interdiction)

Types of Psychological Tests

Many types of psychological tests are available to qualified users.

- Measures of intellectual functioning
- Personality questionnaires
- Projective techniques
- Neuropsychological tests
- Measures of cognitive impairment

Associated tests include:

- Psychodiagnostic screening tests
- Educational diagnostic tests
- Aptitude tests
- Interest inventories

How to Determine the Appropriate Types of Patients for Psychological Testing

- Almost anyone who possesses a reasonable reality orientation and is nonpsychotic is an appropriate candidate for psychological testing.
- Individuals with better mental statuses are capable of participating in more complex psychological testing procedures.
- Not all patients are capable of participating in all psychological tests. Physical handicaps, language barriers, and illiteracy may limit the available testing procedures.
- The willingness of the patient has an influence on the procedure. Angry or deceptive individuals may distort the outcome data. There are specific psychological tests to detect malingering and deception.
- Very specific referral questions allow for the selection of instruments (measures) to specifically address the reason for referral for testing.

How Long Should Psychological Testing Take?

- The time to complete psychological testing depends on the referral questions and the number of testing procedures performed. The time may be as short as 2 hours or as long as 8 hours.
- Testing can be expedited by prearranging appointments, providing relevant records and history, clear referral questions, and, when necessary, preapproval by third-party payers.
- Testing may be delayed when a third-party payer has questions as to the necessity of testing procedures, schedules are full, referral questions are vague, funding is unavailable, or the client is inappropriate for assessment.

Who Performs Psychological Tests?

- A licensed psychologist or a technician under the supervision of a licensed clinical psychologist conducts psychological testing.
- Not all psychologists provide psychological testing and referrals are frequently made to specialists, especially in the case of neuropsychological assessment.
- Some states allow psychological testing to be conducted by nonpsychologists for specific purposes or in limited environments.

Important Issues in Psychological Testing

- Reliability
- Validity
- Cultural bias
- Confidentiality
- Qualified examiners and assistants
- Explaining test results to referral sources

Psychological Tests and Procedures of Importance in Psychiatry

The WAIS-IV

- The gold standard in the assessment of intellectual functioning.
- Cross culturally normed and can be used with any U.S. population over the age of 16.
- Requires 60–90 minutes to administer.
- Provides several IQ and index scores for different realms of intellectual ability.

The MMPI-2

- The most widely investigated and empirically validated personality questionnaire available.
- The self-report format consists of 556 true and false questions requiring 1–2 hours for completion.
- Has built-in validity scales to detect malingering and deception.
- Consists of 10 basic clinical scales and supplemental scales to assess personality.
- Has a number of presentation formats: paper, short form, and computer administration.
- Optic scan options are available, which can then generate a written report for rapid review.

The Rorschach

- The classic inkblot projective technique.
- The patients are instructed to provide a description of what they see in an ambiguous picture.
- The responses have been correlated with personality variables and psychopathology.
- Requires specialized training and supervised practice to administer and interpret.
- Computer programs are available to assist with scoring and interpretation.

Self-Report Instruments

- Typically self-report inventories are pencil-and-paper tests, wherein the patient endorses items either with a true/false or Likert scale format.
- These reports can also be done in an interview format.
- Come in "short" and "long" versions, taking 5–20 minutes to complete.
- Have been empirically validated with various clinical populations and demographic groups.

Common Measures

- The Beck Depression Inventory
- The Beck Anxiety Inventory
- The Hamilton Depression Scales
- The Hamilton Anxiety Scale

Neuropsychological Test Batteries

- A group of tests that describe brain–behavior relationships.
- Some tests are preselected and referred to as structured batteries while others are selected by the neuropsychologist as per the referral question and are known as flexible batteries.
- Individual tests assess psychological functions in different regions of the brain.
- The test results can be assembled to draw conclusions about damaged and persevered cognitive realms and abilities.
- Tests are useful in assessing the loss secondary to neurological insult and making predictions about recovery.
- Neuropsychological testing requires up to 8 hours of testing time.
- Specialized training is required to administer, score, and interpret measures utilized in neuropsychological assessment.

Questions for Referral Sources to Ask in Making a Referral

- Will psychological testing answer the questions I have about my patient?
- How soon will the psychologist see my patient?
- How long will the testing take?
- Is the procedure covered by my patient's insurance?
- Does your office have a payment plan?
- How long will it take to get the results?
- Will the psychologist go over the results with my patient and me?
- If my patient has difficulty in understanding the results, can he/she come see the psychologist for further review?
- Will the results include recommendations that I can implement?
- How will my patient's confidentiality and privacy be protected.

Suggested Readings

American Medical Association. (2009). *AMA physician ICD-9-CM 2009* (Vols. 1 and 2). Chicago: American Medical Association Press.

American Psychiatric Association. (2000). *Diagnostic and statistical manual of mental disorders* (4th ed.). Washington, DC: American Psychiatric Association.

Andronikof, A. (2008). Exneriana-II—The scientific legacy of John E. Exner, Jr. *Rorschachiana, 29,* 81–107.

Carlat, D. J. (2004). *The psychiatric interview: A practical guide to psychiatry* (2nd ed.). Chicago: Lippincott Williams & Wilkins.

Ebert, M. H., Loosen, P. T., Nurcombe, B., & Leckman, J. F. (Eds.). (2008). *Current diagnosis and treatment psychiatry* (2nd ed.). New York: McGraw-Hill.

Gillis, M. M., Haaga, D. A. F., & Ford, G. T. (1995). Normative values for the Beck Anxiety Inventory, Fear Questionnaire, Penn State Worry Questionnaire, and Social Phobia and Anxiety Inventory. *Psychological Assessment, 7,* 450–455.

LeBlond, R. F., DeGowin, R. L., & Brown, D. D. (Eds.). (2009). *DeGowin's diagnostic examination* (9th ed.). New York: McGraw-Hill.

Meyer, G. J., Riethmiller, R. J., Brooks, R. D., Benoit, W. A., & Handler, L. (2000). A replication of Rorschach and MMPI-2 convergent validity. *Psychological Assessment, 74,* 175–215.

Moras, K., di Nardo, P. A., & Barlow, D. H. (1992). Distinguishing anxiety and depression: Reexamination of the reconstructed Hamilton scales. *Psychological Assessment, 42,* 224–227.

Pearson Education, Inc. (2008). Introducing the WAIS-IV.

Scheiber, S. C. (2004). The psychiatric interview, psychiatric history, and mental status examination. In R. A. Hales, S. C. Yukovsky, & J. A. Talbott (Eds.), *Essentials of clinical psychiatry* (2nd ed.). American Psychiatric Press.

Valenstin, M. et al. (1997). Screening for psychiatric illness with a combined screening and diagnostic instrument. *Journal of General and Internal Medicine, 12*(11), 679–685.

Establish a Philosophy of Management

Management of the psychotherapeutic process is a multidimensional endeavor that requires:
- Staff management
- Patient well-being
- Coordination with other professionals
- Time management

Establish a fundamental philosophy guiding both outpatient and inpatient treatment:
- What are the variables that influence service delivery?
- How can you ensure services meet a level of excellence?
- How will staff teamwork be accomplished?
- Selection of the appropriate psychotherapy

- Risk management
- Operations management

The interactions of the above factors with other relevant factors specific to the patient's environment will determine the ultimate process of intervention.

- How can patient outcome be optimal?
- How can the service program become accountable?
- How can the treatment program become flexible and adaptable?
- How can the program achieve total fairness and mutual respect?

Standards of Care in Psychotherapy Management

In the realm of psychotherapy, surrounding issues are not as well-established as in other realms of medicine. This is changing as more becomes known about the process and utility of different forms of intervention. Current influences on the standard of care include:

- Laws and current statutes
- Regulations passed by state licensing boards
- Precedent and case law
- Professional codes of ethics
- Opinions of consumers and other professionals

The three standards of care established in mental health are:

- Duty to report abuse
- The case of *Tarasoff versus the Board of Regents of the University of California*
- Health Insurance Portability and Accountability Act (HIPAA) guidelines

Psychotherapy: Initial Interview

Presentation by the patient:
- Attire
- Overall attitude
- Gross motor skills
- Speech
- Language
- Hygiene

Initial assessment:
- Presenting of the problem
- Secondary problems
- Medical history
- Drug and alcohol history
- Legal history
- Developmental history
- Educational history
- Employment history
- Marital status and history
- Abuse issues

Mental status examination:
- Alertness
- Coherence
- Mental organization

- Thought processing
- Delusions
- Obsessions
- Suicidal/homicidal ideation
- Affect and mood
- Illusions
- Hallucinations
- Orientation
- Memory
- Fund of information
- Abstraction

DSM diagnoses:
- Axis I, major syndromes
- Axis II, personality disorders, mental retardation
- Axis III, concurrent and contributing medical problems
- Axis IV, stressors
- Axis V, general assessment of functioning
  Recommendations:
- Type of therapeutic treatment or intervention
- Therapy setting
- Dangerousness

Psychotherapy Record Management and the Standard of Care

At a minimum, psychotherapy chart or file should include
- Diagnosis
- Presenting of problem
- Mental status examination
- Background information
- Treatment goals
- Progress notes

If appropriate, the chart or notes should display:
- Psychological test results

- Psychiatric consultation
- Relevant medical tests or history
- Consultations
- Unscheduled communications with the patient

Special population notes should include:
- Nature of the condition
- Concurrent problems
- Potential for violence
- Crisis intervention procedures
- Detailed notes concerning abuse or neglect

Psychotherapeutic Management of Disorders

Personality Disorders

The management of personality disorders presents an unusual challenge because many of the maladaptive features that have caused the patient pain and suffering are fundamental components of the personality structure. Key features in management include:

- Maintaining strict boundaries between the patient and the psychotherapist.
- Establishing a clear reimbursement plan.
- In writing, establish the responsibility of the patient and the responsibility of the psychotherapist.
- Setting rules and consequences for tardiness in the outpatient setting.
- Enacting a no-suicide contract.
- Agreeing on a plan of action if the patient becomes suicidal.
- Always promptly addressing patient's threat to discontinue treatment.
- Always assessing secondary issues such as drug and alcohol use.
- Becoming alert to issues of secondary gain and disruptive behavior.
- Addressing self-destructive behaviors.
- Working on enhancing adaptive behaviors and social skills.
- Focusing on educating the patient to cause-and-effect relationships.
- Helping establish personal, spiritual, and vocational goals of a long-term nature.
- Minimizing self-disclosure.
- Not accepting excuses.

Substance Abuse

Substance-abuse disorders require the clinicians to wear many hats and address many different aspects of the patient's experiences.

- Treatment goals should be simple and clear.
- Patients should be actively involved in treatment.
- Therapists should structure a supportive environment.
- Patients must take responsibility for their behavior.
- Therapists should emphasize self-direction.
- Confrontation must be appropriate to the client's tolerance level.
- Empathy should be conditional and measured.
- Avoid arguing with patients.
- Involve the significant other whenever possible.
- Always emphasize the patient's motivation.
- Enhance awareness of problem behaviors.
- Focus on self-destructive cyclic behaviors.
- Educate about the physical destructiveness of substances.
- Engage the family in treatment.
- Help the patient identify feelings and express them appropriately.

Dementia

Management of dementia is achieved in both inpatient and outpatient settings. A multidisciplinary team approach is necessary to manage most cases effectively.

- Address physical safety issues.
- Gauge psychotherapy to the level of impairment.
- Address issues of incontinence in counseling.
- Enhance mobility.
- Educate as to the dangers of falling.
- Address depression in both individual and group sessions.
- Offer orientation counseling to low-functioning patients.
- Offer family consultation and counseling to all family members.
- Address end-of-life issues in group therapy.
- Carefully investigate drug and alcohol issues.
- Consult with family about driving privileges.
- Assess memory repeatedly.
- Stress a wellness model.

- Prepare to address sundowning problems.
- Establish smoking and obesity groups.
- Offer counseling for depression and loss.

Depression

Depression is the most common illness in the general population. There are numerous diagnostic categories for the depressive disorders but some basic management principles apply to all forms of depression.

- Assess the depth of the depression.
- Establish the etiology, duration, and frequency of the depression.
- Assess vegetative signs.
- Assess suicide risk.
- Stabilize the affect and mood with medication management.
- Educate the patient as to the nature of the illness.
- Reduce guilt.
- Initiate a supportive therapy to stabilize.
- Look for cultural influences that maintain depression.
- Reduce stressors.
- Enhance self-esteem.
- Build problem-solving skills.
- Manage self-defeating thoughts.
- Help explore self-defeating behaviors.
- Engage family support.

Psychotic Disorders

A lack of a reality orientation and disorganized thinking are the hallmarks of psychosis. Psychotherapy is unproductive in the acute phase but profitable in the prodromal and residual phases, assisting the client to maintain the medication management program and discover a rewarding life.

- Establish the patient's current level of functioning.
- Encourage compliance with medication management program.
- Reduce stressors.
- Assist with acquiring basic necessities.
- Investigate drug and alcohol use.
- Consistently encourage a balanced life style.
- Discourage self-medication.
- Assist with enrollment in day hospital programs.
- Urge self-exploration of illness.
- Help establish boundaries.
- Assist with financial management.
- Build social skills.
- Teach patient to recognize psychotic features.
- Encourage personal hygiene.
- Teach listening skills.
- Always redirect when patient avoids.
- Enhance independent living skills.
- Prevent self-pity and despondency.
- Directly address noncompliance with treatment.

Suggested Readings

American Psychotherapy Association. (2008). Psychotherapist's oath. Retrieved May 15, 2009, from http://www.americanpsychotherapy.com/about/oath/.

Richmond, R. L. (2009). The psychotherapy process. Retrieved May 15, 2009, from http://www.guideto psychology.com/questions/questions.htm#process.

Richmond, R. L. (2009). Transference issues. Retrieved May 15, 2009, from http://www.guidetopsychology.com/questions/questions.htm#trans.

Richmond, R. L. (2009). Termination issues. Retrieved May 15, 2009, from http://www.guidetopsychology.com/questions/questions.htm#termin.

Zur, O. (2009). The standard of care in psychotherapy and counseling: Bringing clarity to illusive relationships. Retrieved May 15, 2009, from http://www.zurinstitute.com/standardofcaretherapy.html.

Behavioral Therapy and Cognitive-Behavioral Therapy

Definitions

Behavioral Therapy

Any intervention or set of interventions that focuses on the patient behaviors as the primary focus of change. Maladaptive, self-defeating, self-destructive, or otherwise problematic behaviors can be replaced with more effective ones. Learning these new behaviors is a matter of education and reinforcement. Progressive muscle relaxation training and social skills training are the two examples.

Cognitive Therapy

Interventions that target a patient's thinking process. The central principle in cognitive therapy (CT) is that thoughts produce feelings. That is, sadness and anxiety are, in part, the products of the thinking process. Faulty thinking precedes emotional distress. The thinking process is often fraught with faulty assumptions and unexamined tenets that often render the patient unnecessarily constrained and distressed. Through identification and examination of faulty or distorted thinking processes, patients are helped to consider themselves and their circumstances from an alternate perspective and thereby mitigate feelings of distress.

Cognitive-Behavioral Therapy

A body of work in psychotherapy that draws from multiple theorists and focuses on the thoughts and behaviors that shape problematic emotional reactions and consequences.

- In the cognitive-behavioral therapy (CBT) framework, emotional distress is believed to be the result of faulty habits of thought that result in dysfunctional attitudes and behaviors.
- Maladaptive patterns of thinking create the emotional distress.
- In order to alleviate that distress, new objective, evidence-based thought patterns have to be developed and new behavioral skills have to be adopted.
- Through a systematic process of examining, labeling, and analyzing these cognitive errors, patients learn to replace them with more reality based, self-enhancing ones.

Behavioral and Cognitive-Behavioral Processes

Background

- Behavioral therapy is based, in part, on work of B. F. Skinner and others who analyzed how operant conditioning determines behavioral responses and how these responses could be altered through effective environmental reinforcement.
- Reward-based measures, such as token economies, are used to reinforce desired behaviors. Variations in specific theoretical frameworks and treatment techniques exist within behavioral therapy.
- Thought leaders in CT include Albert Ellis (rational emotive therapy) and Aaron Beck (cognitive therapy), who through the 1960s advanced the notion that feelings/emotions were strongly influenced by the habitual patterns people used to make sense of their experiences.
- These thought patterns were considered "automatic" in that they are an innate part of the "self-talk" that seems to be a universal human phenomenon.
- These automatic thoughts are often based on misconceptions, deeply embedded erroneous assumptions (schema), and learned principles that confine the manner in which people respond to all kinds of life problems.
- While psychodynamically oriented approaches look to the origin of feelings in sometimes deeply

conflicted psychosocial, developmental, and cognitive aspects, theorists propose that feelings originate from learned patterns of thinking that create unnecessarily confined mental structures that affect how people learn, grow, and solve problems.

- These false, fixed notions of reality create mental prisons for those who live within them.

Terms and Methods

Fundamental Features

CBT is a relatively short-term psychotherapy process (approximately, 12–28 sessions) that is structured and formalized. Attention to this structure is a hallmark of the approach. The steps of treatment usually include:

1. A thorough diagnostic interview.
2. The partnering of patient and therapist forms an active collaborative team.
3. The therapist–patient team works together to identify problematic areas in the patient's life by identifying cognitive distortions or errors that commonly impose a negative interpretation on everyday events.
4. The therapist–patient team adopts a step-by-step process to examine the underlying assumptions, fundamental beliefs, or "schemas" from which these self-defeating thought patterns and distortions originate. They are often outside the immediate conscious awareness of the patient.
5. The creating and maintaining of a written daily thought record includes the following:
   - Documenting of specific events that evoke emotional distress.
   - Identifying the specific cognitive distortions that are at work in many of these situations.
   - Labeling and analyzing of cognitive distortions.
   - Identifying alternative methods for thinking about these same events (cognitive correction process).
6. The assignment of carefully planned homework so that the patient remains actively engaged in the CBT process outside of the formal sessions.
7. The therapist actively engaging in coaching the patient through a systematic examination of the antecedents and consequences of these errors in thinking.
8. The therapist–patient team designing strategies to examine evidence to determine the validity of these erroneous mental constructs.
9. Prioritization and processing of these problems from a CBT framework.
10. Recording the process of identification of goals in behavioral, measurable terminology.
11. Trying on new behaviors that are outside the patient's usual pattern to explore potential results and sources of reinforcement.
12. Ultimately, the patient becomes his or her own therapist, able to quickly identify erroneous thinking when it occurs and take steps to neutralize or counter it.
13. Coupled with the ability to initiate behavioral measures (relaxation and assertiveness), the patient can choose from a repertoire of skills to meet the demands of the emotionally charged situation and return to a state of emotional equilibrium.

Psychoeducation

- Psychoeducation is a major and ongoing component of the treatment and is usually woven into sessions throughout the course of treatment.
- Patients are introduced to a cognitive conceptualization of their problems and goals from the beginning.
- Psychoeducation teaches patients about the terms, strategies, and processes of CBT and is included in most of the sessions.

Cognitive Distortions

Cognitive distortions are automatic thoughts that are often irrational, illogical, or self-defeating. If occurring regularly, they can result in patterns of ineffective behavior. While different theorists have developed somewhat idiosyncratic terminology to designate similar phenomena, the following are common to many of them.

- Emotional reasoning: the tendency to conclude that if a person feels awkward or uncomfortable after a social event, then the person must actually be socially awkward.

- Dichotomous thinking (all-or-nothing thinking): drawing absolute conclusions. A person whose marriage fails believes that she or he is a "complete loser."
- Discounting the positive: disqualifying all positive experiences or traits as being trivial or unimportant, especially when compared to a seemingly glaring error or shortcoming.
- Personalization: interpreting external data as being related to oneself without evidence for such a conclusion.
- Arbitrary inference: drawing a conclusion without supporting evidence, or even in spite of contradictory evidence.
- Minimization and magnification: overinflating the negative or underestimating the positive in the evaluation of the relative importance of events.
- Catastrophizing: assuming that the worst possible outcome is the most likely.

Interactive Techniques

- Setting an agenda: the agenda for each session is actively negotiated with the patient at the outset.
- Feedback: the therapist deliberately requests feedback to ascertain patient's understanding of, and success with, process and methods. Eliciting and processing patient reactions to, concerns about, and impressions of both the therapy and the therapist are considered essential components of the CBT experience.
- Socratic method: through a series of questions, the therapist gradually advances the nature of a discussion to lead the patient to first uncovering distorted perspective, then drawing more accurate, self-affirming conclusions.
- Guided discovery: examining evidence, weighing the value of alternatives, exploring the advantages, and disadvantages of various options. This is done in an integrated and accepting manner through discussion format.
- Focused attentiveness: focusing on central ideas, relevant thoughts, assumptions, behaviors, and so on, that are germane to the problem being discussed.
- Formulating a strategy for change: plan is actively negotiated with the patient and clearly outlines

CBT strategies to be employed in the change process.

Qualities of the Therapist

- CBT is a methodology that requires its practitioners to be well-grounded in the essential skills of psychotherapy.
- CBT does not replace basic psychotherapeutic practice. Rather, it builds from it.
- The cognitive-behavioral therapist must be well-versed in conceptual and operational underpinnings of psychotherapeutic processes.
- The therapist, while being specifically trained in CBT techniques, must possess and exhibit the fundamental features of any effective therapist including:
  - Graduate education in a mental health field (psychology, psychiatry, social work, nursing, professional counseling, etc.).
  - Formal training in CBT.
  - Deeply embedded commitment to and demonstration of basic therapist skills and attributes like
    - Expression of empathy
    - Professionalism
    - Sound, ethical practice
    - Active listening
    - Authenticity
    - Understanding of complex psychological phenomena that influence human experiences
    - Ability to understand the patient within the social, cultural, environmental context of that patient's lived experience

Evidence-Based Applications

- Among psychotherapy methods, CBT has to its credit the largest body of empirical evidence to support its efficacy.
- Because of the formalized and structured nature of its tenets and interventions, it can be operationalized in a reproducible manner that creates sound reliability and validity.
- Common evidence-based applications include:
  - Anxiety disorders in adults and children
  - Depression

- Addictions
- Personality disorders (especially in the form of dialectical behavioral therapy)
- Examples of newer applications (some still under investigation):
  - Chronic pain
  - Chronic illness
  - Chronic fatigue syndrome
  - Tinnitus
  - Headache, especially with comorbid psychiatric symptoms
  - Schizophrenia
  - Child sexual abuse
  - Treatment of sex offenders
  - Somatoform disorders
  - Anxiety, depression, and insomnia in older adults
  - Psychological adjustment to breast cancer
  - Occupational stress

Related Approach: Dialectical Behavioral Therapy

- Mindfulness and radical acceptance are concepts that complement, draw from, or enhance a CBT.
- These concepts supplement or extend CBT methods and techniques to further target treatment-resistant emotional distress.
- Dialectical behavioral therapy (DBT), for example, provides a systematic and programmed method for dealing with the intense emotional distress that sometimes occurs in patients who struggle with borderline personality disorder.
- Mindful strategies and meditation help to decrease the emotional reactivity that may be, in part, physiologically activated, especially after prolonged periods of intense stress.
- Computer-based, program-driven CBT is now available and these programs claim to provide effective CBT in the absence of a psychotherapist.

Psychoanalysis

Sigmund Freud

Biographical Information

- Born, Moravia in 1856; died in London in 1939.
- Member of the Jewish faith, which had a significant influence on his worldview.
- Trained in neurology, he developed an interest in patients who exhibited neurologic symptoms without any organic etiology.
- Studied with Jean Baptiste Charcot at the Salpetrière in Paris. This greatly affected his thinking about the influence of the unconscious on personality development and behavior.
- After returning to Vienna, he developed the first comprehensive theory of personality.
- His theory of personality led to the development of psychoanalysis.

Freud's Personality Theory

Freud's ideas can be reviewed in two broad sections:

The Topographic Model (1900)

- Saw personality as analogous to an iceberg with three distinct sections.
  - Conscious level: consists of current thoughts and perceptions.
  - Preconscious level: involves memories and stored knowledge that can be retrieved on demand.
  - Unconscious level: inaccessible feelings, urges, drives, desires, and demands. These are driven by a basic biological–sexual need for fulfillment.
- The Topographic Model was represented in Freud's 1900 publication, *The Interpretation of Dreams*, in which he proposed that humans were guided by unconscious sexual energies that lead to conflicts in everyday life.

The Structural Model (ca. 1920)

- As Freud's ideas matured, so did his conceptualization of personality structure.
- Whereas the topographical model was rigid with its three sections, the structural model remained fluid and offered interaction between the realms of one's personality.
- The structural model has three semi-independent realms
  - The id
    - The id is the only part of personality present at birth.
    - The id operates on the pleasure principle.
    - Wants instant gratification—"It wants, what it wants, when it wants it."
    - No frustration tolerance.
    - No empathy or compassion for others; completely egocentric.
    - Goal of the id is to increase pleasure and decrease pain and anxiety.
    - Inappropriate or psychotic behavior results when needs are delayed or denied.
    - The id runs on libido energy (or life energy). The libido energy is a biological energy that drives an individual toward growth and development.
    - Initially, because it is unconscious, the image of an object is just as rewarding as the object itself.
    - The id is forced by the biological necessity to acknowledge the outside world and thus makes arrangements for some libido energy to act as a go-between.
  - The ego
    - The ego begins as a fragile subsection of the id with the goal of satisfying id needs by any practical means.
    - To satisfy id needs, the ego is in communication with reality and guides behavior.
    - Gratifying the id's needs results in greater libido energy being shifted to the ego, which results in a stronger reality reorientation, socialization skills, and frustration tolerance.
    - Failure to meet the id's needs leads to deteriorating ego influence and an increase in primitive, infantile, or psychotic behavior.

- The ego is in touch with reality and operates by the reality principle, which endorses delayed gratification.
- For most people, the ego continues to develop and becomes the executor of personality, balancing the other forces.
- The superego
  - The last portion of personality to develop a relationship with both the unconscious and conscious.
  - The superego begins to develop as the attitudes of authority figures are integrated into the personality structure and a sense of right and wrong is established.
  - As the superego develops, it influences behavior by enhancing self-esteem for appropriate actions and punishing inappropriate behavior through guilt.
  - In a healthy personality, there is a flow of energy among the three realms.
  - If the libido energy becomes focused on the id, psychotic behaviors become prominent in the personality.
  - If the libido energy should become focused on the superego, anxiety disorders become prominent.

In sum: the id is driven by inborn instincts such as anger and sex, while the superego is at the other extreme urging social values and altruism. The ego is the executor and arbitrator, directing and balancing the demands of the id and the superego.

The Psychosexual Stages of Development

Freud adopted a stage theory of psychosexual personality development in his 1905 work, *Three Essays on the Theory of Sexuality* (see Table 3.1).

- The stages are invariant; they cannot be circumvented or skipped.
- The stages represent a shifting of libido energy to different areas of the body. These realms become the center of developmental psychosexual issues and attention.
- Each stage has a psychosexual crisis associated with it that must be successfully resolved before moving on to the next stage of development.

Table 3.1 The Psychosexual Stages of Human Development

Stage	Age (Year[s])	Erogenous Zone	Psychosexual Conflict
Oral	0–1	Mouth	Weaning, sucking, eating
Anal	1–3	Anus	Toilet training, feces
Phallic	3–5	Genitals	Oedipal conflict, sex
Latency	5–6	None	Period of calmness
Genital	Puberty	Mature sexual relationships	

- Failure in resolving the psychosexual crisis associated with the stage results in fixation. Psychosexual energy remains stagnant and the individual (unconsciously) attempts to resolve the crisis. These attempts usually become socially inappropriate as the person ages.

The Oedipal Conflict

- In Greek mythology, Oedipus was the son of the King of Thebes, whose lover, unbeknownst to him, was his mother.
- When Oedipus became aware of the identity of his lover, he gouged out his eyes for violating a sexual taboo.
- The Oedipal conflict provides an explanation of gender orientation and operates unconsciously.
- During this phallic stage, libido energy builds, and the child begins to develop a sexual attraction for the opposite-sex parent.
- The course for boys and girls is different.
  - *Boys*
    - The boy develops affection for his mother and jealously wishes to displace his father as the man in her life. As his psychosexual tension grows, he becomes fearful of reprisal, which leads to a belief that his father may remove him as a contender by removing his genitals, the castration complex.
    - At this point, the anxiety is intolerable and the boy engages two defense mechanisms to reduce anxiety and resolve the psychosexual conflict. He represses his affection for his mother and identifies with his father, leading

to a psychological male orientation that matches his physiology.

- A small proportion of boys fail to resolve this crisis and fail to establish a male identity. This concludes the phallic period and the child enters a period of psychosexual tranquility until puberty.

■ *Girls*
- A girl develops affection for her father and wishes to displace her mother who is now viewed as a rival.
- Eventually the conflict of losing her mother's love and having her mother separate her from the family becomes intolerable.
- Repressing her affection for her father and identifying with her mother successfully resolve the conflict.
- Her psychology now matches her physiology, and she now identifies herself as female.
- A small proportion of females fail to resolve the crisis and experience gender identity issues.

Defense Mechanisms

- The defense mechanisms serve as protection devices for the three mental structures (see Table 3.2).
- Their mission is to mitigate anxiety and stress and enhance stability in the personality structure.
- The defense mechanisms operate unconsciously.
- The implementation of defense mechanisms to manage a stressor is based on efficiency. If unsuccessful, less efficient mechanisms will be implemented and may, unfortunately, lead to a demonstration of age-inappropriate or pathological behavior.
- Psychotic individuals rely heavily on primitive defense mechanisms such as denial and projection.
- Healthy individuals use the most appropriate defense mechanism and can quickly select another when necessary.
- Individuals with personality disorders are unable to select appropriate mechanisms and rely heavily,

Table 3.2 Defense Mechanisms

Defense Mechanism	Activity	Example
Repression	Suppression of anxiety-laden material from consciousness.	A sailor cannot remember the attack on his ship.
Projection	Attributing repulsive attitudes and traits to another.	A student alleges faculty is out to get him.
Denial	Refusal to admit an obvious reality.	Following a divorce, the husband still says he's married.
Rationalization	Substituting a concocted reason rather than the real reason for an event.	Making an excuse using rationale. "If you had a wife like mine, you wouldn't go home either."
Reaction formation	Attesting to the opposite emotion of an impulse or desire.	After breaking up with Mary, Bob says he never really loved her.
Regression	Reverting to a more primitive behavior of an earlier developmental stage.	After losing an argument, Bob assaults his coworker.
Displacement	Substituting a less threatening object for the original object of hostility.	After being fired, Bob returns home and kicks his cat.
Sublimation	Substituting forbidden impulses for socially acceptable activities.	Bob plays tennis when he feels angry with his mother.

even exclusively, on just one defense mechanism, such as paranoia.

The Process of Psychoanalysis

- Freud believed that patients would structure their own emotional resolution if allowed to explore the repressed conflicts that were impeding growth and development.

- The unconscious is both an asset and an impediment to conflict resolution and development. It is, by its nature, protective of the structure by holding an aberrant impulse in abeyance and thus managing anxiety and pain. Simultaneously, it prevents resolution because of this material being inaccessible.
- One of Freud's problems was to develop a mechanism that would prevent overwhelming anxiety to the conscious mind and slowly allow the patient to develop an understanding of unconscious conflicts and developmental failures.
- To address the unconscious, Freud developed psychoanalysis, a procedure by which the client could address repressed issues at his or her own pace in an environment free of ridicule and condemnation.
- The client would recline on a couch and engage in process of free association, a spontaneous discourse of whatever came to mind.
- The psychoanalyst would position himself or herself out of the patient's line of sight and record the process and topics of discourse. Commentary by the psychoanalyst was held to a minimum.
- Occasionally patients were requested to recount dreams. Dream material was given special attention, as Freud believed defense mechanisms were less vigilant during sleep and repressed conflicts and desires would work their way toward consciousness or at least preconsciousness. Even in the sleep state, the repressed material was too anxiety-producing and had to be modified.
- Freud explained the matter as follows:
  - The actual material and recollection of the dream consists of the manifest material. Thus, the content the patient remembers is a defensive modification of the repressed material. To the patient, the material may appear bizarre or nonsense.
  - The latent content is the underlying repressed conflicting material that has been distorted by the manifest content so as to prevent anxiety.
- Periodically, the analyst will interpret the latent content to the patient to facilitate resolution.
- As analysis continues, the client experiences the anxiety of the repressed conflicts. As conflict intensifies, the client will have a catharsis, an outpouring of emotion that facilitates resolution. The analyst's task is to facilitate a controlled release of emotion so the client is not overwhelmed by anxiety and does not suffer a regressive experience.
- The analyst must refrain from addressing specific behaviors or superficial material. Resolving a specific symptom without addressing the underlying conflict might predispose the patient to have symptom substitution, that is, the development of a new symptom to replace the old.
- The process of analysis may be impeded by the patient's unconscious, as the process of investigation will increase anxiety and conflict.
- Patients will develop resistance. They may become dissatisfied with the analyst, skip or be late for appointments, become silent, or fail to report important material.
- The analyst must address resistance as it occurs or it may (will) become self-defeating and prevent deeper understanding of conflict-laden material.
- The patient may develop transference (a specific type of projection), that is, the unconscious association of the analyst with someone of significance in the patient's past. This allows the patient to ascribe to the analyst feelings once attributed to that person.
- Because of the nature of psychoanalysis, the analyst may engage in the same phenomenon, a process known as countertransference.
- Repressed conflicts affect an individual's life in an adverse manner by persistent utilization of inappropriate defense mechanisms. The analyst must interpret and educate the patient about the self-destructiveness of defense mechanisms.

Prominent Ideas of Freud

The role of the unconscious is paramount in personality development and daily behavior.

- Sex, or the enhancement of pleasure, is the driving force in development and behavior.
- Freud possessed a dark view of human nature. He theorized humans as driven by fantasies, conflicts, and sexual urges that were controlled by socialization, training, and religion.

- Freud put tremendous emphasis on early life experiences. He proposed that most of our personality is formed by the age of five.
- Freud outlined set stages of development. These were invariant and could not be circumvented. To obtain adequate psychological growth, the conflict at the end of each stage must be resolved so that libido energy can follow the appropriate developmental path.

The Freudians

Carl Jung, Analytical Psychology

- Jung was a Swiss colleague of Freud and a member of the inner circle until he developed his own theory of personality development.
- Jung believed that the personal unconscious could be understood by studying dreams, folklore, religion and mythology, and symbolism.
- As significant as the personal unconscious was the collective unconscious. He thought that there was a deeper level of the unconscious that was common to the entire species.
- Jung postulated the concept of archetype, a universal concept common to all humans. Many archetypes exist regarding behaviors such as motherhood and physical form. Archetypes are expressed in cultural and religious symbols.
- Mental health is the result of insight and self-realization. Mental illness is the consequence of conflicts that prevent self-exploration and self-realization.

Anna Freud, Ego Psychology

- Daughter of Sigmund Freud, who studied with her father and became an analyst in Vienna and London.
- Though a strong supporter of her father's theoretical positions, Anna came to believe that the ego should be the focus of attention.
- Anna Freud felt that the ego was the executor of personality and that analytical work should be directed at strengthening the ego to mitigate anxiety and stress.

- Anna Freud felt that the ego could become overwhelmed by conflicting demands of the id and the superego.
- Later in life, Anna Freud became a leader in child psychoanalysis and the psychological effects of depravation and poor nurturance.

Otto Rank, Humanistic Psychology

- Rank was Freud's closest associate for 20 years until publication of a paper advocating a different process of development and questioning the importance of early-life psychosexual growth.
- Over time, Rank moved further away from the classic tenets and eventually focused on the "here and now" in psychotherapy, rather than interpreting early-life experiences and repressed conflicts.
- Rank emphasized active learning and continued psychological growth throughout life. Psychotherapy concentrates on discovering give and take, separating and coming together. A patient must find a balance regarding all the forces in his or her environment to achieve mental health. The passiveness of the analysis was changed to an active dialogue with the patient.
- Rank had a profound effect on the professional development of Carl Rogers, Rollo May, and Erik Erikson. His writings are considered the foundation of humanistic and client-centered therapy.

Erik Erikson, Developmental Psychology

- Following his graduation from the Vienna Psychoanalytic Institute, Erikson moved to the United States where he taught at a number of universities and began to work with disadvantaged children and adolescents.
- Erikson revised Freud's five stages of psychosexual development into eight and said that human psychological development continues throughout life and that each stage has its individual challenges.
- Three stages were specific to adulthood and described challenges unique to that period. A ninth stage was later added to account for the challenges of old age.

- Like Anna Freud, Erikson was an ego psychologist and believed that the ego, not the id, was the focal point of personality.
- Social development, and not sexual development, was the underlying force behind growth.

Alfred Adler, Individual Psychology

- Along with Freud, Adler was one of the founders of psychoanalysis and the first colleague to break with Freud and establish his own school of thought.
- Adler believed in the unconscious and held that dream analysis was productive. However, he de-emphasized the role of psychosexual forces in favor of a conflict between inferiority and superiority.
- It was the work of the analyst to bring these two opposing forces into harmony.
- Central to Adler's technique was the concept of holistic treatment, which emphasized all psychological aspects of personal and social functioning of the patient.
- He abandoned the couch and had analyst and patient face each other in chairs. His therapeutic style utilized humor, historical incidents, and paradox.
- Adler's holistic approach led him to address how individuals integrate with society, and he became an advocate of prevention, democratic family structure, parent training, birth order, child psychology, organizational psychology, and women's rights.
- His work has been described as a precursor to modern CT.

Karen Horney, Feminine Psychology and Anxiety

- Psychoanalysis's first female practitioner, teacher, and theoretician, Horney broke with traditional Freudian teachings regarding psychosexual development and neurosis.

- Unlike Freud, who felt neurosis (anxiety) disturbance in mental functioning was the result of conflict, Horney viewed neurosis as a continuous process of managing stressors. All persons possessed some degree of "basic anxiety," which formed the foundation for a lifelong struggle.
- Because of adverse early experiences, some patients were more susceptible to periods of anxiety.
- The management of anxiety was the foundation of development. Horney developed ten basic neurotic needs that were expressed in three categories: moving toward people, moving away from people, and moving against people.
- Horney suggested the "self" was at the core of personality. All persons possess a dual perception of the self: the real self, who we are, and the ideal self, who we wish to be.
- Anxiety is generated when the two selves are in conflict and disharmony.
- The job of the analyst is to resolve the conflict and enhance growth or self-actualization. This is a lifelong process.
- Horney felt Freud had overemphasized male sexual issues.
- She postulated that if women had "penis envy," then men must have "womb envy."
- As such, women had a psychological advantage as self-actualization could be achieved by bearing children.
- Men, unable to bear children, compensated for their feelings of inferiority by seeking self-actualization through external means, such as dominance and aggressiveness.
- Horney felt cultural mores led women to be subservient to men, thereby preventing the attainment of self-actualization. She proposed that both genders had the ability to be productive and was an advocate for gender equality.

Other Resources

Evidence-Based References

American Psychological Association. (2002). Ethical principles of psychologists and code of conduct. Retrieved May 15, 2009, from http://www.apa.org/ethics/code2002.pdf.

American Psychotherapy Association. (2008). Psychotherapist's oath. Retrieved May 15, 2009, from http://www.americanpsychotherapy. com/about/oath/.

Beck, A. T., Rush, A. J., Shaw, B. F., & Emery, G. (1979). *Cognitive therapy of depression.* New York: Guilford Press.

Beck, J. (1995). *Cognitive therapy: Basics and beyond.* New York: Guilford Press.

Burns, D. (1999). *Feeling good: The new mood therapy.* New York: HarperCollins.

Dimeff, L. A., & Koerner, K. (Eds.). (2007). *Dialectical behavioral therapy in clinical practice.* New York: Guilford Press.

Freeman, A., Felgoise, S. H., Nezu, A. M., Nezu, C. M., & Reinecke, M. A. (Eds.). (2005). *Encyclopedia of cognitive behavioral therapy.* New York: Springer Publishing.

Gosch, E. A., Flannery-Schroeder, E., Mauro, C. F., & Compton, S. N. (2006). Principles of cognitive-behavioral therapy for anxiety disorders in children. *Journal of Cognitive Psychotherapy, 20,* 247–262.

Hayes, S. C., Follette, V. M., Linehan, M. (2004). *Mindfulness and acceptance: Expanding the cognitive-behavioral tradition.* New York: Guilford Press.

Kenneth H. K, Vessey, J., Lueger, R., & Schank, D. (1992). The psychotherapeutic delivery system. *Psychotherapy Research, 2,* 164–180.

Kuyken, W., Byford, S., Taylor, R. S., Watkins, E., Holden, E., White, K., et al. (2008). Mindfulness-based cognitive therapy to prevent relapse in recurrent depression. *Journal of Consulting and Clinical Psychology, 76*(6), 966–978.

Linehan, M. (1993). *Cognitive-behavioral treatment of borderline personality disorder.* New York: Guilford Press.

National Institute of Drug Abuse Treatment Manual for Cocaine Abuse. http://www.nida.nih.gov/TXManuals/CBT/CBT1.html.

Richmond, R. L. (2009). The psychotherapy process. Retrieved May 15, 2009, from http://www.guidetopsychology.com/questions/questions.htm#process.

Richmond, R. L. (2009). Transference issues. Retrieved May 15, 2009, from http://www.guidetopsychology.com/questions/questions. htm#trans.

Richmond, R. L. (2009). Termination issues. Retrieved May 15, 2009, from http://www.guidetopsychology.com/questions/questions. htm#termin.

Zur, O. (2009). The standard of care in psychotherapy and counseling: Bringing clarity to an illusive standard. Retrieved May 15, 2009, from http://www.zurinstitute.com/standardofcaretherapy.html.

Web Resources

- Addiction Treatment and CBT: http://www.smartrecovery.org/resources/toolchest.htm.
- Certification Information: Academy of Cognitive Therapy: http://www.academyofct.org/.
- Commercial entities, including Computer-aided Cognitive Behavioral Therapy Ltd.: http://www.ccbt.co.uk/, a UK-based company that provides CBT on-line for panic and phobias, depression and stress, and obsessive-compulsive disorder.
- Other sites that supply online assistance are educational rather than intervention-based and are more research oriented. These provide materials at no cost with the user's agreement to participate in the research process. One such site is the Mood Gym which operates from Centre for Mental Health Research (CMHR) at the Australian National University and is located at http://moodgym.anu.edu.au/.
- Overview of Cognitive Therapy of Depression: http://psychologyinfo.com/depression/cognitive.html.
- Panic and Anxiety Treatment: http://www.paniccenter.net/.

Psychiatric Emergency

Background Information

Definition of Disorder
An emergency is the result of a self-initiated, intentional act of self-harm with fatal outcomes.

Demographics
- Eleventh leading cause of death.
- More than 32,000 people kill themselves each year.
- More than 395,000 individuals are treated in the emergency room each year with self-inflicted injuries.
- Suicide accounts for 1.3% of all deaths in the United States.

Etiology
- The sociological factors include lack of family and social support.
- Psychological factors constitute Freud's and Menninger's theory of aggression turned inward.
- Biological factors focus on low serotonin concentration. Single nucleotide polymorphisms (SNPs) may be related to suicidal thinking and behavior.
- Genetic factors include familial pattern based on twin studies, Danish-American adoption studies, and molecular genetic studies.

Risk Factors
- Gender: the rate of attempt is higher among females, but males succeed four times more than females. Males and females differ in the selected method of suicide. Male veterans have twice the rate of suicide than those of the civilians.
- Age: a higher prevalence rate persists among males below age 25 and above age 45.
- Race: attempts are more common among whites, inner-city dwellers, native Americans, Inuit people, and first-generation immigrants.
- White men older than age 85 have the highest rate of suicide (59%).
- Religion: the rate is highest among Roman Catholics.

- Marital status: the rate is almost double among single, never-married individuals with poor social support.
- Occupation: the rate is higher among professionals—physicians, dentists, law enforcement officers, artists, and insurance agents. Diagnosis of the following medical conditions increases the risk for suicide: cancer, epilepsy, head injury, multiple sclerosis, CVD, dementia, AIDS, Huntington's disease, Cushing's disease, porphyrias, and Klinefelter's syndrome. Ninety-five percent of all attempts have a psychiatric disorder. Schizophrenia or mood disorder substantially increases the rate of suicide among this population. Individuals who have attempted suicide are more likely to successfully complete the attempt in future. Highest risk of completion is within the first year of an attempt, when depression is lifting, and during the first week of hospitalization.

Diagnosis

Assessment
- A thorough assessment comprises a psychiatric history and mental status examination, along with estimate of suicidal severity.
- If patient has attempted to harm self, determine the means utilized to cause harm.
- Physical injury will require an X-ray and suturing with appropriate dressing.
- Overdose attempts and ingestions of foreign bodies will require gastric lavage, administration of charcoal, lab tests, including complete blood count (CBC), comprehensive metabolic panel (CMP), liver function tests (LFTs), acetaminophen and salicilate levels, urine drug screen (UDS), blood alcohol level, and blood gases.
- Assess depressive symptoms, hopelessness, worthlessness, future plans, social support, coping skills, history of past attempts, severity of lethality of past attempts.

- Assess for presence of thoughts of harm, a realistic plan, means and access to means, past attempts at self-harm, lack of future plan, making preparations for death (e.g., giving away belongings).
- Search for weapons and contraband.
- Suicide screening tool for sad persons:

Sex: male	1 point
Age: <19, >45	1 point
Depression	2 points
Previous attempts	1 point
Excessive drug use	1 point
Rational thinking loss	2 points
Separated/divorced	1 point
Organized attempt	2 points
No social support	1 point
Stated future intent	2 points

Scoring: <2—discharge home
Scoring: 3–6—consider hospitalization or
                      close outpatient follow-up
Scoring: >6—admit

ICD Code
ICD 9 Suicide and self-inflicted injury

Treatment
- The treatment of acute psychosis includes administration of antipsychotics. Severe presentations (actively hallucinating) will require injectable form: haloperidol (Haldol) 5 mg, olanzapine (Zyprexa) 10 mg, or ziprasidone (Geodon) 10–20 mg IM. Less severe presentation can be managed by use of PO forms. Olanzapine (Zyprexa Zydis) 10 mg, risperidone (Risperdal) m-tab 1–2 mg are faster-acting POs. Haloperidol (Haldol) 5 mg, olanzapine (Zyprexa) 10 mg, risperidone (Risperdal) 1–2 mg are commonly used.
- A severely depressed individual should be monitored closely. Someone with a realistic plan to harm self should be monitored constantly until condition improves. Follow hospital protocols for documentation of constant observation.
- Substance-induced mood or psychosis requires combination of antipsychotic and benzodiazepine to relieve psychosis, and treatment of withdrawal symptoms. Haldol 5 mg IM and Ativan 2 mg IM are compatible and can be administered as one injection.
- Be supportive of the patient regardless of the presentation.
- If the patient refuses to consider hospitalization in the context of active thoughts of harm to self or others, involuntary commitment must be considered. A thorough documentation of assessment findings should include justification of involuntary commitment, that is, active thoughts of imminent harm to self or others, presence of a plan, and access to means.

Other Resources

Evidence-Based Readings

Cassells, C., Paterson, B., Dowding, D., & Morrison, R. (2005). Long and short term risk factors in the prediction of inpatient suicide: A review of literature. *Crisis: The Journal of Crisis Intervention and Suicide Prevention, 26*(2), 53–63.

DSM-IV-TR. *Diagnostic and statistical manual of mental disorders* (4th ed.).

Emergency Psychiatry, Summer 2005.

Gaynes, B., West, S., Ford, C., et al. (2004, May). Screening for suicide risk in adults: A summary of the evidence for the U.S. Preventive Services Task Force. *Annals of Internal Medicine, 140*(10), 822–835.

Mann, J., Apter, A., Bertolote, J., & Beautrias, A. (2005). Suicide prevention strategies: A systematic review. *Journal of the American Medical Association, 294*(16), 2064–2074.

Muzina, D. (2007). Suicide intervention. *Current Psychiatry, 6*(9), 31–46.

Sadock, B., & Sadock, V. (1996). *Concise textbook of clinical psychiatry* (3rd ed.). Philadelphia: Lippincott, Williams & Wilkins.

Web Resources

- www.bmj.com/cgi/content/abstract/337/ nov18_3/a2205.
- www. cdc.gov.
- www.dmi.columbia.edu.
- National Institute of Mental Health: http://www.nimh. gov.

II

Syndromes and Treatments in Adult Psychiatry

Delirium

Background Information

Definition of Disorder

- Abnormality in cognitive processing affecting thinking, attention, awareness, memory, perception, and orientation to person, place, and time.
- Onset is fairly rapid.
- Delirium is the direct result of an underlying medical condition, illness, or medication.
- Mimics dementia.
- Often the first sign of illness in the elderly.
- An acute confusional state.
- Disturbed attention and lack of environmental awareness.
- May involve visual illusions, hallucinations, and delusions.

Etiology

- One theory is that delirium reflects neuronal dysfunction through excessive neurotransmitter release and abnormal signal conduction.
- Medications—prescription or over-the-counter—are the most common causes of delirium.
- Anticholinergic toxicity from prescribed medications (diphenhydramine [Benadryl]), tricyclic antidepressants (TCAs) (amitriptyline [Elavil], imipramine [Tofranil]), and antipsychotics (chlorpromazine [Thorazine], thioridazine [Mellaril]).
- Benzodiazepines or alcohol.
- Anti-inflammatory agents, including prednisone.
- Cardiovascular (antihypertensives, digitalis).
- Diuretics, if dehydrated.
- Gastrointestional (cimetidine, rentidine).
- Opioid analgesics (especially meperidine).
- Lithium.
- Antipsychotic, sedative, hypnotic drugs often used to treat confusion, agitation, or insomnia may precipitate an episode of delirium.
- Infections: pneumonia, skin, urinary tract.

- Metabolic acute blood loss, dehydration, electrolyte imbalance, organ failure, hyper- or hypoglycemia, hypoxia.
- Heart: arrhythmia, congestive heart failure, myocardial infarction (MI), or shock.
- Neurologic: central nervous system infection, head trauma, seizures, stroke subdural hematoma, transient ischemic accidents, tumors.
- Other: fecal impaction, postoperative recovery, sleep deprivation, urinary retention.

Demographic

- Thirty to forty percent of hospitalized patients over the age of 65 have experienced an episode of delirium.
- Forty to fifty percent of patients are recovering from surgery to repair a hip fracture.
- Thirty to forty percent of patients have acquired immunodeficiency disease (AIDS).
- Forty to seventy percent of patients have cardiac problems.

Risk Factors

- Age: the very old and the very young are at risk for delirium.
- Persons with brain trauma, dementia, cerebrovascular disease, tumor, alcohol dependence, diabetes mellitus, cancer, blindness, or poor hearing are at risk for delirium.
- Persons on multiple medications.
- Another mental disorder, such as depression or substance abuse (alcoholism or drug abuse), increases the risk of developing delirium.
- Another physical disorder: infection, dehydration.
- Metabolic, electrolyte, and endocrine disturbances.

Diagnosis

Differential Diagnosis

- Whether the patient has dementia is the most common issue in the differential diagnosis. Rule out:
- Infection: urinary, pneumonia, skin

- Diabetic-, hyper-, or hypoglycemia
- Cardiac arrhythmias
- Cerebral lesions
- Alcohol withdrawal

ICD-9-CM (2009) Code
293.0 (28 index entries)

Diagnostic Work-Up
- Assume reversibility
- Identify and correct underlying cause(s)
- Physical evaluation
- Blood sugar
- Urinalysis (UA) for culture and sensitivity
- Serum levels of medications
- O$_2$ saturation
- Arrhythmia
- B-12
- Brain imaging tests and measures of serum anticholinergic activity are experimental laboratory tests that show promise

Initial Assessment
- Delirium is often underrecognized by healthcare personnel, especially if the patient has hypoactive delirium, is 80 years of age or older, has vision impairment, or has dementia (Inouye et al., 2001). Periodic application of simple cognitive tests, such as the Mini-Cog, the confusion assessment method for the intensive care unit (CAM-ICU), or the intensive care delirium screening checklist (ICDSC), may improve identification.
- The clock face test is also a simple test of mental status.
- White blood cell count, CBC (complete blood count), electrolytes (potassium, sodium, chloride, bicarbonate).
- Interview.
- Rule out infection and other medical causes.
- Review prescriptions, especially recent ones and over-the-counter medications for anticholinergic delirium.
- HX if drug and alcohol use.
- Electrocardiogram—to identify any arrhythmias.

Clinical Presentation: Symptoms
- Hypervigilance or inattention to the environment
- Disorganized thinking or altered level of consciousness
- Sleep–wake cycle disturbance
- Progressing to anxiety, agitation, flight syndrome—tries to leave hospital
- Perceptual disturbances (visual illusions, hallucinations, delusions)
- Disorientation in regard to time, place, person
- Concomitant physical condition
- Also may exhibit anxiety, fear, depression, irritability, anger
- Symptoms will fluctuate over a 24-hour period

DSM-IV-TR Diagnostic Guidelines
- Delirium is a disturbance in consciousness and/or a change in cognition that cannot be accounted for by a preexisting dementia.

Treatment

Acute Treatment
See the American Psychiatric Association's *Practice Guideline for Treatment of Patients with Delirium.*
- Identifying the underlying cause
- Initiate psychiatric management through therapeutic interaction with the patient to reduce fear
- Educate the family and other clinicians regarding the illness
- Establish therapeutic trust when the patient is stable
- Provide supportive measures that include
- Modifying the environment-orient to environment
- Provide objects to orient patient to day and night (calendar, clock)
- Provide quiet and well-lit surroundings that dampen noise made by machines, overhead pagers, and equipment
- Do not use physical restraints
- Hydrate the patient
- Provide familiar faces of family members, sitters
- Stimulate daytime activity, mobilize the patient
- Correct sensory deficits with eyeglasses, hearing aids, portable amplification devices

- Promote normal sleep with warm milk, massage, nighttime noise reduction
- Prevent dehydration (blood urea nitrogen [BUN] to creatinine ratio > 18) and fecal impaction
- Review risk factors: use of physical restraints, dehydration, and bladder catheter
- For acute agitation, use a high-potency low-anticholinergic, low-arrythmogenic antipsychotic medication, such as haloperidol (Haldol), as needed
- If on antipsychotic medication (risperidone [Risperdal], olanzapine [Zyprexa], and quetiapine [Seroquel, Seroquel XR]), patients should have their electrocardiograms monitored. QTc interval greater than 450 msec or 25% over baseline warrant a cardiology consultation and reduction or discontinuation of the medication
- Morphine (not meperdine) may be required if pain is a factor

Chronic Treatment

- Most people respond well to treatment and can return to normal functioning in hours to days.
- Treatment can be complicated if the patient has another condition at the same time, such as substance abuse, depression, or other anxiety disorders.

Recurrence Rate

If the rate of recurrence is common, the patient needs to be monitored frequently.

Patient Education

- Information regarding delirium may be found in MD Consult: Delirium: Patient Education (http://www.mdconsult. com).
- Advise patients to avoid over-the-counter medications for colds and sleep with high anticholinergic effect, including pseudophedrine or cimedadine.

Medical/Legal Pitfalls

- Delirium is associated with significant morbidity and mortality. Estimated 3-month mortality rate of patient with delirium ranges from 23 to 33%, 1-year mortality rate is as high as 50%.
- Persons with delirium are more likely to have a fall in the hospital or other events that will delay discharge and result in costlier hospital stays.
- Persons with delirium are more susceptible to dehydration or malnutrition because the lack of orientation delays satisfying the urge to eat or drink.
- Pain can also contribute to delirium.
- Alcohol use and withdrawal can cause delirium.

Dementia

Background Information

Definition of Disorder
- Also, Alzheimer's disease.
- Decline in memory beginning with short-term memory loss.
- Decline in other cognitive functions, including performing familiar tasks, language, orientation to time and place, poor or declining judgment, abstract thinking, misplacing objects in unusual places, changes in mood or behavior, loss of initiative sufficient to affect activities of daily living.
- Onset is insidious, progressive over months to years, and is rarely reversible.

Etiology
- A common denominator of all dementia disorders is that memory and cognitive function are impaired due to neuron death. Therefore, it is not reversible.

Demographic
- About 1% of the people of 65 years of age and older and more than 50% of the people of 90 years of age or older have a dementia disorder.
- Worldwide, half of the demented persons (46%) lived in Asia, 30% in Europe, and 12% in North America; 52% live in less-developed regions.
- About 59% of women have Alzheimer's disease.

Risk Factors
- Age: dementia increases with age.
- Genetic changes: Apolipoprotein E (ApoE and E4) allele is a strong risk factor.
- Probable risks: head trauma and genetics.
- Evidence is moderate that low education has a moderate risk effect on dementia.
- The evidence is moderate at midlife that controlling high cholesterol levels and high blood pressure has a protective effect on dementia.
- The evidence is strong that antihypertensive drugs have a protective effect on dementia.

- The evidence is moderate that leisure activities/active lives have a protective effect.
- The evidence is insufficient that social network or personality type has a protective effect.
- Evidence is insufficient that obesity, high homocysteine levels, diet, folate/B12 deficiency, aluminum, and depression are risk factors for dementia.
- Evidence is insufficient that statins, hormone replacement therapy, and nonsteroidal anti-inflammatory drugs (NSAIDs) have a protective effect.
- Evidence is limited that moderate alcohol use has a protective effect on the risk of dementia.

Relationship to Other Diseases
- Dementia is unrelated hypothyroidism or hyperthyroidism, but needs to be diagnosed and treated.
- Studies show variable results in regard to correlation between low vitamin B12 (colbalamin) and dementia or Alzheimer's disease. There is a correlation between low folic acid levels and impaired cognitive function.

Diagnosis

Differential Diagnosis
- Delirium
- Depression
- Thyroid disorders
- Diabetic: hyper- or hypoglycemia
- Cardiac arrhythmias
- Cerebral lesions
- Posttraumatic stress disorder (PTSD)
- Drug interactions or adverse effects

ICD Code
290.0 (8 index entries)—code first the associated neurological condition

Diagnostic Work-Up
- Currently there is no simple, reliable test for diagnosing dementia at an early stage.
- Physical and neurological evaluation is done.

- Evaluate mental status for short- and long-term memory, problem solving, depression.
- CBC with differential.
- Computer tomography (CT scan) and magnetic resonance imaging (MRI) scan can identify people who have Alzheimer's disease.
- Electroencephalography (EEG) brain mapping and apoliprotein levels are currently not recommended for identifying Alzheimer's disease.

Initial Assessment

- History from the family, friends, or caretaker close to the person will supplement the patient's account.
- Clock drawing test or other simple exercise will allow selection for additional testing.
- Assess functional status.
- People with dementia are sometimes stigmatized. Understanding can lead to more compassion among patient, family, and friends.

Clinical Presentation: Symptoms

Early (1–3 Years):
- Disorientation as to date
- Recall problems in relation to recent events
- Naming problems
- Mild language or decision-making problems
- Mild problem in copying figures (example face of a clock)
- Social withdrawal
- Mood change
- Problems managing finances

Middle (2–8 Years):
- Disorientation about date and place
- Getting lost in familiar areas
- Impaired new learning
- Impaired calculating skills
- Agitation and aggression
- Problems with cooking, shopping, dressing, grooming
- Restless, anxious, depressed

Late (6–12 Years):
- Disoriented to time, place, person
- Increasingly nonverbal
- Long-term memory gone

- Unable to copy or write
- Unable to groom or dress
- Incontinent
- Motor or verbal agitation

End Stage:
- Nonverbal
- Not eating or swallowing well
- Not ambulatory
- Incontinent of bowel and bladder
  Depression occurs in 50% of the patients and may cause rapid decline if not treated.

Diagnosis

- *DSM-IV*: Dementia is a syndrome rather than an illness, with a set of signs and symptoms that includes a progressive decline in cognitive function due to damage or disease in the body beyond what might be expected from normal aging. Although dementia is far more common in the geriatric population, it may occur at any stage of adulthood.
- Symptoms of dementia can be classified as either reversible or irreversible, depending on the etiology of the disease. Fewer than 10% of cases of dementia are the result of causes that may presently be reversed with treatment. Without careful assessment of history, the short-term syndrome of delirium can easily be confused with dementia, because they have many symptoms in common. Some mental illnesses, including depression and psychosis, may also produce symptoms that mimic those of dementia.

Treatment

Chronic Treatment

The focus of treatment is to improve the quality of life of the individual and the care provider by maintaining functional ability and by supporting remaining intellectual abilities, mood, behavior, and social support networks such as the Swedish Council on Technology Assessment in Health Care (http://www.sbu.se/en/).

- Treat comorbid physical illnesses, blood pressure, diabetes
- Support the family's setting of realistic goals

- Limit all medications, especially psychotropic or sedatives, to only essential medications
- Maintain functional ability

Nonpharmacologic Approaches
- Care of the family member with dementia requires multilevel resources that increase the caregiver's burden over time.
- Behavior modification, including scheduled activities (e.g., toileting in late stages) and prompted activities (e.g., dressing in middle stages).
- Assistance to meet only what the elder cannot do.
- Familiar music.
- Walking or light exercise.
- Pet therapy.
- Calm and slow approaches.
- Well-lighted areas without shadows.

Pharmacologic Treatment
- Cholinesterase inhibitors such as Aricept, Reminyl, Exelon (benefit for 1–3 years)
- Record functional status and cognitive status
- Treat agitation

Support Caregiver
- Caregiver burden includes isolation and anxiety
- Respite care is

Recurrence Rate
Long-term chronic decline occurs.

Patient Education
- Alzheimer's Association: http://www.alz.org/index.asp
- Family caregiver alliance: http://www.caregiver.org/caregiver/jsp/home.jsp
- National caregiver alliance: http://www.caregiving.org/members/

Medical/Legal Pitfalls
- Dementia affects all areas of life, including physical, social, financial, and social. The issues are complicated and require careful reflection on the human condition and the value of various interventions.
- Dementia affects the lives of family members in a way that requires treatment resources to support the caregiver.
- Legal resources are involved in drawing up living wills and wills before the patient is no longer able to make his or her wishes known.
- Protective services may be involved to protect the patient against financial or physical abuse.

Amnesic Syndrome

Background Information

Definition of Disorder
- Loss of memory from organic or functional causes.
- Organic amnesia is the result of trauma, disease, or certain drugs (usually sedatives).
- Functional causes of amnesia are defense mechanisms and hysterical posttraumatic amnesia.
- Inability to imagine the future from a damaged hippocampus.

Etiology
- Posttraumatic amnesia is usually the result of a head injury and is often, but not always, transient.
- Dissociative amnesia results from psychological trauma rather than direct damage to the brain.
- Repressed memory is the inability to recall information about a traumatic event, such as a mugging or rape. The event is stored in the long-term memory, but access is impaired because of psychological defense mechanisms. People can continue to learn new information, and the repressed memory may eventually return.
- Anterograde amnesia caused by amnestics, such as benzodiazepines or alcohol, in which a memory is never transferred from temporary to permanent storage.
- Dissociative fugue is rare, caused by psychological trauma, and usually temporary. Loss of identity occurs in which there is an inability to recall some or all of one's past.
- Some personality types are at risk for dissociative amnesia. Persons with dissociative disorders have more immature psychological defense mechanisms (Simeon, Guralnik, Knuntelska, & Schmeidler, 2002)
- Posthypnotic amnesia occurs when events during hypnosis are forgotten or when memories cannot be recalled.
- Lacunar amnesia is the loss of memory for one event.

- Childhood amnesia is the common inability to remember events from one's childhood. It is theorized that the brain and language development are immature.
- Transient global amnesia is a form of amnesia reflecting abnormalities in the hippocampus. Symptoms may last for a day, and no clear precipitating factor or concomitant neurological deficit can be identified. Some theorize that the loss of memory is related to a seizure, atypical form of a migraine, or from reduced blood flow.
- Source amnesia occurs when one cannot recall where or how one obtained information.
- Memory distrust syndrome occurs when a person is unable to trust his or her memory.
- Blackout phenomenon is the result of excessive short-term alcohol consumption.
- Korsakoff's syndrome is the result of alcoholism or malnutrition from vitamin B1 deficiency. It may be progressive unless patient receives nutritional treatment. It is connected with confabulation.
- Drug-induced amnesia is often a result of premedication with benzodiazepine, propofol, or scopolamine to help a patient forget a medical procedure that was not performed under full anesthesia.

Demographic
- Can appear in individuals of any age after infancy.

Risk Factors
- Head injury
- Psychological trauma
- Stress: the initial appearance of amnesia often follows a highly stressful event, such as being the victim of a traumatic crime or rape

Diagnosis

Differential Diagnosis
- Diagnosis of exclusion
- Rule out memory loss from seizure disorders
- Alcohol consumption

- Head injuries
- Alzheimer's disease or delirium with fever
- General anesthetics, including halothane, isoflurane, and fentanyl, or drugs, such as barbiturates or benzodiazepines
- Tumors or infection
- Depression
- Stroke or transient ischemic attack (TIA)
- Malingering may be detected because the amnesiac typically exaggerates and dramatizes the symptoms and has obvious financial, legal, or personal reasons for pretending loss of memory
- Inability to recall the first 4–5 years of one's life is a normal feature of human development

ICD-9 Code
780.9 Amnesic Syndrome

Diagnostic Work-Up
- Detailed medical history and physical examination: ask questions as to type, time pattern, or a triggering incident.
- Cerebral angiography.
- Cognitive tests for memory.
- EEG.
- Diagnosis of transient global amnesia may be visualized by MRI of the brain by diffusion-weighted imaging (DWI).

Initial Assessment
- Medical history
- Symptoms experienced
- When the amnesia started
- What effect the amnesia has on the ability to function

Clinical Presentation: Symptoms
- Patient's loss of confidence in his or her own memory and account of past events
- Feeling a loss of control

DSM-IV-TR Diagnostic Guidelines
Amnestic disorder is defined as the loss of ability to recall information that had been previously encoded in memory. This process may be organic or psychogenic in origin.
- Amnesia associated with head trauma is typically both retrograde (the patient has no memory of events shortly before the head injury) and anterograde (the patient has no memory of events after the injury).
- The amnesia that is associated with seizure disorders is sudden onset.
- Amnesia in patients suffering from delirium or dementia occurs in the context of extensive disturbances of the patient's cognition, speech, perceptions, emotions, and behaviors.
- Amnesia associated with substance abuse, which is sometimes called a "blackout," typically affects only short-term memory and is irreversible.
- In dissociative amnesia, in contrast to these other conditions, the patient's memory loss is almost always anterograde, which means that it is limited to the period following the traumatic event(s). In addition, patients with dissociative amnesia do not have problems learning new information.

Treatment

Acute Treatment
- Psychotherapy is supportive by creating an environment of safety. Sometimes, people may regain their memories if they feel safe.
- Most patients have their memories return when they are at home alone or with family or close friends rather than with a therapist. The majority of individuals who recover their memories find evidence of their memories independent of the therapist's suggestions.
- In general, no medications exist for treating most types of amnesic syndromes, although in some instances hypnosis or sodium amytal may prove helpful.
- Neurotransmitters are a class of medications under investigation for memory loss.
- Patients may be given medications for depression, anxiety, and other symptoms that may accompany the loss of memories.
- Treatment consists of strategies to help make up for the loss of memory. For example, the patient may work with an occupational therapist to replace what was lost or work with intact memories as a foundation for learning new information.
- Memory training is also effective.

Chronic Treatment

- After a patient has recalled a great enough number of memories to establish continuity and strengthen his or her sense of self, another phase of psychotherapy may begin. The second phase of recovery focuses on cognitive assimilation of memories within the individual's personality, using the retained memory as the basis.
- Individuals with severe amnesia may find lists, calendars, BlackBerry or personal digital assistants useful to help organize daily schedules and photographs helpful to remember people and places.

Recurrence Rate

- Rate of recurrence is 50% unless patient is involved in CBT.

Patient Education

- International Society for the Study of Dissociation (ISSD); 60 Revere Drive, Suite 500, Northbrook, IL 60062. http://www.issd.org
- National Institute of Mental Health; 6001 Executive Boulevard, Room 8184, MSC 9663, Bethesda, MD 20892–9663. http://www.nimh.nih.gov

Medical/Legal Pitfalls

- Persons with amnesic syndrome are sometimes at the center of lawsuits where recovered memories of abuse are the basis of the case.
- Amnesia has also been the defense in the murder of adults and the murder of infants.
- Judges and attorneys have few guidelines for amnesic cases.

Other Resources

Evidence-Based References

American Psychiatric Association. (1999). Practice guideline for the treatment of patients with delirium. *American Journal of Psychiatry, 156*(5 Suppl), 1–20. Retrieved on June 29, 2009, from http://www.psychiatryonline.com/pracGuide/loadGuidelinePdf.aspx?file = DeliriumPG_05-15-06.

Bourne, R. S., Tahir, T. A., Borthwick, M., & Sampson, E. L. (2008). Drug treatment of delirium: Past, present and future. *Journal of Psychosomatic Research, 65*(3), 273–282.

Chu, J. A., Frey, L. M., Ganzel, B. L., & Matthews, J. A. (1999). Memories of childhood abuse: Dissociation, amnesia, and corroboration. *American Journal of Psychiatry, 156*, 749–755.

Greenaway, M. C., Hanna, S. M., Lepore, S. W., & Smith, G. E. (2008). A behavioral rehabilitation intervention for amnesic mild cognitive impairment. *American Journal of Alzheimer's Disease and Other Dementias, 23*(5), 451–461.

Harrison, M., & Williams, M. (2007). The diagnosis and management of transient global amnesia in the emergency department. *Emergency Medicine Journal, 24*(6), 444–445.

Inouye, S. K., Foreman, M. D., Mion, L. C., Katz, K. H., & Cooney, L. M. (2001). Nurses' recognition of delirium and its symptoms. *Archives of Internal Medicine, 161*, 2467–2473.

Litaker, D., Locala, J., Franco, K., Bronson, D. L., & Tannous, Z. (2001). Preoperative risk factors for postoperative delirium. *General Hospital Psychiatry, 23*, 84–89.

Michaud, M., Bula, C., Berney, A., Camus, V., Voellinger, R., Stiefel, F., Burnand, B., & The Delirium Guidelines Development Group. (2007). Delirium: Guidelines for general hospitals. *Journal of Psychosomatic Research, 62*, 371–383.

Owen, D., Paranandi, B., Sivakumar, R., & Seevaratnam, M. (2007). Classical diseases revisited: Transient global amnesia. *Postgraduate Medical Journal, 83*(978), 236–239.

Pantoni, L., Bertini, E., Lamassa, M., Pracucci, G., & Inzitari, D. (2005). Clinical features, risk factors, and prognosis in transient global amnesia: A follow-up study. *European Journal of Neurology, 12*(5), 350–356.

Simeon, D., Guralnik, O., Knuntelska, M., & Schmeidler, J. (2002). Personality factors associated with dissociation: Temperament, defenses, and cognitive schemata. *American Journal of Psychiatry, 159*, 489–491.

Swedish Council on Technology Assessment in Health Care. (2008). *Dementia—etiology and epidemiology: A systematic review* (Vol. 1). Stockholm: Elanders Infologistics. Retrieved on May 12, 2009, from http://www.sbu.se/en/.

Wilmo, A., Winblad, B., Aguero-Torres, H., & von Stauss, E. (2003). *The magnitude of dementia occurrence in the world.* Stockholm: Aging Research Center.

Web Resources

- http://www.alz.org/index.asp.
- http://www.caregiver.org/caregiver/jsp/home.jsp.
- http://www.caregiving.org/members/.
- American Psychiatric Association: http://www.psych.org.
- Freedom from Fear: http://www.freedomfromfear.org.

Substance Abuse

Background Information

Definition of Disorder
- It is a Maladaptive pattern of substance use.
- The substance used poses a hazard to health.

DSM-IV-TR Classes of Psychoactive Substances
- Alcohol
- Amphetamines
- Caffeine
- Cannabis
- Cocaine
- Hallucinogens
- Inhalants
- Nicotine
- Opioids
- Phencyclidine (PCP)
- Sedatives, hypnotics, and anxiolytics

Etiology
- No single theory can explain the cause of substance abuse/dependence
- Theoretical causes
  - Genetics
  - Biochemical
  - Psychopathological
    - Developmental influences
    - Personality traits
  - Social learning
    - Parental role modeling
    - Cultural and/or ethnic influences

Demographics
- Males are twice as likely to be affected than females
- The use of illegal drugs is most common in young adults (aged 18–25 years)
- More than 100 million Americans, aged 12 years or older, report illicit drug use at least once in their lives
- Fifty to seventy-five percent of those with a mental disorder struggle with substance addiction

- More than 70% of the acquired immune deficiency syndrome (AIDS) cases among women are drug-related
- Over 100,000 deaths in a year in the United States are caused by excessive alcohol consumption
- Approximately, 1 in 10 Americans has an alcohol problem
- Marijuana is the most commonly abused illicit substance in the United States

Risk Factors
- Unemployment
- Poor social coping skills
- History of emotional, physical, or sexual abuse
- Chaotic home environment
- History of mental illness
- Untreated physical pain
- Family history of addiction
- Peer pressure
- Educational level
- Economic status
- Recent incarceration

Diagnosis

Differential Diagnosis
Rule out medical problems that may mimic signs and symptoms of substance intoxication and/or withdrawal:
- Hypoglycemia
- Electrolyte (sodium, potassium, chloride, and sodium bicarbonate) imbalance
- Head injury/trauma
- Stroke
- Psychosis
- Neurological disorder

ICD Code
Diagnostic codes for substance use are classified according to substance. The following code is for unknown substances:
    304.90 Substance Abuse

Diagnostic Work-Up
- Diagnosis of substance abuse/dependence is typically made by detailed subjective history
- Blood, breath, or urine screening for substance(s)

Initial Assessment
- Medical history and examination
- Psychiatric history and examination
- Family and social history
- Cultural history related to substance use
- Detailed history of past and present substance use, tolerance, and withdrawal
- How do the substances affect patient mentally and physically?
- How is the substance use affecting patient's occupational, family, or social life?
  CAGE (cut down, annoyed, guilty, and eye opener), screening questionnaire to assess alcohol dependence
  S-MAST (Short-Michigan Alcoholism Screening Test), screening tool for alcohol use
  CIWA-Ar (Clinical Institute Withdrawal Assessment for Alcohol) is a validated 10-item assessment tool to evaluate alcohol withdrawal symptoms
  COWS (clinical opiate withdrawal scale), assessment tool to evaluate opioid withdrawal symptoms

Clinical Presentation
Signs and symptoms will vary with individuals/substances used, but include:
- Sudden weight loss/gain
- Periods of excessive sleep or inability to sleep
- Periods of excessive energy
- Chronic nosebleeds
- Chronic sinusitis
- Chronic cough or bronchitis
- Increased periods of agitation, irritability, or anger
- Depressed mood
- Temporary psychosis
- Inability to perform task at work, school, or home

DSM-IV-TR Diagnostic Guidelines for Substance Abuse
- Maladaptive pattern of substance use may occur
- Leads to adverse consequences

- Recurrent substance use within a 12-month period
- Symptoms have never met criteria for substance dependence

Treatment

Treatment for Substance Use
- Psychosocial
  - Cognitive-behavioral therapy (CBT)
  - Motivational enhancement therapy (MET)
  - Behavioral therapy
  - Psychotherapy
- Pharmacological
  - Treatment of withdrawal states is used
  - Medication is given to decrease reinforcing effects of substance(s)
  - Maintenance medication management (agonist therapy)
  - Medication for relapse prevention
  - Treatment of comorbid conditions
- Self-help groups
  - Alcoholics Anonymous
  - Narcotics Anonymous
  - Cocaine Anonymous

Pharmacological Treatment for Use of Specific Substances
- Nicotine
  - Nicotine replacement: patch, gum, spray, lozenge, and inhaler
  - Bupropion (Wellbutrin)
  - Varenicline
- Alcohol
  - Symptoms of withdrawal may occur within 4–12 hours after cessation or reduction
  - Thiamine replacement and fluids are given
  - Benzodiazepine is tapered to prevent withdrawal
  - Clonidine (Catapres) as needed for hypertensive episode due to withdrawal
  - Naltrexone (Nalorex) (oral or intramuscular [IM]) or acamprosate (Campral) is given to decrease craving
  - Disulfiram (Antabuse) is a deterrent to drinking
- Marijuana
  - No recommended pharmacologic treatment

- Cocaine
    - Pharmacological treatment is not indicated
    - Topiramate (Topamax), disulfiram (Antabuse), modafinil (Provigil) with psychosocial treatment may be effective
- Opioids
    - Opioid overdose: naloxone is given to reverse respiratory depression
    - Maintenance treatment: methadone (Dolophone) or buprenorphine (Subutex) is gradually tapered
    - Alternative maintenance: naltrexone (Nalorex)

Recurrence Rate
- Rate of relapse for those who have been in treatment is approximately 90%
- Majority of relapses take place within 3 months following treatment

Patient Education
- Educate on importance of joining a support group. Information available online for worldwide support groups, including Narcotics Anonymous, Alcoholic Anonymous, and Cocaine Anonymous.
- Teach about relapse prevention. Encourage CBT to increase coping skills and individual therapy to enhance personal insight.
- Patients taking disulfiram (Antabuse) must be advised to avoid alcohol and any substances that contain alcohol. This includes mouthwash, colognes, cough syrups, etc.

Medical/Legal Pitfalls
- Rates of suicide are three to four times more prevalent in people who abuse alcohol or drugs as compared to the general population.
- Individuals withdrawing from substances are at great risk for depression. When not properly treated, depression can lead to suicide.
- Individuals being treated for addiction may have a history of seeing multiple healthcare professionals obtain medications ("doctor shopping"). Such practice may lead to accidental and/or intentional overdose.

Substance Dependence

Background Information

Definition of Disorder
- It is commonly known as addiction.
- Tolerance to substance is examined.
- Leads to withdrawal when substance is eliminated or significantly reduced.

DSM-IV-TR Classes of Psychoactive Substances
- Alcohol
- Amphetamines
- Caffeine
- Cannabis
- Cocaine
- Hallucinogens
- Inhalants
- Nicotine
- Opioids
- PCP
- Sedatives, hypnotics, and anxiolytics

Etiology
- No single theory can explain the cause of substance abuse/dependence
- Theoretical causes
  - Genetics
  - Biochemical
  - Psychopathological
    - ◆ Developmental influences
    - ◆ Personality traits
  - Social learning
- Parental role modeling
- Cultural and/or ethnic influences

Demographics
- Males are twice as likely to be affected than females
- The use of illegal drugs is most common in young adults (aged 18–25 years)

- More than 100 million Americans, aged 12 years or older, report illicit drug use at least once in their lives
- About 50–75% of people with a mental disorder struggle with substance addiction
- More than 70% of the AIDS cases among women are drug related
- More than 100,000 deaths in the United States each year are caused by excessive alcohol consumption
- Approximately, 1 in 10 Americans has an alcohol problem
- Marijuana is the most commonly abused illicit substance in the United States

Risk Factors
- Unemployment
- Poor social coping skills
- History of emotional, physical, or sexual abuse
- Chaotic home environment
- History of mental illness
- Untreated physical pain
- Family history of addiction
- Peer pressure
- Educational level
- Economic status
- Recent incarceration

Diagnosis

Differential Diagnosis
Rule out medical problems that may mimic signs and symptoms of substance intoxication and/or withdrawal:
- Hypoglycemia
- Electrolyte imbalance (sodium, potassium, chloride, and bicarbonate)
- Head injury/trauma
- Stroke
- Psychosis
- Neurological disorder

ICD Code

Diagnostic codes for substance use are classified according to the substance. The following codes are for unknown substances:

Substance Abuse
Substance Dependence
Substance Withdrawal
Substance Intoxication

Diagnostic Work-Up

- Diagnosis of substance abuse/dependence is typically made by detailed subjective history
- Blood, breath, or urine screening for substance(s)

Initial Assessment

- Medical history and examination
- Psychiatric history and examination
- Family and social history
- Cultural history related to substance use
- Detailed history of past and present substance use, tolerance, and withdrawal
- How do the substances affect patient mentally and physically?
- How is the substance use affecting patient's occupational, family, or social life?
- CAGE questionnaire or S-MAST, a screening tool for alcohol use
- CIWA Ar, an assessment tool to evaluate alcohol withdrawal symptoms
- COWS, an assessment tool to evaluate opioid withdrawal symptoms

Clinical Presentation

Signs and symptoms will vary with individuals/substances used, but include:

- Sudden weight loss/gain
- Periods of excessive sleep or inability to sleep
- Periods of excessive energy
- Chronic nosebleeds
- Chronic sinusitis
- Chronic cough or bronchitis
- Increased periods of agitation, irritability, or anger
- Depressed mood
- Temporary psychosis
- Inability to perform tasks at work, school, or home

DSM-IV-TR Diagnostic Guidelines for Substance Dependence

- Maladaptive pattern of substance use may occur
- Characterized by behavioral and physiological symptoms:
  - Physical dependence is due to tolerance to substance being used
  - Psychological dependence, overwhelming desire to repeat use of substance to achieve desired effect

Treatment for Substance Dependence

- Psychosocial
  - CBT
  - MET
  - Behavioral therapy
  - Psychotherapy
- Pharmacological
  - Treat withdrawal states
  - Medication is given to decrease reinforcing effects of substance(s)
  - Maintenance medication management (agonist therapy)
  - Medication for relapse prevention
  - Treatment of comorbid conditions
- Self-help groups
  - Alcoholics Anonymous
  - Narcotics Anonymous
  - Cocaine Anonymous

Pharmacological Treatment for Use of Specific Substances

- Nicotine
  - Nicotine replacement: patch, gum, spray, lozenge, and inhaler
  - Bupropion (Wellbutrin)
  - Varenicline
- Alcohol
  - Symptoms of withdrawal may occur within 4–12 hours after cessation or reduction
  - Thiamine replacement and fluids
  - Benzodiazepine tapered to prevent withdrawal
  - Clonidine (Catapres) as needed for hypertensive episode due to withdrawal
  - Naltrexone (Nalorex) (oral or IM) or acamprosate (Campral) to decrease craving
  - Disulfiram (Antabuse) as deterrent to drinking

- Marijuana
  - No pharmacologic treatment is recommended
- Cocaine
  - Pharmacological treatment is not indicated
  - Topiramate (Topamax), disulfiram (Antabuse), modafinil (Provigil) with psychosocial treatment may be effective
- Opioids
  - Opioid overdose: naloxone is given to reverse respiratory depression
  - Maintenance treatment: methadone (Dolophone) or buprenorphine (Subutex) is gradually tapered
  - Alternative maintenance: naltrexone (Nalorex)

Recurrence Rate
- Rate of relapse, for those who have been in treatment, is approximately 90%
- Majority of relapses take place within 3 months following treatment

Patient Education
- Educate on importance of joining a support group. Information is available online for worldwide support groups, including Narcotics Anonymous, Alcoholics Anonymous, and Cocaine Anonymous.
- Teach about relapse prevention. Encourage CBT to increase coping skills and individual therapy to enhance personal insight.
- Patients taking disulfiram (Antabuse) must be advised to avoid alcohol and any substances that contain alcohol. This includes mouthwash, colognes, cough syrups, etc.

Medical/Legal Pitfalls
- Rates of suicide are three to four times more prevalent in those who abuse alcohol or drugs as compared to the general population.
- Individuals withdrawing from substances are at great risk for depression. When not properly treated, depression can lead to suicide.
- Individuals being treated for addiction may have a history of seeing multiple healthcare professionals to obtain medications ("doctor shopping"). Such practices may lead to accidental and/or intentional overdose.

Intoxication

Background Information

Definition of Disorder
- An altered physical or mental state due to use of substance
- A physical and mental state of euphoria, exhilaration, or excitement occurs

DSM-IV-TR Classes of Psychoactive Substances
- Alcohol
- Amphetamines
- Caffeine
- Cannabis
- Cocaine
- Hallucinogens
- Inhalants
- Nicotine
- Opioids
- PCP
- Sedatives, hypnotics, and anxiolytics

Etiology
- No single theory can explain the cause of substance abuse/dependence
- Theoretical causes
  - Genetics
  - Biochemical
  - Psychopathological
    - Developmental influences
    - Personality traits
  - Social learning
    - Parental role modeling
    - Cultural and/or ethnic influences

Demographics
- Males are twice as likely to be affected than females
- The use of illegal drugs is most common in young adults (aged 18–25 years)
- More than 100 million Americans, aged 12 years or older, report illicit drug use at least once in their lives

- About 50–75% of those with a mental disorder struggle with substance addiction
- More than 70% of the AIDS cases among women are drug related
- More than 100,000 deaths in the United States each year are caused by excessive alcohol consumption
- Approximately, 1 in 10 Americans has an alcohol problem
- Marijuana is the most commonly abused illicit substance in the United States

Risk Factors
- Unemployment
- Poor social coping skills
- History of emotional, physical, or sexual abuse
- Chaotic home environment
- History of mental illness
- Untreated physical pain
- Family history of addiction
- Peer pressure
- Educational level
- Economic status
- Recent incarceration

Diagnosis

Differential Diagnosis
Rule out medical problems that may mimic signs and symptoms of substance intoxication and/or withdrawal:
- Hypoglycemia
- Electrolyte (sodium, potassium, chloride, and sodium bicarbonate) imbalance
- Head injury/trauma
- Stroke
- Psychosis
- Neurological disorder

ICD Code
Diagnostic codes for substance use are classified according to substance. The following code is for unknown substances:

292.89 Substance Intoxication

Diagnostic Work-Up

- Diagnosis of substance abuse/dependence is typically made by detailed subjective history
- Blood, breath, or urine screening for substance(s)

Initial Assessment

- Medical history and examination
- Psychiatric history and examination
- Family and social history
- Cultural history related to substance use
- Detailed history of past and present substance use, tolerance, and withdrawal
- How do the substances affect patient mentally and physically?
- How is the substance use affecting patient's occupational, family, or social life?
- CAGE questionnaire or S-MAST, a screening tool for alcohol use
- CIWA-Ar, an assessment tool to evaluate alcohol withdrawal symptoms
- COWS, an assessment tool to evaluate opioid withdrawal symptoms

Clinical Presentation

Signs and symptoms will vary with individuals/substances used, but include:

- Slurred speech
- Poor psychomotor coordination
- Impairment in attention and concentration
- Nystagmus
- Stupor or coma
- Pupil changes

DSM-IV-TR Diagnostic Guidelines for Substance Intoxication

- Reversible syndrome is due to recent exposure to substance
- Clinically significant and maladaptive psychological and behavioral changes occur, affecting the central nervous system (CNS)

Treatment for Substance Use

- Psychosocial
  - CBT
  - MET
  - Behavioral therapy
  - Psychotherapy
- Pharmacological
  - Treat withdrawal states
  - Medication is given to decrease reinforcing effects of substance(s)
  - Maintenance medication management (agonist therapy)
  - Medication is given for relapse prevention
  - Treatment of comorbid conditions is given
- Self-help groups
  - Alcoholics Anonymous
  - Narcotics Anonymous
  - Cocaine Anonymous

Pharmacological Treatment for Use of Specific Substances

- Nicotine
  - Nicotine replacement: patch, gum, spray, lozenge, and inhaler
  - Bupropion (Wellbutrin)
  - Varenicline
- Alcohol
  - Symptoms of withdrawal may occur within 4–12 hours after cessation or reduction
  - Thiamine replacement and fluids
  - Benzodiazepine is tapered to prevent withdrawal
  - Clonidine (Catapres) is used as needed for hypertensive episode due to withdrawal
  - Naltrexone (Nalorex) (oral or IM) or acamprosate (Campral) is used to decrease craving
  - Disulfiram (Antabuse) is a deterrent to drinking
- Marijuana
  - No recommended pharmacologic treatment
- Cocaine
  - Pharmacological treatment is not indicated
  - Topiramate (Topamax), disulfiram (Antabuse), modafinil (Provigil) with psychosocial treatment may be effective
- Opioid
  - Opioid overdose: naloxone is used to reverse respiratory depression
  - Maintenance treatment: methadone (Dolophone) or buprenorphine (Subutex) is gradually tapered
  - Alternative maintenance: naltrexone (Nalorex)

Recurrence Rate

- Rate of relapse, for those who have been in treatment, is approximately 90%
- Majority of relapses take place within 3 months following treatment

Patient Education

- Educate on importance of joining a support group. Information is available online for worldwide support groups, including Narcotics Anonymous, Alcoholic Anonymous, and Cocaine Anonymous
- Teach about relapse prevention. Encourage CBT to increase coping skills and individual therapy to enhance personal insight
- Patients taking disulfiram (Antabuse) must be advised to avoid alcohol and any substances that contain alcohol. This includes mouthwash, colognes, cough syrups, etc.

Medical/Legal Pitfalls

- Rates of suicide are three to four times more prevalent in those who abuse alcohol or drugs as compared to the general population.
- Individuals withdrawing from substances are at great risk for depression. When not properly treated, depression can lead to suicide.
- Individuals being treated for addiction may have a history of seeing multiple healthcare professionals to obtain medications ("doctor shopping"). Such practices may lead to accidental and/or intentional overdose.

Substance Withdrawal

Background Information

Definition of Disorder
- Physiological and cognitive changes with cessation or reduction of substance
- Follows period of heavy or prolonged drug use

DSM-IV-TR Classes of Psychoactive Substances
- Alcohol
- Amphetamines
- Caffeine
- Cannabis
- Cocaine
- Hallucinogens
- Inhalants
- Nicotine
- Opioids
- PCP
- Sedatives, hypnotics, and anxiolytics

Etiology
- No single theory can explain the cause of substance abuse/dependence
- Theoretical causes
  - Genetics
  - Biochemical
  - Psychopathological
    - Developmental influences
    - Personality traits
  - Social Learning
    - Parental role modeling
    - Cultural and/or ethnic influences

Demographics
- Males are twice as likely to be affected than females
- The use of illegal drugs is most common in young adults (aged 18–25 years)
- More than 100 million Americans, aged 12 years or older, report illicit drug use at least once in their lives
- About 50–75% of those with a mental disorder struggle with substance addiction

- More than 70% of the AIDS cases among women are drug related
- More than 100,000 deaths in the United States each year are caused by excessive alcohol consumption
- Approximately, 1 in 10 Americans has an alcohol problem
- Marijuana is the most commonly abused illicit substance in the United States

Risk Factors
- Unemployment
- Poor social coping skills
- History of emotional, physical, or sexual abuse
- Chaotic home environment
- History of mental illness
- Untreated physical pain
- Family history of addiction
- Peer pressure
- Educational level
- Economic status
- Recent incarceration

Diagnosis

Differential Diagnosis
Rule out medical problems that may mimic signs and symptoms of substance intoxication and/or withdrawal:
- Hypoglycemia
- Electrolyte (sodium, chloride, potassium, sodium bicarbonate) imbalance
- Head injury/trauma
- Stroke
- Psychosis
- Neurological disorder

ICD Code
Diagnostic codes for substance use are classified according to substance. The following code is for unknown substances:

292.00 Substance Withdrawal

Diagnostic Work-Up

- Diagnosis of substance abuse/dependence is typically made via a detailed subjective history
- Blood, breath, or urine screening for substance(s)

Initial Assessment

- Medical history and examination
- Psychiatric history and examination
- Family and social history
- Cultural history related to substance use
- Detailed history of past and present substance use, tolerance, withdrawal
- How do the substances affect patient mentally and physically?
- How is the substance use affecting patient's occupational, family, or social life?
- CAGE questionnaire or S-MAST, a screening tool for alcohol use
- CIWA-Ar, an assessment tool to evaluate alcohol withdrawal symptoms
- COWS, an assessment tool to evaluate opioid withdrawal symptoms

Clinical Presentation

Signs and symptoms will vary with individuals/substances used, but include:

- CNS depressants:
  - Restlessness, anxiety
  - Sleep disturbances
  - Diaphoresis
  - Vital changes: increase in blood pressure heart rate, and temperature
- CNS stimulants:
  - Depressed mood, fatigue
  - Anxiety
  - Intense cravings
- Opioids:
  - Runny nose
  - Diaphoresis
  - Yawning
  - Anxiety
  - Intense cravings
  - Vital changes: increase in blood pressure and pulse
  - Muscle and bone pain
  - Abdominal cramps
  - Tremors
  - Nausea, vomiting, diarrhea

Diagnosis

DSM-IV-TR Definition of Substance Withdrawal

- Substance-specific syndrome is due to cessation or reduction of substance use that has been heavy and/or prolonged
- Syndrome produces significant clinical distress or diminished functioning

Treatment for Substance Abuse or Dependence

- Psychosocial
  - CBT
  - MET
  - Behavioral therapy
  - Psychotherapy
- Pharmacological
  - Treat withdrawal states
  - Medication is used to decrease reinforcing effects of substance(s)
  - Maintenance medication management (agonist therapy)
  - Medication is used for relapse prevention
  - Treatment of comorbid conditions
- Self-help groups
  - Alcoholics Anonymous
  - Narcotics Anonymous
  - Cocaine Anonymous

Pharmacological Treatment for Use of Specific Substances

- Nicotine
  - Nicotine replacement: patch, gum, spray, lozenge, and inhaler
  - Bupropion (Wellbutrin)
  - Varenicline
- Alcohol
  - Symptoms of withdrawal may occur within 4–12 hours after cessation or reduction
  - Thiamine replacement and fluids
  - Benzodiazepine is tapered to prevent withdrawal
  - Clonidine (Catapres) is used as needed for hypertensive episode due to withdrawal
  - Naltrexone (Nalorex) (oral or IM) or acamprosate (Campral) is used to decrease craving
  - Disulfiram (Antabuse) is a deterrent to drinking

- Marijuana
  - No pharmacologic treatment is recommended
- Cocaine
  - Pharmacological treatment is not indicated
  - Topiramate (Topamax), disulfiram (Antabuse), modafinil (Provigil) with psychosocial treatment may be effective
- Opioid
  - Opioid overdose: naloxone is used to reverse respiratory depression
  - Maintenance treatment: methadone (Dolophone) or buprenorphine (Subutex) is gradually tapered
  - Alternative maintenance: naltrexone (Nalorex)

Recurrence Rate

- Rate of relapse, for those who have been in treatment, is approximately 90%
- Majority of relapses take place within 3 months following treatment

Patient Education

- Educate on importance of joining a support group. Information is available online for worldwide support groups, including Narcotics Anonymous, Alcoholics Anonymous, and Cocaine Anonymous
- Teach about relapse prevention. Encourage CBT to increase coping skills and individual therapy to enhance personal insight
- Patients taking disulfiram (Antabuse) must be advised to avoid alcohol and any substances that contain alcohol. This includes mouthwash, colognes, cough syrups, etc.

Medical/Legal Pitfalls

- Rates of suicide are two to three times more prevalent in those who abuse alcohol or drugs as compared to the general population
- Individuals withdrawing from substances are at greater risk for depression. When not properly treated, depression can lead to suicide
- Individuals being treated for addiction may have a history of seeing multiple healthcare professionals to obtain medications ("doctor shopping"). Such practices may lead to accidental and/or intentional overdose

Other Resources

Evidence-Based References

American Psychiatric Association (APA). (2000). *Diagnostic and statistical manual of mental disorders (DSM-IV-TR)* (4th ed.). Washington, DC: American Psychiatric Association.

American Psychiatric Association (APA). (2006). *Practice guidelines for the treatment of patients with substance use disorders* (2nd ed.). Retrieved February 10, 2009, from http://www.Psychiatryonline.com/contenc.aspx?aID=14079.

Cleary, M., Hunt, G. E., Matheson, S. L., Siegfried, N., & Walter, G. (2008). Psychosocial interventions for people with both severe mental illness and substance misuse. *Cochrane Database of Systematic Reviews*, (1).

Ferri, M. M. F., Amato, L., & Davoli, M. (2006). Alcoholics Anonymous and other 12-step programmes for alcohol dependence. *Cochrane Database of Systematic Reviews*, (3).

Fox, C., Loughlin, P., & Cook, C. (2003). Disulfiram for alcohol dependence (Protocol). *Cochrane Database of Systematic Reviews*, (3).

Gowing, L., Ali, R., & White, J. M. (2006). Buprenorphine for the management of opioid withdrawal. *Cochrane Database of Systematic Reviews*, (2).

Naegle, M. (2008). Substance misuse and alcohol use disorders. In E. Capezuti, D. Zwicker, M. Mezey, & T. Fulmer (Eds.), *Evidence-based geriatric nursing protocols for best practice* (3rd ed., pp. 649–676). New York: Springer Publishing Company.

Substance Abuse and Mental Health Services Administration (SAMHSA). (2007). *2007 National survey on drug use & health: National results*. Retrieved February 13, 2009, from http://www.oas.samhsa.gov/nsduh/2k7nsduh/2k7Results.cfm#TOC.

Vaz de Lima, F. B., da Silveira, D. X., & Andriolo, R. B. (2008). Effectiveness and safety of topiramate for drug dependents (Protocol). *Cochrane Database of Systematic Reviews*, (4), 431–435.

Web Resource

- The Substance Abuse and Mental Health Services Administration: http://www.samhsa.gov/.

7. PSYCHOTIC DISORDERS
Brief Psychotic Disorder

Background Information

Definition of Disorder
- Sudden onset of psychotic symptoms occurs
- These include delusions, hallucinations, disorganized speech, or grossly disorganized or catatonic behavior
- Episode lasts from 1 day to less than 1 month, with return to premorbid level of functioning
- Symptoms may or may not meet the definition of schizophrenia

Etiology
- Often precipitated by extremely stressful life events
- Cause is unknown
- Patients with personality disorder may have predisposition toward development of psychotic symptoms
- May have prevalence of mood disorders in family
- May have poor coping skills along with secondary gains for psychotic symptoms
- May have defense against a prohibited fantasy, fulfillment of unattained wish, or escape from a distasteful situation

Demographics
- It is generally considered uncommon
- More likely to occur in young rather than older patients
- It generally first occurs in early adulthood (ages: 20s and 30s) and is more common in women than in men
- More frequent in lower socioeconomic classes
- Patient may have prior personality disorder
- May predispose to survivors of disasters or major cultural changes

Risk Factors
- Major life events that cause significant emotional stress
- Severity must be in relation to patient's life

Age
- Young rather than old

Gender
- No differentiation, although women may be affected more than men

Family History
More common in families with history of mood (bipolar) disorders. This suggests a genetic link.
- Stressful events in susceptible people:
  - Usually follows life-altering stressor
  - May present after series of less overtly stressful events
  - Rarely, stressor could be unrelated to the psychotic episode having another mental disorder
  - Paranoia is often predominant

Diagnosis

Differential Diagnosis
- Factitious disorder with mainly psychological symptoms
- Malingering
- Psychotic disorder with medical causation
- Substance-induced psychotic disorder
- Seizure disorders
- Delirium
- Dissociative identity disorder
- Borderline personality disorder symptoms
- Schizotypal personality disorder symptoms

ICD Code
298.8 Brief Psychotic Disorder

Diagnostic Work-Up
- Always includes at least one major symptom of psychosis
- Delusions with rapidly changing delusional topics
- Abrupt onset occurs
- Affective symptoms, confusion, and impaired attention are presented
- Emotional lability is observed
- Inappropriate dress or behavior is seen
- Patient is screaming or mute
- Impaired recent memory occurs

- Organic work-up includes complete blood count (CBC) with differentials, complete serum chemistry, thyroid function studies, and thyroid-stimulating hormone, serum alcohol and illegal substance levels (including anabolic steroids, cannabis, alcohol, tobacco, termazepam, opium, heroine/morphine, and methamphetamines)
- No imaging studies are required to diagnose brief psychotic disorder

Initial Assessment
- Medical history is obtained
- Psychiatric history is obtained
- In-depth mental status exam (a careful mental status examination can distinguish this disorder from delirium, dementia, or other organic brain syndromes, such as meningitis, transient ischemic attack, and epilepsy).
- Family history is obtained
- History may need to be obtained from significant others in acutely ill patients
- Symptoms are observed

Clinical Presentation
- Psychotic symptoms are seen, most likely paranoia
- Sudden onset occurs
- May not include entire spectrum of schizophrenia
- Mood variability occurs
- Reactive confusion
- Reactive depression
- Impaired attention span
- Reactive excitation
- Screaming or silence
- Impaired short-term memory
- Changes in sleep or eating habits, energy level, or weight
- Inability to make decisions
- Garish style of dress

Diagnosis

DSM-IV-TR Diagnostic Guidelines
Presence of one or more of the following symptoms (when the possibility of a cultural and/or culturally sanctioned expression or response has been excluded):
- Delusions
- Hallucinations
- Disorganized speech
- Grossly disorganized or catatonic behavior is seen
- Duration is at least 1 day but less than 1 month, with eventual return to premorbid functioning
- The disturbance is not better described as a mood disorder with psychotic features, schizoaffective disorder, or schizophrenia, and not directly a result of substance or medication use or a general medical condition
- Individuals with brief psychotic disorder are likely to experience emotional turmoil

Treatment

Acute Treatment
- In the acute phase, inpatient hospitalization may be necessary for safety and evaluation. This includes close monitoring of symptoms and assessment of danger to self and others.
- Mental status examination: patients usually present with severe psychotic agitation that may be associated with strange or bizarre behavior, uncooperativeness, physical or verbal aggression, disorganized speech, screaming or muteness, labile or depressed mood, suicidal and/or homicidal thoughts or behaviors, restlessness, hallucinations, delusions, disorientation, impaired attention, impaired concentration, impaired memory, poor insight, and poor judgment.
- A quiet, structured hospital setting may assist in regaining reality.
- Administration of antipsychotic medication as indicated, most frequently a high-potency dopamine receptor agonist. Conventional (typical) antipsychotic medications most commonly used in this disorder include haloperidol (Haldol) and chlorpromazine (Thorazine).
- Newer medications, called atypical antipsychotic drugs, include olanzapine (Zyprexa), ziprasidone (Geodon), quetiapine (Seroquel), and risperidone (Risperdal).
- Benzodiazepine medication may be given to patients who present or are at high risk for excitation, as they also are beneficial in the treatment of brief psychosis. Lorazepam (Ativan) or diazepam (Valium) may be used if the person has a very high level of anxiety or insomnia.

- While waiting for the milieu or pharmaceutical effects to take effect, one-to-one, seclusion or physical restraint of the patient may be necessary for safety.
- If symptoms are only minimally impairing the patient's function and a specific stressor is identified, removing the stressor should suffice.
- Further inpatient care is unnecessary once the acute attack has ended.

Chronic Treatment
- Following the resolution of the episode, hypnotic medications may be useful.
- Long-term use of medications should be avoided. If maintenance medications are necessary, reevaluation of the diagnosis is indicated.
- Individual, family, and group psychotherapies are essential to integrate the experience psychologically into the lives of the patient and/or significant others.
- Therapies should include discussion of the precipitating stressors, the psychotic episode itself, and development of successful coping strategies. Sessions should be at least weekly, once the patient is discharged from the hospital, and last 6–8 weeks or longer.
- The length of acute and residual symptoms is usually less than a week.
- Depressive symptoms may present following cessation of psychosis.
- Risk for suicide can escalate in the postpsychotic depressive stage.

Recurrence Rate
Good prognosis can be predicted if:
- Prior good adjustment occurs
- Few premorbid schizoid tendencies occur
- The precipitating stressor is severe
- Onset of symptoms is sudden
- Affective symptoms are present
- During acute phase, manifestation of confusion and bewilderment is seen
- Minimal affective blunting occurs

- There is a short duration of symptoms
- There is an absence of schizophrenic relatives

In general, 50–80% of all patients have no further major psychiatric episodes.

Patient Education
- Information for patients and families is available in easy-to-understand language at www.webmd.com
- Signs, symptoms, and treatment information can be obtained from www.healthline.com
- Data on foundations and support groups are available at www.organizedwisdom.com
- The National Alliance on Mental Illness—at www.nami.org—is the government-sponsored organization for information regarding mental illness
- Specific information regarding this disorder is presented at www.medicinenet.com/brief_psychotic_disorder

There is no known way to prevent brief psychotic disorder. However, early diagnosis and treatment can help decrease the disruption to the person's life, family, and friendships. Both the patient and the family must be educated about the illness and the potential adverse effects of the medications.

Medical/Legal Pitfalls
Risk of suicide or harm to others may occur if no immediate safety measures are taken:
- Misdiagnosis may be the result of symptoms similar to those of other psychiatric/medical disorders. General recommendations include serious consideration of medical causes in any acute-onset new psychosis. This does not necessarily mean ordering every possible test, but history and the physical examination often alert the clinician to the need for additional medical evaluation.
- Physical or chemical restraints may be necessary in cases of severe uncontrolled agitation to provide safety to self and/or others.

Delusional Disorder

Background Information

Definition of Disorder

- It is a psychiatric disorder in which primary symptoms are delusions (formerly called paranoia or paranoid disorder)
- Delusions can include those of paranoia, grandiosity, erotica, jealousy, somatic and mixed responses
- Delusions are nonbizarre (situations that may occur in everyday life), such as being followed, spousal infidelity, or illness
- Incorrect inference about external reality persists despite the evidence to the contrary, and these beliefs are not ordinarily accepted by other members of the person's culture or subculture

Etiology

- Cause is unknown
- Distinctness from schizophrenia and mood disorders is seen
- Later onset in life occurs
- Predominance varies depending on source reviewed
- Increased prevalence occurs with personality traits of suspiciousness, jealousy, and secretiveness
- Relatively stable diagnosis, with less than a quarter of delusional patients rediagnosed as schizophrenic, and less than 10% as mood disordered, can be made
- Delusional disorder may involve the limbic system or basal ganglia when intact cerebral cortical function is present

Demographics

- Prevalence in the United States is estimated to be 0.025–0.03%
- Annually, new cases account for one to three cases per 100,000 people
- Four percent of all first admissions to psychiatric hospitals are for psychoses not due to a general medical condition or substance
- Average age of onset is 40, with a range of from 18 to the 90s
- Slightly more females than men are affected
- Many patients are married or employed
- Some association with recent immigration or low socioeconomic status, celibacy among men, and widowhood among women is noted
- Because of poor insight into their pathological experiences, patients with delusional disorder may rarely seek psychiatric help and often may present to internists, surgeons, dermatologists, police officers, and lawyers rather than to psychiatric professionals
- Men are more likely than women to develop paranoid delusions; women are more likely than men to develop delusions of erotomania
- Patients often do not present for treatment, and thus they do not commonly make themselves available for research studies

Risk Factors

Age
- Eighteen to forty years

Gender
- Slightly more males than females

Family History
- A hostile family environment is observed, usually with an overcontrolling mother and a distant or sadistic father

Stressful Events in Susceptible People
- Social isolation
- Less-than-expected levels of achievement
- Hypersensitivity
- Specific ego function including reaction formation, projection, and denial
- Distrust in relationships evolving from hostility, abuse

Having Another Mental Disorder
- May have a mood component, but not severe enough to be classified as a mood disorder

Diagnosis

Differential Diagnosis

- Delusions can transpire simultaneously with many medical and neurological illnesses.
- Most common sites for lesions are the basal ganglia and limbic system.
- Toxicology screening and routine lab studies, including CBC with differential, serum chemistries, and thyroid function, are done.
- Differs from malingering and factitious disorder.
- Separated from schizophrenia by the absence of other schizophrenic symptoms and nonbizarre qualities of delusions, impairment of functioning.
- Differs from depressive disorders in that somatic features are not pervasive.
- Differences from somatoform disorders, due to which patients with delusional disorders cannot admit their symptoms, do not exist.
- In differentiating delusional disorder from paranoid personality disorder, it is necessary to determine the distinction between extreme suspiciousness and delusion. If in doubt that a symptom is a delusion, diagnosis of delusional disorder should not be made.

ICD Code

297.1 Bipolar and Depressive Disorders

Diagnostic Work-Up

By psychiatric presentation:

- Delusions are characterized as nonbizarre, therefore possible, if unlikely.
- Symptoms have to occur without other symptoms of schizophrenia, except for tactile or olfactory hallucinations, if part of the delusional belief.
- Mild impairment of function occurs as compared to other major psychiatric diagnoses.
- Presence of delusions is seen for at least 1 month.
- Medical evaluation is done.
- Laboratory studies: toxicology screening, CBC with differential, serum chemistries, thyroid function studies (triiodothyronine [T3], thyroxine [T4], thyroid-stimulating hormone [TSH]).
- CT scan of the brain is done to visualize the lesions.

Initial Assessment

- Psychiatric history and presentation are assessed to establish whether pathology is present.
- Determining the presence or absence of important characteristics often associated with delusions is important.
- Delusional disorder should be seen as a diagnosis of exclusion.
- Medical history is obtained.
- Veracity of symptoms should be checked before automatically considering the content to be delusional.
- Assessment of homicidal or suicidal ideation is extremely important in evaluating patients with delusional disorder. The presence of homicidal or suicidal thoughts related to delusions should be actively screened for and the risk of carrying out violent plans should be carefully assessed.

Clinical Presentation

Mental status examination reveals patients as usually well-groomed, remarkably normal except for the specific delusional system:

- Patients may attempt to engage clinicians to agree with their delusions
- Moods and affects are congruent with the delusions
- No significant hallucinations occur unless strictly pertaining to the delusions presented
- Disorder of thought content is primary symptom
- Delusions are characterized as being possible, and may be simple or complex
- Sudden onset occurs
- Below-average intelligence is seen
- Intact memory and orientation
- No insight
- Poor impulse control

Diagnosis

DSM-IV-TR criteria for delusional disorder include:

- Nonbizarre delusions (i.e., involving situations that occur in real life) of at least 1 month's duration.

- Functioning is not markedly impaired, and behavior is not obviously odd or bizarre.
- If mood episodes have occurred simultaneously with delusions, their total duration has been brief relative to the duration of the delusions.
- The disturbance is not a direct physiological effect of a substance (e.g., a drug of abuse or a medication) or a general medical condition.

Subtypes are defined, including erotomanic, grandiose, jealous, persecutory, somatic, and mixed disorders.

Treatment

Acute Treatment
- Hospitalization should be considered if a potential for harm or violence exists.
- A complete neurological and medical work-up may be indicated to determine an organic cause for the symptoms.
- Delusional disorder is challenging to treat for various reasons, including patients' frequent denial that they have any problem, especially of a psychological nature, difficulties in developing a therapeutic alliance, and social/interpersonal conflicts.
- Avoiding direct confrontation of the delusional symptoms enhances the possibility of treatment compliance and response.
- Treatment of delusional disorder often involves both psychopharmacology and psychotherapy.
- Polypharmacy is common, most often including a combination of antipsychotic and antidepressant medications. No difference in response is noted between typical and atypical antipsychotic agents.
- Antidepressants, particularly the selective-serotonin reuptake inhibitors (SSRIs), have been successfully used for the treatment of the somatic-type delusional disorder.
- Establishing a therapeutic alliance, establishing acceptable symptomatic treatment goals, and educating the patient's family are of paramount importance.
- Avoiding direct confrontation of the delusional symptoms enhances the possibility of treatment compliance and response.
- Outpatient treatment is preferred.

Chronic Treatment
- The chronic nature of delusional disorders suggests treatment strategies should be tailored to the individual needs of the patients and focus on maintaining social function and improving quality of life.
- For most patients with delusional disorder, some form of supportive therapy is helpful. The goals of supportive therapy include facilitating treatment adherence and providing education about the illness and its treatment.
- Educational and social interventions can include social skills training (e.g., not discussing delusional beliefs in social settings) and minimizing risk factors.
- Providing realistic guidance and assistance in coping with problems stemming from the delusional system may be very helpful.
- Cognitive therapeutic approaches may be useful for some patients by identifying delusional thoughts and then replacing them with alternative, more adaptive ones.
- It is important that goals be attainable, since a patient who feels pressured or repeatedly criticized by others will probably experience stress that may lead to a worsening of symptoms.
- Insight-oriented therapy is rarely indicated.

Recurrence Rate
- Delusional disorder has a relatively good prognosis when adequately treated: 52.6% of the patients recover, 28.2% achieve partial recovery, and 19.2% do not improve
- Less than 25% of all cases are later diagnosed with schizophrenia
- Less than 10% develop mood disorders
- Good prognosis is predicted with high levels of occupational and social functioning, the female sex, onset before age 30, sudden onset, and short duration of illness

Patient Education
- Educating the family about the symptoms and course of the disorder is helpful. This is especially true since the family frequently feels the impact of the disorder the most.

- In addition to involvement with seeking help, family, friends, and peer groups can provide support and encourage the patient to regain his or her abilities.

Medical/Legal Pitfalls
- Patients with delusional disorder are more susceptible to becoming dependent on alcohol, tobacco, and drugs.

- It is not uncommon for people with delusional disorder to make repeated complaints to legal authorities.
- Patients with delusional disorder may encounter legal or relationship problems as a result of acting on their delusions.
- Civil commitment in patients with delusional disorder who may be dangerous focuses on being a preventive measure against potential harm to self or others.

Schizoaffective Disorder

Definition of Disorder
- This disorder has features of both schizophrenia and mood disorder.
- Specifically, schizoaffective disorder is a combination of symptoms of a thought disorder or other psychotic symptoms such as hallucinations or delusions (schizophrenia component) and those of a mood disorder (depressive or manic component).

Etiology
- May either be a type of schizophrenia or a mood disorder, or both occurring at the same time, or not related to either.
- Most theories agree that schizoaffective disorder comprises all three possibilities.
- May encompass bipolar and depressive types and may have a genetic component.
- Relatives of the persons with the depressed type of schizoaffective disorder have a higher incidence.
- There is a tendency to respond to lithium and have a better course outcome.
- Balance of dopamine and serotonin in the brain may contribute to development of the disease. Other theories consider that it may be due to in utero exposure to viruses, malnutrition, or even birth complications.
- Abnormalities of the neurotransmitters serotonin, norepinephrine, and/or dopamine could all contribute to this disorder.

Demographics
- There is a lifetime prevalence rate of less than 1%.
- Diagnosis may be used when clinician is unsure of the classification of symptoms.
- The prognosis for patients with schizoaffective disorder is thought to be between that of patients with schizophrenia and that of patients with a mood disorder, with the prognosis better for schizoaffective disorder than for schizophrenic disorder but worse than for a mood disorder alone.

- The incidence of suicide is estimated to be 10%. Caucasians have a higher rate of suicide than African Americans. Immigrants have higher suicide rates than natives.
- As in other psychiatric disorders, women attempt suicide more than men, but men complete suicide more often.
- Schizoaffective disorder affects more women than men, with more women in the depressive type as compared with the bipolar type.
- A poor prognosis in patients with schizoaffective disorder is generally associated with a poor premorbid history, an insidious onset, no precipitating factors, a predominant psychosis, negative symptoms, an early onset, an unremitting course, or their having a family member with schizophrenia.

Risk Factors
Age
- Young people with schizoaffective disorder tend to have a diagnosis with the bipolar subtype, whereas older people tend to have the depressive subtype
- Age of onset is later in women than for men

Gender
- Prevalence is lower in men, and less in married women
- Men with schizoaffective disorder may exhibit antisocial behavior and flat or inappropriate affect

Family History
- Patients may have a genetic predisposition
- Inconsistent study results, although relatives with the depressed type may be at higher risk

Stressful Events in the Lives of Susceptible People
- No studies provide data

Having Another Disorder
- Not studied

Diagnosis

Differential Diagnosis

- All mood and schizophrenic disorders should be considered in the differential diagnosis of schizoaffective disorder.
- Testing is done for use of amphetamines, phencyclidines (PCPs), hallucinogens, cocaine, alcohol, and steroids, as these can present with similar symptoms.
- Seizure disorders of the temporal lobe can mimic schizoaffective signs, as can human immunodeficiency virus (HIV)/autoimmune deficiency syndrome, hyperthyroidism, neurosyphilis, delirium, metabolic syndrome, or narcolepsy.

ICD Code

295.70 Schizophrenia

Diagnostic Work-Up

- Schizoaffective disorder must meet *DSM-IV-TR* criteria for components of schizophrenia and mood disorders (depressed) concurrently.
- Delusions or hallucinations for at least 2 weeks may be seen in the absence of mood symptoms.
- Laboratory studies a include sequential multiple analysis, CBC, rapid plasma reagent, thyroid function, drug and alcohol screens, lipid panel, Elisa test results, and the Western Blot test.
- If the patient's neurologic findings are abnormal, computed tomography or magnetic resonance imagery may be ordered to rule out any suspected intracranial pathology. Findings include decreased amounts of cortical gray matter and increased fluid-filled spaces.

Initial Assessment

- Medical work-up, including neurological history and evaluation of laboratory data.
- Psychiatric assessment, including mental status examination and history.
- Mental status examination may reveal appearances ranging from well-groomed to disheveled; possible psychomotor agitation or retardation; euthymic, depressed, or manic mood; eye contact ranging from appropriate to flat affect; speech which ranges from poverty to flight of ideas or pressured; suicidal or homicidal ideation may or may not be present; presence of delusions and/or hallucinations.
- Psychological testing may assist with diagnosis and in rating the severity of the disease. These scales may be useful in assessing the patient's progress positive and negative symptoms scale (PANSS), Hamilton depression scale, and Young mania scale. The cut down, annoyed, guilty, and eye opener (CAGE) questionnaire is helpful in determining alcohol consumption in patients with schizoaffective disorder.

Clinical Presentation: Symptoms

- All the signs and symptoms of schizophrenia, manic episodes, and depressive disorders occur
- Symptoms can appear in concert or alternating
- May be mood incongruent, which has a poor prognosis
- Suicidal ideation or attempt(s) may occur

DSM-IV-TR Diagnostic Guidelines

- An uninterrupted period of illness occurs during which a major depressive episode, a manic episode, or a mixed episode occurs with symptoms that meet criteria for schizophrenia. The major depressive episode must include a depressed mood.
- Symptoms that meet the criteria for mood episodes are present for a substantial portion of the active and residual periods of the illness.
- The disturbance is not the direct physiologic effect of a substance (e.g., illicit drugs, medications) or a general medical condition.
- The bipolar type is diagnosed if the disturbance includes a manic or a mixed episode (or a manic or mixed episode and a major depressive episode).
- The depressive type is diagnosed if the disturbance includes only major depressive episodes.

Treatment

Acute Treatment

- The major treatments include in-patient psychiatric hospitalization, medication, and psychosocial therapies. Inpatient treatment is mandatory for patients who are dangerous to themselves or others and for patients who cannot take care of themselves.

- Activity should be restricted if patients represent a danger to themselves or to others.
- Pharmaceutical treatment involves use of medications, antipsychotics to treat aggressive behavior and psychosis, along with antidepressants, and/or mood stabilizers. Agent selection depends on whether the depressive or manic subtype is present.
- In the depressive subtype, combinations of antidepressants plus an antipsychotic are used.
- In refractory cases, clozapine (Clozaril, FazaClo ODT) has been used as an antipsychotic agent. In the manic subtype, combinations of mood stabilizers plus an antipsychotic are used.
- Early treatment with medication along with good premorbid functioning often improves outcomes.

Chronic Treatment

- Patients who have schizoaffective disorder can greatly benefit from psychotherapy as well as psychoeducational programs and regularly scheduled outpatient medication management.
- When making the transition to outpatient, stressing the importance of medication compliance is crucial.
- If possible, select once-daily or long-acting medications to help with patient compliance.
- Therapy is most effective if it involves their families, develops their social skills, and focuses on cognitive rehabilitation.
- Psychotherapies should include supportive therapy and assertive community therapy in addition to individual and group forms of therapy and rehabilitation programs.
- Family involvement is needed in the treatment of this particular disorder.
- Treatment includes education about the disorder and its treatment, family assistance in compliance with medications and appointments, and maintenance of structured daily activities.
- Otherwise, encourage patients who are schizoaffective to continue their normal routines and strengthen their social skills whenever possible.

Recurrence Rate

- A good outcome is predicted in the presence of a good premorbid history, acute onset, a specific precipitating factor, few psychotic symptoms, a short course, and no family history of schizophrenia.
- The prognosis for patients with schizoaffective disorder is thought to lie between that of patients with schizophrenia and that of patients with a mood disorder. Therefore, the prognosis is better with schizoaffective disorder than with a schizophrenic disorder but worse than with a mood disorder alone.
- Individuals with the bipolar subtype are thought to have a prognosis similar to those with bipolar type I, whereas the prognosis of people with the depressive subtype is thought to be similar to that of people with schizophrenia.
- Overall, determination of the prognosis is difficult.

Patient Education

- Discuss compliance with patients as well as the family members. Always discuss all the risks, benefits, adverse effects, and alternatives of each medication.
- Stress-reduction techniques are employed to prevent relapse and possible rehospitalization.
- Education should also include social skills training and cognitive rehabilitation.
- Family education should involve reduction of expressed emotions, criticism, hostility, or overprotection of the patient.

Medical/Legal Pitfalls

- Patients with schizoaffective disorder often lack judgment and insight into their illness. They commonly refuse to continue the medications started in the hospital after they are discharged. Noncompliance may also be the result of adverse effects of the medication, such as sedation and weight gain.
- Patients may begin to feel better as a result of their medications and believe that they no longer

need to take them. This thinking leads to the discontinuation of medication and can result in rehospitalization.

- Be familiar with local mental health laws as patients with schizoaffective disorder, who represent a danger to self or others or are unwilling to seek help on a voluntary basis, may need to be committed for further evaluation and treatment.
- If noncompliance with medications is an issue, a court order may be necessary to force the patient to take medications.
- Physical restraints may also be indicated for protection of self and/or others.

Schizophrenia

Background Information

Definition of Disorder

- This is a chronic, severe, and disabling brain disorder characterized by disordered thoughts, delusions, hallucinations, and bizarre or catatonic behavior.

Etiology

- Several genes are found to be strongly associated with schizophrenia. However, genes alone are not sufficient to cause this disorder.
- Imbalance of the neurotransmitters dopamine and glutamate (and possibly others) are found to play a role in schizophrenia.
- Scientists believe that interactions between genes and the environment are necessary to develop schizophrenia. Environmental risk factors (e.g., exposure to viruses or malnutrition in the womb, problems during birth), and psychosocial factors (e.g., stressful conditions) are found to increase the risk of schizophrenia.
- Research shows that schizophrenia runs in families. People who have first-degree relatives (a parent, sibling) or second-degree relatives (grandparents, aunts, uncles, cousins) with this disorder develop schizophrenia more often than the general population. The identical twin of a person with schizophrenia has the highest risk (40–65%) of developing this disorder.

Demographics

- Schizophrenia occurs in 1% of the general population.
- Schizophrenia affects men and women equally and occurs at similar rates in all ethnic groups worldwide.
  - Patients with schizophrenia are found to abuse alcohol and/or drugs more often than the general population. Abusing a substance can reduce the effectiveness of treatment.
  - Patients with schizophrenia are more likely to be addicted to nicotine as compared with the general population (75–90% vs. 25–30%).

Patients may need higher doses of psychotropic medication if they smoke.
- Patients with schizophrenia attempt suicide much more often than people in the general population; approximately, 10% succeed, especially among young adult males.

Risk Factors

Age
- Onset of symptoms typically emerges in men in their late teens and early 20s and in women in their mid-20s to early 30s.
- Psychotic symptoms seldom occur after age 45 and only rarely before puberty (although cases of schizophrenia in children as young as 5 have been reported).

Gender
- The prevalence of schizophrenia among men and women is about the same.
- Pregnancy can worsen mental health in a subset of women with schizophrenia. Women are found to be especially susceptible for acute exacerbation of symptoms in the postpartum period. Compared to men, women tend to experience more pronounced mood symptoms.
- The gender differences in course and outcome is probably due to the effect of estrogen in women before menopause.

Family History
- Patients with immediate family members diagnosed as schizophrenic have approximately a 10% risk of developing the disorder.

Factors Associated with Birth
- Infants who experience a complication while in mothers' wombs or who experience trauma during delivery are at higher risk for developing schizophrenia.
- Intrauterine viral infection may occur in the womb.

Environmental Stressors
- Environmental stressors are found to be associated with the development of

schizophrenia, including problems with interpersonal relationships, difficulties at school/work, and substance abuse.

Substance Abuse

- Most researchers do not believe that substance abuse causes schizophrenia; however, patients with schizophrenia abuse alcohol and/or drugs more often than the general population.

Diagnosis

Differential Diagnosis

- Psychotic disorder due to a general medical condition, delirium, or dementia
- Substance-induced psychotic disorder, substance-induced delirium, substance-induced persisting dementia, and substance-related disorders may be seen
- Brief psychotic disorder
- Delusional disorder
- Schizophreniform disorder
- Psychotic disorder may not be otherwise specified
- Schizoaffective disorder
- Mood disorder with psychotic features
- Mood disorder with catatonic features
- Depressive disorder may not be otherwise specified
- Bipolar disorder may not be otherwise specified
- Pervasive developmental disorders (e.g., autistic disorder)
- Childhood presentations combining disorganized speech (from a communication disorder) and disorganized behavior (from attention-deficit/hyperactivity disorder)
- Schizotypal personality disorder
- Schizoid personality disorder
- Paranoid personality disorder

ICD Code

295.10 Disorganized type
295.20 Catatonic type
295.30 Paranoid type
295.60 Residual type
295.90 Unspecified type

Diagnostic Work-Up

- Physical and mental status examination

- CBC, including hemoglobin, hematocrit, red blood cell (RBC) count, white blood cell (WBC) count, WBC differential count, and platelet count
- Hepatic and renal function tests, including alanine transaminase (ALT), aspartate transaminase (AST), alkaline phosphatase (ALP), blood urea nitrogen (BUN), and creatinine
- Thyroid function tests (T3, T4, and TSH)
- Electrolytes (potassium, chloride, sodium, bicarbonate), glucose, B12, folate, and calcium level
- For patients with a history of suspicion, check for HIV, syphillis, ceruloplasmin, antinuclear antibody test, urine for culture and sensitivity and/or drugs of abuse, and 24-hour urine collections for porphyrins, copper, or heavy metals
- Alcohol and drug screening
- Pregnancy test for female patients at childbearing age

Initial Assessment

- Current physical status and physical history
- Current mental status and mental health history, including symptoms patient experiences, how long patient has been having symptoms, when the symptoms started, how often the symptoms occur, when and where symptoms tend to occur, how long symptoms last, and what effect symptoms have on patient's ability to function
- Drug history including prescribed and over-the-counter drugs
- Safety needs

Clinical Presentation: Symptoms

- Positive symptoms are extreme or exaggerated behaviors, including:
  - Delusions (somatic, ideas of reference, thought broadcasting, thought insertion, and thought withdrawal)
  - Hallucinations (visual, auditory, tactile, olfactory, and gustatory)
  - Inappropriate or over-reactive affect
- Negative symptoms:
  - Blunted or flat affect, unable to experience pleasure or express emotion (anhedonia)
  - Inability to carry out goal-directed behavior (avolition)

- Limited speech (alogia)
- Lack of energy and initiative
- Poor coordination and self-care
- Thought disorganization
  - Abnormal thoughts
  - Tangential, incoherent, or loosely associated speech

DSM-IV-TR Diagnostic Guidelines

- The diagnosis is given if two or more of the following signs and symptoms are present for a significant portion of time during a 1-month period, and persisting for at least 6 months:
  - Delusions
  - Hallucinations
  - Disorganized speech
  - Grossly disorganized or catatonic behavior
  - Negative symptoms
- Only one symptom is required for schizophrenia if delusions are bizarre or hallucinations consist of voice hallucinations. One or more major areas of functioning (e.g., work, interpersonal relations, self-care, school) are markedly reduced relative to prior levels of functioning.
- Continuous signs of the disturbance for at least 6 months.
- Schizoaffective disorder and mood disorder have been excluded.
- Substance abuse and other general medical condition have been excluded.
- Schizophrenia subtypes are defined by the predominant symptomatology at the time of evaluation. The five subtypes of schizophrenia are paranoid type, disorganized type, catatonic type, undifferentiated type, and residual type.
- The first signs for the adolescent population may include drops in academic performance, changes of friends, sleep problems, or irritability. A diagnosis of schizophrenia can be difficult to make for members of this age group since many normal adolescents also exhibit these behaviors.

Treatment

Acute Treatment

- Inpatient treatment is necessary for patients with a serious suicidal or homicidal ideation and plan, whose behavior can unintentionally be harmful to self or others, who is incapable of providing self-care, or who is at risk for behavior that may lead to long-term negative consequences.
- The goal of acute-phase treatment, usually lasting for 4–8 weeks, is to alleviate the most severe psychotic symptoms, such as agitation, frightening delusions, and hallucinations.
- Low-dose, high-potency antipsychotics have been found to be safe and effective in managing agitated psychiatric patients. For instance:
  - Haloperidol (Haldol) IM is used to clam patients with moderately severe to very severe agitation. Subsequent doses may be needed within 1 hour depending on the responses.
- Ziprasidone (Geodon) IM is recommended.
- A low dose of a short-acting benzodiazepine (e.g., lorazepam [Ativan]) is also found to be effective in decreasing agitation during the acute phase, and may reduce the amount of antipsychotic needed to control patients' psychotic symptoms.
- Atypical antipsychotic drugs are suggested to be used as a first-line treatment of schizophrenia because of their fewer side effects than with conventional or typical antipsychotic medications.
  - Aripiprazole (Abilify)
  - Clozapine (Clozaril, FazaClo ODT)
  - Olanzapine (Zyprexa)
  - Risperidone (Risperdal)
  - Long-acting risperidone (Risperdal Consta)
  - Quetiapine (Seroquel)
  - Ziprasidone (Geodon)
- Electroconvulsive therapy (ECT), in combination with antipsychotic medications, can be considered for patients with schizophrenia who do not respond to antipsychotic agents. The rate and number vary from patient to patient depending on their clinical responses and side effects.
- Substantial improvement of symptoms is seen in many patients by the sixth week of treatment. Providers may switch to other antipsychotic medications if patients are not responding to an adequate trial of a prescribed medication, are not able to tolerate a medication, or have poor medication adherence.

Chronic Treatment

- The treatment goals are to prevent relapse and to improve patient's level of functioning.
- It is estimated that 40–50% of patients are not adherent to treatment within 1–2 years. Long-acting medications are found to increase treatment adherence as compared to oral medications.
- It is important to monitor and manage side effects of antipsychotic medications, including extrapyramidal side effects (mostly common in patients treated with first-generation antipsychotics), tardive dyskinesia (TD), sedation, postural hypotension, weight gain, disturbances in sexual function. Using standardized rating scales (e.g., the Abnormal Involuntary Movement Scale) to access TD can help monitor medication-induced side effects.
- If patients develop extrapyramidal symptoms, give bromocriptine as directed.
- For dystonic reaction (especially of head and neck), give diphenhydramine (Benadryl).
- For pseudoparkinsonism reaction, use trihexyphenidyl (Artane) or benztropine (Cogentin).
- The neuroleptic malignant syndrome (NMS), characterized by fever (hyperthermia), muscular rigidity, altered mental status, and autonomic dysfunction, is a rare but potentially fatal reaction to neuroleptic medications. If a parent has hyperthermia, or stops antipsychotic medications, give dantrolene and continue as needed until cumulative total dose is up to 10 mg/kg. After the acute phase, give dantrolene to prevent recurrence.
- Body Mass index (BMI), fasting blood glucose, and lipid profiles are important health indicators to monitor since weight gain has occurred with most antipsychotic agents. It is recommended to weigh patients and check BMI for every visit for 6 months after a change in medications.
- Clozapine (Clozaril, FazaClo ODT) is the drug of choice for treatment-resistant schizophrenia patients (little or no symptomatic response to at least 2 antipsychotic trials of an adequate duration [at least 6 weeks] and at a therapeutic dose range) and it has a lower risk of TD. However, due to the potential side effect of agranulocytosis (loss of WBCs), a blood test is required weekly for the first 6 months, and biweekly for the next 6 months. Monitoring can be done monthly if no hematological problems are found after 1 year of clozapine (Clozaril, FazaClo ODT) treatment.
- Social skills training, aimed at improving the way patients with schizophrenia interact with others (e.g., poor eye contact, odd facial expressions, inaccurate or lack of perceptions of emotions in other people), has been found to be effective in reducing the relapse rate.
- Cognitive-behavioral therapy (CBT) helps patients with schizophrenia to learn some insight into their illness and appears to be effective in reducing the severity of symptoms and decreasing the risk of relapse.
- Dialectical behavior therapy (DBT) combines cognitive and behavioral theories. Patients with schizophrenia may benefit from DBT to improve interpersonal skills.
- Individual psychotherapy focuses on forming a therapeutic alliance between therapists and patients with schizophrenia. A good therapeutic alliance is likely to help patients with schizophrenia remain in the therapy, increase adherence to treatments, and have positive outcomes at 2-year follow-up evaluations.
- Personal therapy, a recently developed form of individual treatment, uses social skills and relaxation exercises, self-reflection, self-awareness, exploration of vulnerability and stress, and psychoeducation to enhance personal and social adjustment of patients with schizophrenia. Patients who receive personal therapy have shown better social adjustment and a lower rate of relapse after 3 years than those not receiving it.
- Many patients with schizophrenia benefit from art therapy because it helps them communicate with and share their inner word with others.
- Employment programs that include individualized job development, rapid placement, ongoing job supports, and integration of mental health and vocational services have been found to be effective in helping patients with schizophrenia to achieve employment.

- Family-oriented therapies that help family and patients with schizophrenia understand the disorder, and encourage discussions of psychotic episode and events leading up to it may be effective in reducing relapses.
- Treatment for co-occurring substance abuse. Substance abuse is the most common co-occurring disorder in patients with schizophrenia. Integrated treatment programs for schizophrenia and substance use produce better outcomes.
- Many studies show that integrating psychosocial and medication treatment produces the best results in patients with schizophrenia.

Recurrence Rate

The reported recurrence rates range from 10–60%; approximately, 20–30% of patients with schizophrenia can have somewhat normal lives, 20–30% continue to experience moderate symptoms, and 40–60% of them remain significantly impaired for their entire lives.

Patient Education

- Information regarding schizophrenia is available from the National Institutes for Mental Health Web site at http://www.nimh.nih.gov/health/publications/schizophrenia/index.shtml.
- Antipsychotic medications can produce dangerous side effects when taken with certain drugs. It is important for patients to tell health care providers about all medications, including over-the-counter medications, prescribed medications, vitamins, minerals, and herbal supplements that patients take. *Note*: Medications should be used with particular caution in children, pregnant/breastfeeding women, and older adults.
- It is important to teach patients about the importance of medication adherence and to avoid using alcohol and other substances.
- For excellent patient education resources, visit eMedicine's Mental Health and Behavior Center. See also eMedicine's patient education article on schizophrenia.

Medical/Legal Pitfalls

- Misdiagnosis.
- Patients with schizophrenia are addicted to nicotine at three times the rate of the general population (75–90% vs. 25–30%).
- Approximately, 20–70% of patients with schizophrenia have a comorbid substance abuse problem, which is associated with increased violence, suicidality, nonadherence with treatment, hostility, crime, poor nutrition, etc.
- Mental health providers should inform patients being treated with conventional antipsychotic medications about the risk of TD. AIMS (Abnormal Involuntary Movement Scale) is recommended for detecting TD early.
- Patients with schizophrenia are found to have a higher risk for acquiring obesity, diabetes, cardiovascular disease, HIV, lung diseases, and rheumatoid arthritis. It is important for mental health care providers to monitor their physical conditions regularly.

Schizophreniform Disorder

Background Information

Definition of Disorder
- This is characterized by the presence of the principal symptoms of schizophrenia, including delusions, hallucinations, disorganized speech, disorganized or catatonic behavior, and negative symptoms.
- An episode of the disorder (including prodromal, active, and residual phases) lasts at least 1 month but less than 6 months.

Etiology
- The cause of schizophreniform remains unknown.
- Current biological and epidemiological data suggest that some of the schizophreniform patients are similar to those with schizophrenia, whereas others have a disorder similar to mood disorder.

Demographics
- The lifetime prevalence rate of schizophreniform is 0.2%, and a 1-year prevalence rate is 0.1%.

Risk Factors
Age
- Schizophreniform is most common in adolescents and young adults.

Gender
- The prevalence of schizophreniform disorder is equally distributed between men and women, with peak onset between the ages of 18 and 24 in men and 24 and 35 in women.

Family History
- Studies show that relatives of individuals with schizophreniform disorder are at higher risk of having mood disorders than are relatives of individuals with schizophrenia.
- Relatives of individuals with schizophreniform disorder are more likely to have a psychotic mood disorder than are relatives of individuals with bipolar disorders.

Diagnosis

Differential Diagnosis
- Schizophrenia
- Brief psychotic disorder
- Substance-induced psychotic disorder
- Bipolar disorder and major depression with mood-incongruent features

ICD Code
295.40 Schizophreniform Disorder

Diagnostic Work-Up
- Physical and mental status examination
- Electrolytes (potassium, chloride, bicarbonate)
- Thyroid function tests (TSH, T3, and T4)
- Screen for alcohol and drugs, including amphetamines, methamphetamines, barbiturates, phenobarbital, benzodiazepines, cannabis, cocaine, codeine, cotinine, morphine, heroin, lysergic acid diethylamide (LSD), methadone, and PCP

Initial Assessment
- Current physical status and physical history
- Current mental status and mental health history, including symptoms patient experiences, how long patient has been having symptoms, when the symptoms started, how often the symptoms occur, when and where symptoms tend to occur, how long symptoms last, and what effect symptoms have on patient's ability to function
- Drug history, including prescribed and over-the-counter drugs
- Safety needs

Clinical Presentation: Symptoms
- Delusions (somatic, ideas of reference, thought broadcasting, thought insertion, and thought withdrawal)
- Hallucinations (visual, auditory, tactile, olfactory, and gustatory)
- Disorganized speech (e.g., frequent derailment or incoherence)

- Grossly disorganized or catatonic behavior
- Negative symptoms (e.g., flat affect, lack of energy and initiative)

DSM-IV-TR Diagnostic Guidelines

The essential features of schizophreniform disorder and those of schizophrenia are the same, with two exceptions: duration (an episode of schizophreniform disorder lasts at least 1 month but less than 6 months), and personal functioning (in schizophreniform disorder impaired social or occupational functioning need not always be present).

Treatment

Acute Treatment

- Inpatient treatment is often necessary for patients with schizophreniform disorder for effective assessment and treatment. Patients who are at risk of harming themselves or others require hospitalization to allow comprehensive evaluation and to ensure their safety as well as others'.
- The pharmacotherapy for schizophreniform disorder is similar to that for schizophrenia. Atypical antipsychotics are mostly used at this time. See details in the schizophrenia discussion.
- Antidepressants may help reduce mood disturbances associated with schizophreniform disorder, but patients need to be monitored carefully for possible exacerbations of psychotic symptoms.

Chronic Treatment

- Long-acting medications are found to increase treatment adherence. Paliperidone (Invega), a major active metabolite of risperidone (Risperdal Consta) and the first oral agent allowing once-daily dosing (6 mg PO in the morning), has been approved by the FDA in 2006.
- Ziprasidone (Geodon) and aripiprazole (Abilify) are available in injection form to help control acute psychotic symptoms. The injections are less likely to cause acute extrapyramidal side effects.
- It is critical to monitor and manage side effects of antipsychotic medications (e.g., extrapyramidal side effects, TD, sedation, postural hypotension,

weight gain, disturbances in sexual function). See details in the schizophrenia section.
- Psychotherapeutic treatment modalities used in the treatment of patients with schizophrenia may be helpful in treating patients with schizophreniform disorder. However, patients with schizophreniform disorder can become frightened in groups in which they are mixed with patients who have chronic schizophrenia.
- Family therapy is proven to be appropriate for patients with schizophreniform disorder and their families.
- In patients with schizophreniform disorder exhibiting impairments in social functioning, rehabilitative strategies similar to those described for patients with schizophrenia may be helpful.

Recurrence Rate

It is estimated that 60–80% of patients with schizophreniform disorder will progress to full-blown schizophrenia despite treatment.

Patient Education

- Antipsychotic medications can produce dangerous side effects when taken with certain drugs. It is important for patients to tell health care providers about all medications, including over-the-counter medications, prescribed medications, vitamins, minerals, and herbal supplements that patients take.
- It is important to teach patients about the importance of medication adherence and to avoid using alcohol and other substances.
- For excellent patient education resources, visit eMedicine's Mental Health and Behavior Center. See also eMedicine's patient education article, "Schizophrenia."

Medical/Legal Pitfalls

- Misdiagnosis.
- Mental health care providers should inform patients being treated with conventional antipsychotic medications about the risk of TD. AIMS is recommended for detecting TD early.
- Use medications with particular caution in children, pregnant/breastfeeding women, and older adults.

Shared Psychotic Disorder

Background Information

Definition of Disorder

- It is also called "folie à deux" (the folly of two); it is a rare disorder characterized by the apparent movement of delusions from one person (primary) to another person (secondary) with whom the first has close emotional ties.

Etiology

- The individual who first has delusion (the primary case) is often chronically ill and is the influential member of a close relationship with a more suggestible individual (the secondary case) who also develops delusion.
- Occurrence of delusion in the secondary case is attributed to the strong influence of the more dominant member.

Demographics

- The epidemiology remains unclear since most data have been extrapolated from case reports.
- Inconsistent with an earlier hypothesis, recent studies suggest that females and males are equally affected, the secondary person can be either younger or older than the primary person, and the incidence rate in married couples is equal to that in siblings.

Risk Factors

- A close association contributes more to the development of shared psychotic disorder than age.
- The shared psychotic disorder is equally distributed between men and women.
- A psychosocial stressor, such as social conflict with family members or friends, social isolation, or recent immigration, may be associated with onset of shared psychotic disorder.

Diagnosis

Differential Diagnosis

- Medical conditions associated with the development of delusions, such as toxic-metabolic

conditions affecting the limbic system and basal ganglia, Huntington's disease, etc.
- Delirium
- Dementia
- Substance-related disorders
- Schizophrenia
- Mood disorders
- Obsessive-compulsive disorder
- Somatoform disorders
- Paranoid personality disorder

ICD Code

297.3 Shared Psychotic Disorder

Diagnostic Work-Up

- Physical and mental status examination
- Chest X-ray
- CBC, electrolyte analysis (potassium, chloride, bicarbonate), BUN, creatinine
- Drug screen should include alcohol, amphetamines, barbiturates, benzodiazepines, cocaine, codeine, heroin, hydromorphone, methadone, morphine, PCP, propoxyphene, and tetrahydrocannabinol (THC)

Initial Assessment

- Current physical status and physical history
- Current mental status and mental health history
  - Symptoms patient experiences
  - How long patient has been having symptoms
  - When the symptoms started
  - How often the symptoms occur
  - When and where symptoms tend to occur
  - How long symptoms last
  - What effect symptoms have on patient's ability to function
  - Family history of mental disorder
- Drug history including prescribed and over-the-counter drugs
- Safety needs

Clinical Presentation: Symptoms

- Delusions that are similar to those of someone close who has a well-established delusion.

DSM-IV-TR Diagnostic Guidelines

- A delusion develops in the context of a close relationship.
- The secondary instance of delusion is similar in content to that of the person who has an established delusion.
- The disturbance is not better accounted for by another psychotic disorder, a mood disorder with psychotic features, or as the direct physiological effect of a substance or a general medical condition.

Treatment

Acute Treatment

- Hospitalization may be required if patients need an assessment of violent impulses (e.g., commit suicide or homicide) related to their delusions, or the delusions have significantly affected patients' self-care and social functioning. Hospitalization also allows a complete medical and neurological evaluation to rule out medical conditions that cause delusional symptoms.
- Separating the primary and secondary cases is insufficient. The definition of primary and secondary cases is described above. The primary case is often chronically ill and is the influential member of a close relationship with a more suggestible individual (the secondary case) who also develops delusion. Antipsychotic medications are required for effective treatment besides separation.
- Newer generation anticonvulsants are found to be highly effective in treating patients with shared psychotic disorder.
  - Antipsychotic medications are reported to be effective and should start with low doses in these patients—for instance, aripiprazole (Abilify) and quetiapine (Seroquel).

Chronic Treatment

- Nonadherence to the medications is a common cause of treatment failure. It is critical to monitor and manage side effects of antipsychotic medications.
- Psychotherapy (e.g., cognitive behavioral therapy) is recommended; individual therapy has been found to be more effective than group therapy.

Recurrence Rate

It is estimated that 50% of patients with shared psychotic disorder recover at a long-term follow-up, 20% show improved symptoms, and 30% have no change in symptoms.

Patient Education

- Antipsychotic medications can produce dangerous side effects when taking with certain drugs. It is important for patients to tell health care providers about all medications, including over-the-counter medications, prescribed medications, vitamins, minerals, and herbal supplements that patients take.
- It is important to teach patients about the importance of medication adherence and to avoid using alcohol and other substances.
- For excellent patient education resources, visit eMedicine's Mental Health and Behavior Center. See also eMedicine's patient education article on schizophrenia.

Medical/Legal Pitfalls

- Misdiagnosis.
- Mental health care providers should inform patients being treated with conventional antipsychotic medications about the risk of TD. AIMS is recommended for detecting TD early.
- Use medications with particular caution in children, pregnant/breastfeeding women, and older adults.

Other Resources

Evidence-Based References

American Psychiatric Association. (2006). *Practice guidelines for treatment: compendium 2006.* Washington, DC: American Psychiatric Press.

Azorin, J. M., Kaladjian, A., & Fakra, E. (2005). Current issues on schizoaffective disorder. *Encephale, 31*(3), 359–365.

Bond, G. R., & Drake, R. E. (2008). Predictors of competitive employment among patients with schizophrenia. *Current Opinions in Psychiatry, 21*(4), 362–369.

Cervini, P., Newman, D., Dorian, P., et al. (2003). Folie a deux: an old diagnosis with a new technology. *Canadian Journal of Cardiology, 19*(13),1539–1540.

Emsley, R., Oosthuizen, P., Koen, L., Niehaus, D. J., Medori, R., & Rabinowitz, J. (2008). Oral versus injectable antipsychotic treatment in early psychosis: Post hoc comparison of two studies. *Clinical Therapy, 30*(12), 2378–2386.

Etter, M., & Etter, J. F. (2004). Alcohol consumption and the CAGE test in outpatients with schizophrenia or schizoaffective disorder and in the general population. *Schizophrenia Bulletin, 30*(4), 947–956.

Fennig, S., Fochtmann, L. J., & Bromet, E. J. (2005). Delusional and shared psychotic disorder. In H. I. Kaplan & B. J. Sadock (Eds.), *Kaplan and Sadock's comprehensive textbook of psychiatry* (8th ed., pp. 1525–1533). New York: Lippincott, Williams & Wilkins.

Fochtmann, L. J. (2005). Treatment of other psychotic disorders. In *Kaplan and Sadock's comprehensive textbook of psychiatry* (8th ed., pp. 1545–1550). New York: Lippincott, Williams & Wilkins.

Harrow, M., Grossman, L. S., Herbener, E. S., & Davies, E. W. (2000). Ten-year outcome: Patients with schizoaffective disorders, schizophrenia, affective disorders and mood-incongruent psychotic symptoms. *British Psychiatry, 177*, 421–426.

Jones, R. T., & Benowitz, N. L. (2002). Therapeutics for nicotine addiction. In K. L. Davis, D. Charney, J. T. Coyle, & C. Nemeroff (Eds.), *Neuropsychopharmacology: The fifth generation of progress* (pp. 1533–1544). Nashville, TN: American College of Neuropsychopharmacology.

Kaplan, H. I., & Sadock, B. J. (Eds.). (2003). *Kaplan and Sadock's synopsis of psychiatry: Behavioral sciences/clinical psychiatry* (9th ed., pp. 508–511). New York: Lippincott, Williams & Wilkins.

Kwon, J. S., Jang, J. H., Kang, D. H., Yoo, S. Y., Kim, Y. K., & Cho, S. J., APLUS study group. (2009). Long-term efficacy and safety of aripiprazole in patients with schizophrenia, schizophreniform disorder, or schizoaffective disorder: 26-week prospective study. *Psychiatry and Clinical Neuroscience, 63*(1), 73–81.

Marder, S. R. (2000). Integrating pharmacological and psychosocial treatments for schizophrenia. *Acta Psychiatrica Scandinavica Supplementum, 102*(407), 87–90.

Meltzer, H. Y., Alphs, L., Green, A. I., Altamura, A. C., Anand, R., Bertoldi, A., Bourgeois, M., Chouinard, G., Islam, M. Z., Kane, J., Krishnan, R., Lindenmayer, J. P., & Potkin, S.; International Suicide Prevention Trial Study Group. (2003). Clozapine treatment for suicidality in schizophrenia: International Suicide Prevention Trial (InterSePT). *Archives of General Psychiatry, 60*(1), 82–91.

Meltzer, H. Y., & Baldessarini, R. J. (2003). Reducing the risk for suicide in schizophrenia and affective disorders. *Journal of Clinical Psychiatry, 64*(9), 1122–1129.

Möller, H. J. (2005). Occurrence and treatment of depressive comorbidity/cosyndromality in schizophrenic psychoses. Conceptual and treatment issues. *World Journal of Biology and Psychiatry, 6*(4), 247–263.

Morken, G., Widen, J. H., & Grawe, R. W. (2008). Nonadherence to antipsychotic medication, relapse and rehospitalisation in recent-onset schizophrenia. *BMC Psychiatry, 8*, 32.

Mueser, K. T., & McGurk, S. R. (2004). Schizophrenia. *Lancet, 363*(9426), 2063–2072.

Pharoah, F. M., Mari, J. J., & Streiner, D. (2003). Family intervention for schizophrenia. *Cochrane Database of Systemic Reviews, 4*, CD000088.

Reif, A., & Pfuhlmann, B. (2004). Folie a deux versus genetically driven delusional disorder: case reports and nosological considerations. *Comprehensive Psychiatry, 45*(2), 155–160.

Sadock, B. J., & Sadock, V. A. (2008). Delusional disorder and shared psychotic disorder. In B. J., Sadock & V. A. Sadock (Eds.). *Kaplan and Sadock's concise textbook of clinical psychiatry.* (3rd ed., pp. 182–190). Philadelphia: Wolters Kluwer/Lippincott Williams & Wilkins.

Sadock, B. J., & Sadock, V. A. (2008). Schizophrenia. In B. J. Sadock & V. A. Sadock (Eds.), *Kaplan and Sadock's concise textbook of clinical psychiatry* (3rd ed., pp. 156–177). Philadelphia: Lippincott, Williams & Wilkins.

Sadock, B. J., & Sadock, V. A. (2008). Schizophreniform disorder. In B. J., Sadock & V. A. Sadock (Eds.). *Kaplan and Sadock's concise textbook of clinical psychiatry* (3rd ed., pp. 178–180). Philadelphia: Wolters Kluwer/Lippincott Williams & Wilkins.

Shimizu, M., Kubota, Y., Toichi, M., & Baba, H. (2007). Folieà deux and shared psychotic disorder. *Current Psychiatry Report, 9*(3), 200–205.

Silveira, J. M., & Seeman, M. V. (1995). Shared psychotic disorder: a critical review of the literature. *Canadian Journal of Psychiatry, 40*(7), 389–395.

Solari, H., Dickson, K. E., & Miller, L. (2009). Understanding and treating women with schizophrenia during pregnancy and postpartum—Motherisk Update 2008. *Canadian Journal of Clinical Pharmacology, 16*(1), e23–32.

Suzuki, K., Awata, S., Takano, T., Ebina, Y., Takamatsu, K., Kajiwara, T., et al. (2006). Improvement of psychiatric symptoms after electroconvulsive therapy in young adults with intractable first-episode schizophrenia and schizophreniform disorder. *Tohoku Journal of Experimental Medicine, 210*(3), 213–220.

Wenning, M. T., Davy, L. E., Catalano, G., & Catalano, M. C. (2003). Atypical antipsychotics in the treatment of delusional parasitosis. *Annals of Clinical Psychiatry, 15*(3–4), 233–239.

Web Resources

- American Psychiatric Association: http://www.psych.org.
- Cleveland Clinic: http://www.ClevelandClinic.org.
- National Alliance on Mental Illness (NAMI): http://www.nami.org.
- National Mental Health Information Center: http://mentalhealth.samhsa.gov/.
- Psych Central: http://psychcentral. com/.

8. MOOD DISORDERS
Major Depressive Disorder

Background Information

Definition of Disorder

- Overwhelming sadness or lack of enjoyment, sometimes with anxiety and irritability, are the primary indicators.
- Hopelessness and a sense of feeling overwhelmed or helpless are common.
- Fatigue or somatic symptoms are also usually present.
- Often follows chronic stress or significant acute stressor(s).
- May complicate the treatment of other medical conditions such as stroke, diabetes, etc. For example, people with depression are four times more likely to develop a heart attack than those without a history of the illness. After a heart attack they are at a significantly increased risk of death or a second heart attack.
- Negatively impacts social functioning, such as getting out of bed, going to work, and having positive relationships.
- Is a recurrent illness. Risk for relapse after one episode is 50%. After two episodes, risk for relapse is 80–90%. Average number of lifetime episodes is four.

Etiology

- Although heterogeneous in nature and poorly understood, the chronic stress response and the subsequent continuous activation of the hypothalamic-pituitary-adrenal axis results in chronic brain changes, such as a smaller hippocampus and changes in neurotransmitters.
- Corticotropin-releasing hormone (CRH) is a neuropeptide released by the hypothalamus to activate the pituitary in response to acute stress, but is hypersecreted in depression.
- Serotonin and norepinephrine are thought to be the primary neurotransmitters involved in depression, although dopamine can also be related to depression.
- Cognitive and personality factors, such as how people view their influence, their ability to

change, and their interpretation of stressors, also play a role. The depressive thinks that good things are temporary, limited in scope, and the result of sheer luck. Bad things are considered permanent, pervasive in impact, and his or her fault.
- Major depressive disorder (MDD) has been found to run in families, and this may mean that inheritance (genes) plays a strong role in determining who will get it. However, people who have no family history of the disorder also develop it.
- Often, depression occurs in the context of chronic illness or major life stressors.

Demographics

- Affects approximately 14.8 million American adults, or about 6.7% of the U.S. adult population.
- Affects 17.6 million Americans annually.
- Prevalence is 3–6% with a 2:1 female-to-male ratio.
- As many as 1 in 33 children and 1 in 8 adolescents have clinical depression.
- Individuals with MDD use 2–3 times the amount of health care services as nondepressed patients.
- MDD is the leading cause of disability in the United States for ages 15–44 and the leading cause of disability in the world for adolescents and adults.
- Suicide results in 32,000 deaths annually in the United States, and two-thirds of these suicides are related to MDD.
- About 4.5 times more men than women die from suicide. White men complete more than 78% of all suicides and 56% of suicide deaths among men involve firearms. Poisoning is the predominant method among females.
- An estimated 8–25 attempted suicides occur for every completion. The majority of suicide attempts are expressions of extreme distress, not merely bids for attention.
- The rate of substance abuse (especially of stimulants, cocaine, and hallucinogens) in persons with MDD is 7–28%, a risk 4–14 times greater than that of the general population.

- Pregnant mothers with MDD are more likely to have infants of smaller birth weight for gestational age.

Risk Factors

Age

- First occurrence is often between the ages of 20 and 40.
- The prevalence of major depression seems to be increasing in younger generations.

Gender

- Major depression is twice as common in women as in men.
- Pregnancy can either improve the condition or make it worse.
- The postpartum period is a time of especial susceptibility to major depression.

Family History

- Many studies have shown an increased incidence of major depression when there is a history of depression, alcoholism, or other psychiatric illnesses in first-degree relatives.
- The disorder is two times more common in first-degree relatives with MDD.

Past Medical History

- Comorbidities with chronic disease are common, with conditions such as prior myocardial infarction, multiple sclerosis (MS), Parkinson's, and chronic pain having a greater than 40% prevalence.
- Current alcohol or substance abuse incidence of MDD may have occurred.

Stressful Events in Susceptible People

- The initial appearance of MDD may follow a highly stressful event, such as being the victim of a crime, or the loss of a job, a loved one, or an important relationship.

Social History

- There is often a lack of social support
- Frequent use of medical resources in the absence of serious illness may be seen
- Past or current history of abuse (childhood, sexual, or domestic violence) increases the incidence of MDD

Having Another Mental Disorder

- A previous episode of depression may increase the risk of subsequent episodes of depression by as much as 90%.
- A history of dysthymic disorder precedes MDD in 10–25% of individuals.
- Having another mental disorder, such as substance abuse (alcoholism or drug abuse) or a sleep disorder, may increase the risk of developing MDD.
- Past history of suicide attempt.

Risk Factors for Suicide

- Elderly
- Male gender
- Widows/widowers/unmarried people
- Unemployed
- People living alone
- History of previous psychiatric hospitalization
- Substance abuse
- Recent loss of significant relationship
- Recent loss of financial security
- Previous suicide attempt(s)

Diagnosis

Differential Diagnosis

- Common
  - Thyroid disease
  - Anemia
  - Menopause
  - Chronic fatigue syndrome
  - If an underlying chronic health condition such as MS or stroke is the physiologic *cause* of the depressed mood, the diagnosis is mood disorder due to a general medical condition
  - Bipolar disorder
  - Bereavement
  - Adjustment disorder with depressed mood
  - Anxiety disorders
  - Dementia
  - Drug interactions or adverse effects
  - Infectious disease, such as autoimmune disorder, mononucleosis, or hepatitis C
  - Fibromyalgia
  - Personality disorder
- Less common
  - Amphetamine or cocaine withdrawal
  - Parathyroid disease

- ▪ Adrenal disease
- ▪ Cancer
- ▪ Neurologic disease, such as cerebrovascular accident (CVA), MS, subdural hematoma, normal pressure hydrocephalus, or Alzheimer's disease
- ▪ Cardiovascular disease such as congestive heart failure (CHF) or cardiomyopathy
- ▪ Nutritional deficiency, such as B vitamin, folate, or iron deficiency
- ▪ Pulmonary disease, such as chronic obstructive pulmonary disorder (COPD)
- ▪ Heavy metal poisoning

ICD Code
296.20 Major Depressive Disorder, single episode, unspecified degree

296.30 Major Depressive Disorder, recurrent episodes, unspecified degree

311 Depressive Disorder (NOS, or not otherwise specified)

Diagnostic Work-Up
- ▪ Physical and mental evaluation
- ▪ Labs as needed to evaluate physical complaints
  - ▪ Thyroid function studies (triiodothyronine [T3], thyroxine [T4], thyroid-stimulating hormone [TSH]).
  - ▪ CMP (complete metabolic panel), including glucose, calcium, and albumin; total protein analysis; and levels of sodium, potassium, CO_2 (carbon dioxide, bicarbonate), chloride, blood urea nitrogen (BUN), creatinine, alkaline phosphatase (ALP), alanine amino transferase (ALT, also called SGPT), aspartate amino transferase (AST, also called SGOT), and bilirubin.
  - ▪ Complete blood count (CBC) with differentials: hemoglobin, hematocrit, red blood cells, white blood cells, white blood cell differential count, and platelet count.
  - ▪ Testing for infectious diseases such as hepatitis C or HIV, if applicable.

Initial Assessment
- ▪ Screening question: In the past month, have you felt down or depressed? In the past month, have you lost interest in the things you usually do?
- ▪ Use of a standard screening tool, such as:

1. SIG E CAPS
   - ▪ Depressed mood
   - ▪ Sleep decreased (insomnia with 2 A.M. to 4 A.M. awakening)
   - ▪ Interest decreased in activities (anhedonia)
   - ▪ Guilt or worthlessness (not a major criterion)
   - ▪ Energy decreased
   - ▪ Concentration difficulties
   - ▪ Appetite disturbance or weight loss
   - ▪ Psychomotor retardation/agitation
   - ▪ Suicidal thoughts
2. Beck Depression Inventory: twenty-one question survey completed by patient
3. Zung Self-Rating Scale: twenty-question survey completed by patient, Likert scale format
4. PHQ 9: brief survey completed by patient
- ▪ Past medical history
- ▪ Family medical history, with emphasis on psychiatric history
- ▪ Social history, including safety of relationships, family support, recent or ongoing stressors
- ▪ Past suicide attempts or past psychiatric hospitalizations
- ▪ Any prior manic/hypomanic episodes (*any* history suggests bipolar or cyclothymia diagnosis). Mood Disorder Questionnaire is a helpful tool.
- ▪ What effect symptoms have had on ability to function (any missed work, etc.?)
- ▪ Assess for suicide ideation, suicide plan, and suicide intent

Clinical Presentation: Symptoms
- ▪ Somatization: often, presentation of depression is through complaints of (often multiple) physical symptoms which do not have clearly identifiable causes
- ▪ Sadness
- ▪ Lack of enjoyment of usual activities (anhedonia)
- ▪ Fatigue
- ▪ Sleep problems (early-morning awakening with difficulty or inability to fall back asleep is typical)
- ▪ Feelings of guilt
- ▪ Feeling overwhelmed
- ▪ Difficulty concentrating, focusing, or remembering

- Appetite disturbances (lack of appetite, or excessive eating)
- Irritability, agitation, or slowed movements
- Thoughts of suicide or wanting to "escape"
- Obsessive rumination about problems

Signs
- Flattened affect
- Slowed speech and movements, sighs, long pauses
- Tearfulness
- Lack of eye contact
- Memory loss, poor concentration, or poor abstract reasoning
- Sometimes irritability, belligerence, or defiance (more common in adolescence)

DSM-IV-TR Diagnostic Guidelines
The *DSM-IV-TR* distinguishes between major depressive disorder, single episode; and major depressive disorder, recurrent.

For major depressive disorder—single episode:
- At least five of the following symptoms have been present for at least 2 weeks in duration: depressed mood, anhedonia, change in eating habits, sleep disturbance, psychomotor agitation or retardation, fatigue, excessive guilt or feelings of worthlessness, difficulty concentrating, and recurrent thoughts of death or suicide (at least one of the symptoms being depressed mood or anhedonia).
- Symptoms must cause a significant social or occupational dysfunction or subjective distress.
- Symptoms cannot be caused by a medical condition, medications, drugs, or bereavement.
  For major depressive disorder—recurrent:
- Two or more major depressive episodes occur.
- Absence of manic, hypomanic, or "mixed" episodes.

Treatment

Acute Treatment
- Patients with MDD must be evaluated for suicide risk.
- Depressed patients with suicidal ideation, plan, and intent should be hospitalized, especially if they have current psychosocial stressors and access to lethal means.
- Depressed patients with suicidal ideation and a plan, but without intent, may be treated on an outpatient basis with close follow-up, especially when they have good social support and no access to lethal means.
- Depressed patients who express suicidal ideation but deny a plan should be assessed carefully for psychosocial stressors. Remove weapons from the environment.
- Pay careful attention in the first 1–4 weeks of treatment to a sudden lift of depression, or to worsening mood as an initial response to antidepressant therapy as these could be signs of increased risk for suicide.
- Most patients are started on long-term (e.g., 6–9 months) therapy with selective serotonin reuptake inhibitors (SSRIs), serotonin and norepinephrine reuptake inhibitor (SNRIs), or atypical antidepressants. Assist patients with side effects, which are more likely to occur early in treatment.
- The combination of pharmacological therapy and cognitive-behavioral therapy (CBT), individually or in combination, is effective in more than 85% of cases.
- The goal during the acute phase of treatment, which can last up to 12 weeks, is to assist the patient in achieving full remission of symptoms.

Chronic Treatment
- Pharmacotherapy with or without individual counseling, particularly CBT, is the treatment of choice, and should be considered for patients.
- Cognitive restructuring involves substituting positive perceptions for negative perceptions and assistance with problem solving and stress management.
- The continuation phase begins once remission has been achieved. Relapse is common during this time, so ensure that patient understands the importance of continuing pharmacologic therapy for at least 6 months.
- Maintenance of therapy preferred for first-time episodes for 9 months. Will need to discuss tapering of therapy when appropriate (avoid winter months, stressful times).

- Consider long-term treatment in patients with two or more episodes. A history of three or more episodes of depression indicates a very high risk for recurrence, and the need for continuous treatment.
- Stress management and lifestyle changes, such as regular exercise, which has been found to decrease depression, are essential to ongoing prevention.
- Behavioral therapy involves various relaxation techniques, self-care strategies, and cognitive and dialectical may also be helpful. Studies suggest that augmentation of antidepressant effect occurs with adjunct use of omega-3 fish oil supplements, 1000 mg twice daily. B vitamin supplementation has also been used in some studies, with equivocal results.
- Treatment can be complicated by having another condition at the same time, such as substance abuse, depression, or other anxiety disorders.

Recurrence Rate
Rate of recurrence is 50% after 1 episode, 80% after 2 episodes, and >90% after 3 episodes

Patient Education
- Information regarding MDD and support groups can be obtained from the National Institute for Mental Health (see further outpatient care).
- Advise patients with MDD to avoid nicotine and avoid excess alcohol intake (no more than 1 svg/day for a woman, 2 svg/day for a man).
- Thirty minutes of daily exercise has been found beneficial for MDD patients and daily exposure to outdoor light may be beneficial.

Medical/Legal Pitfalls
- Failure to monitor for suicide risk.
- Failure to screen for bipolar disorder (any history of mania/hypomania).
- Pay careful attention in the first 1–4 weeks of treatment to a sudden lift of depression, or to worsening mood as initial response to antidepressant therapy as these could be signs of increased risk for suicide.
- When initiating treatment, see patients on a more frequent basis until response to antidepressant is clear.
- Have a follow-up system to ensure that there are calls to patients who fail to schedule follow-up appointments or fail to show up for scheduled appointments.
- Patients with MDDs are more likely than the general population to use alternative therapies. Use of dietary supplements (e.g., herbs) should be discussed to avoid drug interactions.

Bipolar Disorder

Background Information

Definition of Disorder
- Historically has been referred to as manic depression or manic-depressive illness.
- Neurobiological psychiatric disorder is characterized by sustained extreme mood swings from extremely low (depression) to extremely high (mania).
- Both phases of this disorder are deleterious in that they adversely affect thoughts, behaviors, judgment, and relationships.
- Patients with Bipolar I Disorder have episodes of sustained mania, and often experience depressive episodes.
- Patients with Bipolar II Disorder have one or more major depressive episodes (MDEs), with at least one hypomanic episode.
- Extreme mood swings that occur hourly or daily are very rarely associated with this disorder and other medical and/or psychiatric diagnoses should be considered and ruled out first.
- An age of onset of mania after the age of 40 alerts the practitioner that the symptoms are most likely due to a medical condition or substance use, and newly diagnosed mania is uncommon in children and adults over the age of 65.
- It is not uncommon for bipolar disorder to go undetected.
- Patients in the manic phase of the disorder often do not seek psychiatric or medical attention.
- Patients experiencing the depressive phase of the disorder often initially present to a primary care setting due to an increase in health issues, somatic complaints, or chronic pain that do not appear to have an objective or identifiable etiology.

Etiology
- The exact cause of bipolar disorder is not known.
- The "kindling theory" is the current predominant theory, meaning the disorder is likely caused by multiple factors that potentially interact and lower the threshold at which mood changes occur. Eventually, a mood episode can start itself and thus become recurrent.
  - Environmental factors:
    - Sleep deprivation can trigger episodes of mania while hypersomnia can trigger MDEs.
    - Traumatic and/or abusive events in childhood.
    - Approximately, one-fifth of individuals with bipolar disorder, mostly those with Bipolar II, have mood symptoms that wax and wane with the seasons. It is hypothesized that those with a diurnal pattern are mostly affected by both fluctuating light and temperature.
  - Biological perspectives
- Genetics:
  - Twin studies consistently show that identical twins (40–70%) are far more concordant for mood disorders than fraternal twins (0–10%).
  - The overall heritability of bipolar spectrum disorders has been put at 0.71.
  - Between 4 and 24% of first-degree relatives of individuals with Bipolar I Disorder are also diagnosed with Bipolar I Disorder.
- Neural processes:
  - Hypersensitivity of melatonin receptors
  - Structural abnormalities in the amygdala, hippocampus, and prefrontal cortex
  - Larger lateral ventricles
  - White matter hyperintensities
- Endocrine models:
  - Hypothyroidism can cause depression and/or mood instability.
  - Abnormalities have also been found in the hypothalamic-pituitary axis due to repeated stress.

Demographics
- True prevalence is not known due to misdiagnosis or undetected episodes of mania.
- Bipolar disorder affects approximately 2.3 million American adults annually.

- Lifetime prevalence is 1% for Bipolar I, and between 0.5 and 1% for Bipolar II.
- First-degree biological relatives of individuals with Bipolar I Disorder are more likely to have an earlier onset of bipolar spectrum disorders.
- Forty percent or more of patients with this disorder experience mixed episodes (MDE + manic episode).
- Men and women are equally likely to develop bipolar disorder.
- The World Health Organization identified bipolar disorder as the sixth leading cause of disability-adjusted life years worldwide among people aged 15–44 years.
- Cardiovascular disease, obesity, type 2 diabetes mellitus, and other endocrine disorders occur more often in patients with bipolar spectrum disorders.
- Patients with bipolar disorder have higher rates of comorbid neurological disorders and migraine headaches.

Risk Factors

Age
- The average age of onset is 20.
- Late adolescence and early adulthood are peak years for the onset of bipolar disorder.
- Approximately, 10–15% of adolescents with recurrent MDEs are more likely to develop Bipolar I Disorder.
- Mixed episodes appear more likely in adolescents and young adults than in older adults.
- Often, the cycling between depression and mania accelerates with age.

Gender
- Men and women are affected equally.
  - Men:
    - The first episode in males is most likely to be a manic episode.
    - Early-onset bipolar disorder tends to occur more frequently in men and it is associated with a more severe condition.
    - Men with bipolar spectrum disorders tend to have higher rates of substance abuse (drugs, alcohol).
    - The number of manic episodes equals or exceeds the number of MDEs in men.

- Women:
  - The first episode in females is most likely to be an MDE.
  - There is a higher incidence of rapid cycling, and mixed mood episodes among women.
  - Women have higher incidences of Bipolar II Disorder.
  - The number of MDEs exceeds the number of manic episodes in women.
  - Women with Bipolar I Disorder appear to have an increased risk of developing mood episodes in the immediate postpartum period.
  - Women in the premenstrual period may have worsening of ongoing major depressive, manic, mixed, or hypomanic episodes.

Family History
- Genetic factors account for 60% of the cases of bipolar disorder.
- The approximate lifetime risk in relatives of a bipolar proband is 40–70% for a monozygotic twin and 5–10% for a first-degree relative.
- Family members of patients with bipolar disorder also have a higher-than-average incidence of other psychiatric problems.
  - Schizophrenia
  - Schizoaffective disorder
  - Anxiety disorders
  - Attention-deficit hyperactivity disorder
  - Major depression
  - Obsessive-compulsive disorder

Stressful Events in Susceptible People
- There have been repeated findings that about one-third to one-half of adults diagnosed with bipolar disorder report traumatic/abusive experiences in childhood. Particularly events stemming from a harsh environment rather than from the child's own behavior. This is generally associated with earlier onset, a worse course, and more co-occurring mental disorders such as posttraumatic stress disorder (PTSD) or other anxiety-related disorders.
- Ongoing psychosocial stressors have been shown to destabilize moods in patients with bipolar spectrum disorders.

Having Another Mental Disorder

- Anxiety disorders
  - There is a greater than 50% lifetime comorbidity of anxiety disorders with bipolar illness and these patients appear to have a more difficult course of their illness.
  - Decreased likelihood of recovery.
  - Poorer role functioning and quality of life.
  - Greater likelihood of suicide attempts.
- Substance-use disorders
  - Sixty-one percent of patients diagnosed with Bipolar I Disorder and 48% of patients diagnosed with Bipolar II Disorder also have coexisting substance-use disorders.
  - The most common substance-use disorder appears to be alcohol abuse/dependence.
  - Lifetime prevalence of alcohol abuse/dependence is 49% of men and 29% of women diagnosed with bipolar spectrum disorders.
  - Attention-deficit hyperactivity disorder; a diagnosis of attention-deficit hyperactivity disorder as a child may be a marker for a bipolar spectrum diagnosis as an adult.
- Personality disorders
  - Approximately, one-third of patients with bipolar disorder also have a cluster B (borderline, narcissistic, antisocial, and histrionic) personality disorder.
  - Marked personality disorder symptoms negatively influence treatment-related outcomes in patients with bipolar disorder.

Risk Factors for Suicidal Behavior in Bipolar Spectrum Disorders

- Completed suicide occurs in 10–15% of individuals with Bipolar I Disorder.
- Personal or family history of suicidal behavior.
- Severity and number of depressive episodes or mixed mood states.
- Alcohol or substance abuse/dependence.
- Level of pessimism and hopelessness.
- Level of impulsivity and/or aggression.
- Younger age of onset of the disorder.
- A concomitant personality disorder diagnosis.
- Patients with remitting depressive symptoms are thought to be at an increased risk for suicide.

Risk Factors for Harm to Others in Bipolar Spectrum Disorders

- A history of violent behavior has consistently been shown to be the best single predictor of future violence.
- The presence of symptoms that increase the risk of violence in the absence of overt threats includes presenting as guarded and/or paranoid, psychosis, command hallucinations, cognitive disorders, and substance use. Child abuse, spouse abuse, or other violent behavior may occur during severe manic episodes or during mood episodes with psychotic features.
- Younger age.
- Gender is not a factor and the rates of violence among the genders are equal in patients who are acutely mentally ill.
- A history of victimization as a child or witnessing or experiencing violence after the age of 16.
- Level of impulsivity.
- More than a half of victims of violence by persons with mental disorders are family members.
- The availability of firearms and/or weapons.

Diagnosis

Differential Diagnosis

There is a broad differential diagnosis for bipolar spectrum disorders that includes the following:

- Thyroid or other metabolic disorders
- Epilepsy (partial complex seizures)
- Diabetes mellitus
- Sleep apnea
- Brain lesions
- MS
- Systemic infection
- Tertiary syphilis
- Systemic lupus erythematosus
- Cerebral vascular accident
- Human immunodeficiency virus
- Steroid-induced mood symptoms
- Vitamin B_{12} deficiency
- Vitamin D deficiency
- PTSD
- Attention-deficit hyperactivity disorder
- Cyclothymic disorder
- MDD
- Dysthymic disorder

- Schizoaffective disorder
- Schizophrenia
- Personality disorders
- Eating disorder
- Drug interactions or adverse effects that can cause mood symptoms (e.g., baclofen, bromide, bromocriptine, captopril, cimetidine, corticosteroids, cyclosporine, disulfiram (Antabuse), hydralazine, isoniazid, levodopa, methylphenidate (Ritalin), metrizamide, procarbazine, procyclidine (Kemadrin))
- Drug or alcohol intoxication or withdrawal

ICD-10 Code

296.80 Bipolar Disorder Not Otherwise Specified (NOS)

296.00 Bipolar I Disorder, single manic episode, unspecified degree

296.40 Bipolar I Disorder, most recent episode manic

296.60 Bipolar I Disorder, most recent episode mixed

296.50 Bipolar I Disorder, most recent episode depressed

296.89 Bipolar II Disorder (specify if most recent episode is hypomanic/depressed)

Diagnostic Work-Up

- There are no biological tests that confirm bipolar disorder. Rather, tests are carried out to rule in/out medical issues that may be mimicking a mood disorder.
  - Antinuclear antibody (ANA): ANAs are found in patients whose immune system may be predisposed to cause inflammation against their own body tissues. Antibodies that are directed against one's own tissues are referred to as autoantibodies.
  - Thyroid and other metabolic function studies suggest hyperexcitability or hypoexcitability symptoms.
  - Blood glucose level rules out diabetes.
  - Serum proteins.
  - Lithium levels are measured if patient has history of diagnosis and taking this medication.
  - Complete blood count with differential to rule out anemia or other blood dyscrasias.

- Urine toxicology screening for drug and alcohol screening (see previous data).
- Urine copper level.
- Venereal disease research lab test (RPG).
- HIV testing (Elisa and Western Blot test).
- Electrocardiogram (ECG).
- Electroencephalogram (EEG) to exclude epilepsy.
- Sleep study.
- Magnetic resonance imagery.
- Computed tomography scan of head.
- Clinical history
- Collateral information from close friends and family

Initial Assessment

- It is important to gain a complete history and carefully assess for historical and/or current episodes of mania and/or hypomania as well as depression.
- Physical examination with a focus on neurological and endocrine systems and infectious diseases.
- Specific screening questions to assess for manic episodes, mixed episodes, or hypomanic episodes:
  - Have you ever experienced periods of feeling uncharacteristically energetic?
  - Have you had periods of not sleeping but not feeling tired?
  - Have you ever felt that your thoughts were racing and that there was nothing you could do to slow them down?
  - Have you ever experienced periods where you were doing more risky activities, more interested in sex than usual, or spending more than you usually would?
- Uses of standardized screening tools:
  - Bipolar Spectrum Diagnostic Scale (BSDS)
  - Mood Disorder Questionnaire (MDQ)
  - Violence Screening Checklist (VSC): reliably indicates the level of risk during the next 24-hour period
  - The short-term assessment of risk and treatability (START): assesses risk and guides treatment for violence, suicide, self-neglect, substance use, and victimization
- Psychiatric assessment with a focus on current symptoms, date of onset, potential precipitating

factors, and perpetuating factors (e.g., drug or alcohol use), traumatic events in childhood and substance use.

■ Family history with an emphasis on psychiatric history and suicide attempts and completed suicides.

■ Social history with an emphasis on current social support and safety issues in relationships, recent psychosocial stressors, ability to maintain employment, and financial concerns.

■ Assessment of safety risk with an emphasis on history of harm to self or others, history of childhood abuse or victimization, plan and intent, and access to firearms and/or weapons.

■ Level of functional impairment and need for hospitalization (e.g., assess ability to work, engage in self-care activities, ability to conduct activities of daily living, and ability to get along with others).

Clinical Presentation: Signs and Symptoms

■ Manic episode:
  ▪ Affect/moods
    ◆ Euphorically elevated, overly happy, outgoing
    ◆ Irritable mood, agitation, jumpy, "wired"
    ◆ Inappropriately joyous
  ▪ Behaviors
    ◆ Increased goal-directed activity
    ◆ Excessive involvement in high-risk activities
    ◆ Impulsivity
    ◆ Restlessness
    ◆ Energized behavior
    ◆ Clothing may look disorganized or disheveled
    ◆ Increased psychomotor changes
    ◆ Religiosity
    ◆ Decreased need for sleep
    ◆ Behavior may become aggressive, intrusive, or combative
    ◆ No patience or tolerance for others
    ◆ Increased talkativeness or rapid, pressured speech
  ▪ Thoughts
    ◆ Inflated self-worth
    ◆ Expansive and optimistic thinking
    ◆ Flight of ideas and/or loose associations

    ◆ Racing thoughts and feeling that their minds are active
  ▪ Perceptions
    ◆ Approximately, three-fourths have delusions.
    ◆ Manic delusions reflect perceptions of power, prestige, position, self-worth, and glory.
    ◆ Some have auditory hallucinations and delusions of persecution.

■ Hypomanic episode:
  ▪ Affect/moods
    ◆ Up
    ◆ Expansive
    ◆ Irritable
  ▪ Behaviors
    ◆ Busy
    ◆ Active
    ◆ Overinvolved
    ◆ Increased energy
    ◆ Increase in planning and doing things
    ◆ Others notice their increase in activity but the patient often denies that anything about him or her has changed
  ▪ Thoughts
    ◆ Optimistic
    ◆ Future focused
    ◆ Positive attitude
  ▪ Perceptions
    ◆ Patients with hypomania typically do not experience perceptual changes.

■ Major depressive episode:
  ▪ Affect/moods
    ◆ Sadness dominates affect and is often blunted or flattened
    ◆ Feeling sad, depressed, empty, isolated
    ◆ Hopelessness
    ◆ Helplessness
    ◆ Worthlessness
    ◆ Easily overwhelmed
  ▪ Behaviors
    ◆ Poor grooming
    ◆ Increase in tearfulness
    ◆ Poor eye contact or no eye contact
    ◆ Psychomotor changes: move slowly or move very little and psychomotor retardation
    ◆ Social withdrawal, shyness, or increase in social anxiety

- Decreased interest in sexual activity and/or difficulty enjoying sexual activity
- Somatization (e.g., increase in physical or somatic complaints without objective, identified able cause)
- Difficulty with attention and concentration
- Appetite disturbances (increase or decrease)
- Sleep disturbance
- Decrease in energy and increase in fatigue regardless of amount of sleep
- Attempts at suicide
- Thoughts
  - Increased thoughts of death or morbid thoughts, and/or suicidal thoughts or specific plans for committing suicide
  - Thoughts that reflect their sadness (negative thoughts about self, world, and future)
  - Nihilistic concerns
  - Short-term memory deficits
  - Increase in worry and rumination; also referred to as brooding
  - Inappropriate guilt
- Perceptions
  - In severe episodes, psychotic symptoms may be present (e.g., auditory hallucinations).
  - Delusions, for example, that they have sinned.
- Mixed episodes:
  - Affect/Moods
    - Marked irritability
    - Agitation
    - Anxiety
    - Rage
  - Behaviors
    - Aggressiveness
    - Belligerence
    - Impulsiveness
    - Sleep disturbance
    - Rapid and pressured speech
    - Psychomotor agitation
    - Fatigue
  - Thoughts
    - Confusion
    - Morbid thoughts and/or suicidal ideation
    - Paranoia and/or persecutory delusions
    - Racing thoughts
    - Increased worry and rumination

- Perceptions
  - Patients may exhibit hallucinations and/or delusions congruent with either depression or mania or both.

DSM-IV-TR Diagnostic Guidelines
Manic Episode
- The patient's mood is disturbed and characterized as high, irritable, or expansive for at least one week.
- The patient exhibits three or more of the following:
  - Grandiose thinking
  - Diminished sleep
  - Volubility, or rapid and pressured speech
  - Racing thoughts
  - Distractibility, trouble concentrating
  - Expanded pleasurable activities that have potential for adverse outcomes (e.g., spending sprees)
  - Psychomotor agitation
  - Psychotic features (e.g., delusions of grandeur, hallucinations)
- Symptom severity results in one or both of the following:
  - Reduced social functioning (social, marital, occupational)
  - Hospitalization (owing to the presence of safety risk)
- The symptoms do not fulfill criteria for a mixed episode.
- The symptoms are not more easily ascribed to other medical diagnoses, other medical conditions, substance use, or withdrawal from prescription medications.

Major Depressive Episode
- The patient has experienced 5 or more of the following in a 2-week period:
  - Depressed mood
  - Anhedonia
  - Change in eating habits, weight loss, or weight gain
  - Psychomotor agitation or retardation
  - Fatigue
  - Feelings of guilt, feelings of worthlessness
  - Problems with concentration, short-term memory deficits

- Suicidal ideation
- Psychotic features (hallucinations)
  Note: Depressed mood or anhedonia must be one of the 5.
- Symptom severity results in one or both of the following:
  - Reduced social functioning (social, marital, occupational)
  - Hospitalization (owing to the presence of safety risk)
- The symptoms do not fulfill the criteria for a mixed episode.
- The symptoms cannot be more easily ascribed to other medical diagnoses, other medical conditions, substance use, or withdrawal from prescription medication.

Mixed Episode

- The patient manifests signs and symptoms of both poles (of mania and depression) every day or nearly every day for one week or more.
- Symptom severity yields at least one of the following:
  - Disrupted social functioning
  - Hospitalization (owing to the presence of safety risk)
  - Psychotic features
- The symptoms cannot be more easily ascribed to other medical diagnoses, other medical conditions, substance use, or withdrawal from prescription medication.

Hypomanic Episode

- Elevated, expansive, or irritable mood for at least 4 days.
- During this same period the patient has had three or more of the following:
  - Grandiose thinking, inflated self-esteem
  - Diminished sleep
  - Volubility
  - Racing thoughts
  - Problems with concentration
  - Psychomotor agitation
  - A focus on goal-directed activities
  - Poor judgment and increased engagement in activities that have potential for adverse consequences (e.g., spending sprees)
- Psychotic features are absent.

- Social functioning is not impeded.
- Hospitalization is not required.
- The symptoms are not more easily ascribed to other medical diagnoses, other medical conditions, substance use, or withdrawal from prescription medication.

Bipolar I

- Criteria for one manic episode, one major depressive episode, or one mixed episode have been met. A history of one or more manic episodes or one or more mixed episodes in the absence of major depressive episodes also fulfills criteria for Bipolar I.
- If the patient is experiencing a hypomanic episode, he or she must have had at least one prior manic episode or one prior mixed episode.
- Markedly reduced social or occupational functioning.
- For a majority of patients, depression is present more often than mania.
- The symptoms cannot be ascribed to other medical diagnoses, other medical conditions, substance use, or withdrawal from prescription medication.

Bipolar II

- The patient has had one or more major depressive episodes.
- The patient has had one or more hypomanic episodes.
- A history of manic episodes or mixed episodes is absent.
- The symptoms cause significant distress for the patient or significantly reduced functioning.
- The symptoms cannot be more easily ascribed to other medical diagnoses (including other psychiatric diagnoses), other medical conditions, substance abuse, or withdrawal from prescription medication.

Rapid Cycling

- The patient has experienced 4 or more of: major depressive episodes, manic episodes, or hypomanic episodes (any combination) within a 12-month period.
- Episodes are generally separated by periods of at least 2 months of full or partial remission, or

there is a switch to an episode of the opposite polarity.

Treatment

Acute Treatment

- The primary goal of the acute phase is to manage acute mania, hypomania, mixed or depressive episodes, and associated safety risk issues.
- Diagnostic tests should be performed to rule out potential medical etiologies for mood symptoms, especially if this is the first episode of mania, hypomania, mixed mood symptoms, or depression.
- How to handle suicidal ideation:
  - Patient with suicidal ideation with plan and intent should be hospitalized (voluntarily or involuntarily) due to acute safety risk.
  - Patient with suicidal ideation with plan but no intent may be treated on an outpatient basis with close follow-up if they do not have access to the means to carry out their plan and adequate social support.
  - Patient with suicidal ideation without plan and no intent requires careful assessment of current psychosocial stressors, access to weapons and other lethal means, substance use, and impulse control issues. Any lethal means should be removed.
- How to handle aggression and potential harm to others:
  - If patients have access to firearms and or weapons, they should be removed.
  - Those with thoughts of harming others with plan and intent should be hospitalized (voluntarily or involuntarily).
  - Antipsychotics are often used for the management in emergent situations, which the patient presents as possibly psychotic, agitated, and making overt threats.
  - Those with thoughts of harming others with plan but no intent can be treated on an outpatient basis, with increased intensity of treatment with an established provider, depending on risk factors.
  - Those with thoughts of harming others without plan or intent do require increased intensity of treatment and perhaps increased dosages of medications.
- Acute manic episode or mixed mood episode:
  - Hospitalization is necessary in patients that present with significant suicide risk, increased aggressiveness and significant risk of violence of others, the potential for serious alcohol withdrawal symptoms, or when the differential includes other medical disorders that warrant admission.
  - Antidepressants, if the patient has been prescribed, should be discontinued if the patient is presenting with an acute manic episode or mixed mood episode.
  - Patient should be advised to decrease alcohol, caffeine, and nicotine use.
  - Most patients are started on long-term mood stabilizers and also are given antipsychotic medications if agitated and/or experiencing psychotic symptoms.
  - Medications in the acute phase are commonly used to induce remission in acute mania or hypomania.
- Acute hypomanic episode:
  - Treatment for hypomania, which can lead to either a manic or depressive episode, may decrease symptom progression.
- Acute MDE:
  - Hospitalization is necessary if patient presents with a significant suicide risk, if there is potential for serious withdrawal symptoms, or when the differential includes other medical disorders that warrant admission.
  - Antidepressant medications have not been shown to be an effective adjunctive therapy, and as a monotherapy, they can precipitate mania in individuals with Bipolar I Disorder.
  - Antidepressants are used for those with Bipolar II Disorder.
  - Be alert to sudden decreases of depressed mood, or to worsening mood as initial response to antidepressant therapy as these could be signs of increased risk for suicide.
- Medication noncompliance is common because mania and hypomania may be a desired state for many individuals with bipolar disorder, and many are reluctant to take medications.

- Because bipolar disorder is a lifelong and recurrent illness, long-term treatment is needed to manage and control mood symptoms.
- Cardiovascular mortality is almost twice as high in patients with bipolar disorder. The risk of sudden death may also theoretically be increased due to reduced heart-rate variability.

Chronic Treatment

- The continuation phase of treatment lasts weeks to months and the primary goal is to reach full remission of symptoms and restoration of functioning.
- The primary goal of the maintenance phase of treatment is to achieve full and sustained symptom remission for at least 1 year after resolution of symptoms.
- Long-term life maintenance is recommended for patients who have suffered three or more manic episodes.
- Study results from a large-scale National Institute of Mental Health–funded clinical trial found patients treated with both medications and intensive psychotherapy (30 sessions over 9 months of therapy) demonstrated the following:
  - Fewer relapses
  - Lower hospitalization rates
  - Better ability to stick to treatment plans
  - More likely to get well faster and stay well longer
- Medications:
  - Long-term management of bipolar disorder should be treated with a mood stabilizer.
  - For patients who fail to respond to one mood stabilizer, they may need to be switched to another mood stabilizer, or the addition of another mood stabilizer or an atypical antipsychotic may be required.
  - Risk of suicide is reduced 13-fold with long-term maintenance therapy with lithium.
  - There is limited research on all of the atypical antipsychotics in the maintenance phase of treatment; however, any of the atypical antipsychotics may be considered when other treatments are unsuccessful.
  - Antidepressant medications have not been shown to be an effective adjunctive therapy, and as a monotherapy, they can precipitate mania.
- Electroconvulsive therapy (ECT) is used only as a last resort if the patient does not adequately respond to medications and/or psychotherapy.
  - Psychotherapy
  - CBT: helps individuals with bipolar disorder learn to change harmful and negative thought patterns and behaviors, as well as learn coping skills such as stress management, identifying triggers for mood symptoms, and relaxation techniques.
  - Family therapy: this therapy includes family members. By doing so, it helps family members enhance coping strategies, such as recognizing new episodes and how to help their loved one. Therapy also focuses on communication skills and problem solving.
  - Interpersonal therapy: helps people with bipolar disorder improve their relationships with others.
  - Social rhythm therapy: therapy focuses on maintaining and managing their daily routines such as regular sleep/wake cycles, eating patterns, and social routines.
  - Psychoeducation: focuses on teaching individuals with bipolar disorder about the illness and its treatment. This form of treatment helps people realize signs of relapse so that they can access treatment early before a full episode occurs. This is usually in a group format and it may also be helpful for family members and caregivers.
- Follow-up care by a chemical dependence treatment specialist is recommended when indicated.
- Patients with cardiac comorbidity, abnormal findings on cardiac examination, or significant risk factors for heart disease should be referred to a cardiologist.
- Patients with endocrine dysfunction, such as hyperthyroidism or hypothyroidism, should be referred to an endocrinologist.
- Treatment can be complicated or have a poorer course by having another condition at the same time, such as substance abuse, depression, anxiety disorders, or a personality disorder.

- Concomitant substance abuse/dependence is correlated with increased hospitalizations and a worse course of the illness and increases safety risk.

Recurrence Rate
- Bipolar I Disorder
  - The course of Bipolar I Disorder is marked by relapses and remissions, often alternating manic with depressive episodes.
  - Ninety percent of individuals who have a single manic episode go on to have future manic or hypomanic episodes within another 5 years.
  - Approximately, 60–70% of manic episodes occur immediately before or after an MDE.
  - The majority of individuals with Bipolar I Disorder experience symptom reduction among episodes; however, between 20 and 30% continue to have mood lability and other symptoms.
  - Sixty percent of sufferers experience chronic interpersonal and occupational difficulties among acute episodes.
  - Patients with Bipolar I fare worse than patients with a major depression. Within the first 2 years after the initial episode, 40–50% of patients experience another manic episode.
  - Psychotic symptoms can develop after days or weeks after a previous nonpsychotic manic or mixed episode.
  - Individuals who have manic episodes with psychotic features are more likely to have subsequent manic episodes with psychotic features.
  - Ninety percent of individuals with Bipolar I Disorder have at least one psychiatric hospitalization and two-thirds have two or more hospitalizations in their lifetime.
- Bipolar II Disorder
  - This disorder is studied less and the course is less well understood.
- Patient behaviors that can lead to a recurrence of depressive or manic symptoms:
  - Discontinuing or lowering one's dose of medication.
  - An inconsistent sleep schedule can destabilize the illness. Too much sleep can lead to depression, while too little sleep can lead to mixed states or mania.
  - Inadequate stress management and poor lifestyle choices. Medication raises the stress threshold somewhat, but too much stress still causes relapse.
  - Using drugs or alcohol can either trigger or prolong mood symptoms.

Patient Education
- Advise patients that it is important to deal with mania early in the episode, and thus recognizing the early warning signs is the key so that more intensive treatment can be administered before symptoms escalate.
- Advise patient to stay on all medications and to not decrease or stop any medications without medical supervision. This is especially important when experiencing mania or hypomania.
- Also advise patients that sometimes several medications trials are needed to find ones that will be efficacious in controlling mood symptoms.
- Advise patients that symptoms will improve gradually, not immediately as they begin to remit.
- In general, there is little research about herbal or natural supplements for bipolar spectrum disorders and not much is known about their efficacy, however, St. John's Wort may cause a switch to mania, and can make other medications less effective (e.g., antidepressants and anticonvulsants). Additionally, the effects of Sam-E or omega-3 fatty acids are not known. All herbal and natural remedies for mood symptoms should be discussed with a medical provider.
- The best approach to treatment is a combination of psychotherapy and medications. This helps prevent relapses, reduces hospitalizations, and helps the patient get well faster and stay well longer.
- If patients plan extensive travel into other time zones, advise them to call their doctor before leaving to determine if any changes in their medicines should be made and what to do if they have a manic or depressive episode while away.
- Women who are pregnant or would like to become pregnant and have been diagnosed with a bipolar spectrum disorder should speak with their doctor about the risks and benefits of all

treatments during pregnancy. Mood stabilizing medications used today can cause harm to the developing fetus or a nursing infant. Additionally, stopping or reducing medications during pregnancy can cause a recurrence of mood symptoms.

- Helping the individual identify and modify stressors provides a critical aspect of patient and family awareness.

- Changes in sleep patterns can sometimes trigger a manic or depressive episode. Advise patients to keep a regular routine such as eating meals at the same time every day, and going to sleep at the same time nightly and waking up at the same time daily.

- Patients should be encouraged to keep a chart of daily mood symptoms, treatments, sleep patterns, and life events to both help themselves and their providers treat the illness most effectively. This is often referred to as a "life chart."

- Advise patients with bipolar spectrum disorders to avoid nicotine, sympathomimetic or anticholinergic drugs, caffeine, alcohol, illicit drugs.

- For excellent patient education resources, visit eMedicine's Mental Health and Behavior Center and Bipolar Center. See also eMedicine's patient education articles on bipolar disorder.

Medical/Legal Pitfalls

- Failure to assess, monitor, and treat safety risk issues.
- Failure to assess for history of manic or hypomanic episodes when patient presents with a depressive symptoms.
- Failure to assess for coexisting substance-use disorders.
- Failure to discontinue antidepressants if individual presents with acute mania or mixed mood symptoms.
- Failure to monitor for toxicity or metabolic changes associated with prescribed lithium and atypical antipsychotics.
- Prescribing and not properly monitoring valproic acid (Depakote) for girls and women of childbearing age. This medication may increase the levels of testosterone, which can lead to polycystic ovary syndrome (PCOS). Most PCOS symptoms begin after stopping treatment with valproic acid (Depakene).
- Prescribing an antidepressant during an MDE and not also prescribing a mood-stabilizing agent in patients with known bipolar spectrum disorders. Only taking an antidepressant increases the risk of switching their mood to either mania or hypomania, or developing rapid cycling symptoms.

Cyclothymic Disorder

Background Information

Definition of Disorder

- Cyclothymia is considered a mild, subthreshold form of bipolar disorder and is often referred to as a "soft" bipolar spectrum disorder.
- The main difference between cyclothymic disorder and Bipolar I Disorder is the severity of the mania in that the symptoms do not meet the criteria for a manic episode.
- The main difference between cyclothymic disorder and Bipolar II Disorder is the severity of the depressive symptoms in that the depressive symptoms do not meet the full criteria for an MDE.
- Mood changes in cyclothymic disorder can be abrupt and unpredictable, short and with infrequent euthymic episodes.
- Both phases of the disorder appear deleterious to their psychosocial functioning; however, they can also have high levels of achievement and creativity, which can be socially advantageous due to hypomania.
- Hypomania or subthreshold depressive symptoms can last for weeks or days. In between up and down moods, a person may have normal moods or they may continue to cycle continuously from hypomanic to depressed with no normal periods in between.
- The mood swings in this disorder appear to be biphasic.
- Cyclothymia symptoms are typically chronic, often do not appear to be related to life events, and appear to an observer as a personality trait.
- Although the mood symptoms are milder than those of Bipolar I and Bipolar II disorders, they can be disabling due to unstable moods and the unpredictability of the mood pattern can cause significant distress.
- Some patients with cyclothymic disorder were characterized as being interpersonally sensitive, hyperactive, or moody as young children.
- Onset of cyclothymic disorder after the age of 65 is rare and alerts the practitioner to rule out organic reasons for the mood fluctuations.
- It is not uncommon for cyclothymic disorder to go undetected.
- Patients rarely seek treatment during the periods of hypomania because it is often considered a desired state.

Etiology

- The exact cause of cyclothymic disorder is not known.
- The "kindling theory" is the current predominant theory, meaning that the disorder is likely to be caused by multiple factors that potentially interact and lower the threshold at which mood changes occur. Eventually, a mood episode can start itself and thus become recurrent.
- Environmental factors:
  - Irregular sleep/wake patterns have been shown to trigger mood symptoms.
- Biological perspectives:
  - Genetics
    - Cyclothymic disorder appears more common in first-degree biological relatives of individuals with bipolar disorder.
    - An individual appears 2–3 times more likely to have cyclothymic disorder if first-degree biological relatives also have the disorder.
- Neural processes:
  - There does not appear to be research investigating the underlying molecular or neurotomical etiology for cyclothymic disorder.
  - The disorder appears to have a circadian component. Some patients state, for example, that they can go to bed in a good mood and wake up with subthreshold depressive symptoms.
  - Declines in REM period latency during the sleep cycle have been noted in patients with cyclothymia.

- Reduced skin conductance has been found in patients with cyclothymic disorder.
- Endocrine models:
  - Endocrine studies in cyclothymia are very limited.
  - Hypothyroidism can cause depression and/or mood instability.
  - Cortisol hypersecretion and poor regulation of cortisol have been noted in patients with cyclothymia when faced with an experimental stressor.

Demographics

- True prevalence is not known due to misdiagnosis or undetected episodes of hypomania.
- At this time, it does not appear that epidemiological studies have been specifically conducted for cyclothymic disorder; however, lifetime prevalence of cyclothymic disorder is estimated to range from 0.3 to 6%, depending on the criteria used.
- Women and men are affected equally, but women typically present for treatment more often then men.
- Medically, research has shown the following related to dysthymia, the subthreshold depression associated with this disorder:
  - Due to the subthreshold depression, patients with this disorder are approximately 2.6 times more likely to suffer a cerebral vascular accident and are at greater risk for cardiovascular disorders.
    - The presence of depressive symptoms in the absence of MDEs is associated with greater risk for cardiac events.
    - The aspect of depression, hopelessness, has been linked to sudden death.
    - The presence of vital exhaustion (fatigue, irritability, and demoralized feelings) has been reported to predict progression of coronary artery disease and/or cardiac events.
    - Cardiovascular mortality is almost elevated for individuals who have dysthymia. The risk of sudden death may also theoretically be increased due to reduced heart-rate variability.

- Overall, 28% of patients who have mild depressive symptoms suffer from incapacitating medical conditions.
  - Forty-five percent of patients have chronic insomnia.
  - Four to eighteen percent have comorbid diabetes mellitus.
  - Fourteen to twenty percent have human immunodeficiency virus infection.
  - Three to thirty-one percent have significant premenstrual syndrome.
  - Fourteen percent have Parkinson's disease.
  - Twenty-eight percent experience chronic pain.
- Individuals with dysthymia use medical treatment to a higher degree than the general population.

Risk Factors

Age

- Cyclothymic disorder usually begins in adolescence or in early adulthood.
- True age of onset is typically difficult to ascertain due to the insidious nature of the mood symptoms and its chronic course.
- Incidence rates are rare before puberty, and hypomanic episodes are not known in children.
- Cyclothymia and dysthymia appear common in adolescents where the depressive onsets outnumber the nondepressive onsets.
- Often, the cycling between moods accelerates with age.

Gender

- Some studies indicate that men and women are affected equally and others state that women are affected more than men.
- Women in the premenstrual period may have worsening of ongoing hypomanic episodes or depressive symptoms.

Family History

- Individuals who have first-degree relatives diagnosed with bipolar disorder are at greater risk of cyclothymic disorder.

Stressful Events in Susceptible People

- Often patients with cyclothymic disorder cannot identify an environmental precipitant to their moods.

- Ongoing psychosocial stressors have been shown to destabilize moods.
- Major life changes have also been shown to destabilize moods.

Having Another Mental Disorder
- Substance-use disorders
  - Individuals with cyclothymia are at heightened risk for substance-abuse issues due to high frequency of their mood symptoms.
  - Substance abuse is common in cyclothymic disorder and it is hypothesized that the individual is attempting to self-medicate the dysthymic mood symptoms and/or sleep disturbance or to precipitate and sustain hypomania.
- Bipolar I or Bipolar II disorder
  - This disorder has a 15–50% risk that the individual will eventually develop Bipolar I or Bipolar II disorder.
- A diagnosis of attention deficit hyperactivity disorder
  - The diagnosis for a child may be a marker for a bipolar spectrum diagnosis as an adult.
- Personality disorders
  - Differentiating between individuals with cyclothymic disorder and particularly cluster B personality disorders (borderline personality disorder, histrionic personality disorder, and antisocial personality disorder) is difficult because the affective instability is similar.
  - Mood symptoms from cyclothymic disorder can be so flagrant that a personality disorder may be erroneously diagnosed.
  - Marked personality disorder symptoms negatively influence treatment-related outcomes in patients with bipolar disorder.

Risk Factors for Suicidal Behavior in Bipolar Spectrum Disorders
- Patients with cyclothymic disorder are at higher risk for suicide due to frequently changing mood episodes.
- Personal or family history of suicidal behavior.
- Severity and number of depressive episodes.
- Alcohol or substance abuse/dependence.
- Level of pessimism and hopelessness.
- Level of impulsivity and/or aggression.

- Younger age of onset of the disorder.
- A concomitant personality disorder diagnosis.
- Patients with remitting depressive symptoms are thought to be at an increased risk for suicide.

Risk Factors for Harm to Others in Bipolar Spectrum Disorders
- A history of violent behavior has consistently been shown to be the best single predictor of future violence.
- The presence of symptoms that increase the risk of violence in the absence of overt threats includes presenting as guarded and suspicious.
- Younger age.
- Gender is not a factor and the rates of violence among genders are equal in patients who are acutely mentally ill.
- A history of victimization as a child or witnessing or experiencing violence after the age of 16.
- Level of impulsivity.
- More than a half of victims of violence by persons with mental disorders are family members.
- The availability of firearms and/or weapons.

Diagnosis

Differential Diagnosis
There is a broad differential diagnosis for bipolar spectrum disorders that includes the following:
- Thyroid or other metabolic disorders
- Epilepsy (partial complex seizures)
- MS
- Diabetes mellitus
- Sleep apnea
- Brain lesions
- Systemic infection
- Systemic lupus erythematosus
- Cerebral vascular accident
- Human immunodeficiency virus
- Steroid-induced mood symptoms
- Vitamin B_{12} deficiency
- Vitamin D deficiency
- PTSD
- Attention-deficit hyperactivity disorder
- Bipolar I or II disorder with rapid cycling
- MDD
- Dysthymic disorder
- Borderline personality disorder

- Eating disorder
- Drug interactions or adverse effects that can cause mood symptoms (e.g., baclofen, bromide, bromocriptine, captopril, cimetidine, corticosteroids, cyclosporine, disulfiram [Antabuse], hydralazine, isoniazid, levodopa, methylphenidate [Ritalin], metrizamide, procarbazine, procyclidine [Kemadrin]).
- Drug or alcohol intoxication or withdrawal

ICD Code

301.13 Cyclothymic Disorder

Diagnostic Work-Up

- There are no biological tests that confirm cyclothymic disorder. Rather, tests are carried out to rule in/out medical issues that may be mimicking a mood disorder.
  - Antinuclear antibody: ANAs are found in patients whose immune system may be predisposed to cause inflammation against their own body tissues. Antibodies that are directed against one's own tissues are referred to as autoantibodies.
  - Thyroid and other metabolic function studies suggest hyperexcitability or hypoexcitability symptoms
  - Blood glucose level rules out diabetes
  - Serum proteins
  - Lithium levels should be measured if patient has history of diagnosis and taking this medication
  - Complete blood count with differential is used to rule out anemia or other blood dyscrasias
  - Urine toxicology screening for drug and alcohol screening (see previous data)
  - Urine copper level, high levels indicate toxic exposure
  - Venereal disease research lab test (RPG)
  - HIV testing (Elisa and Western Blot test)
  - Electrocardiogram determines cardiac anomolities
  - Electroencephalogram may exclude epilepsy
  - Sleep study: sleep apnea
  - Magnetic resonance imagery determines presence of aneurysms, past head trauma, brain tumors

- Computed tomography scan of head is used to rule out head injury
- Clinical history
- Diagnosis is difficult to establish without a prolonged period of observation or obtaining an account from others about their moods and functioning across their lifespan. Thus, collateral information from close friends and family is important.

Initial Assessment

- It is important to gain a complete history and carefully assess for historical and/or current episodes of mania and/or hypomania as well as major depression and episodes of subclinical depression.
- Physical examination with a focus on neurological and endocrine systems and infectious diseases.
- Differentiation of cyclothymic disorder from personality disorders:
  - Periods of elevation and depression that typify affective disorders tend to be endogenous in cyclothymic disorder. This means that the mood symptoms come out of the blue with little external provocation.
  - Diurnal variations with worsening symptoms in the morning are typical in cyclothymic disorder.
  - The disturbances in cyclothymia are biphasic (see Signs and Symptoms for Biphasic Symptoms of Cyclothymia).
- Specific screening questions to assess for and rule out manic episodes, mixed episodes, or hypomanic episodes:
  - Have you ever experienced periods of feeling uncharacteristically energetic?
  - Have you had periods of not sleeping but not feeling tired?
  - Have you ever felt that your thoughts were racing and that there was nothing you could do to slow them down?
  - Have you ever experienced periods where you were doing more risky activities, more interested in sex than usual, or spending more than you usually would?

- Uses of standardized screening tools:
  - BSDS
  - MDQ
  - VSC: reliably indicates the level of risk during the next 24-hour period
  - The START: assesses risk and guides treatment for violence, suicide, self-neglect, substance use, and victimization
- Psychiatric assessment with a focus on current symptoms, date of onset, potential precipitating factors, and perpetuating factors (e.g., drug or alcohol use), traumatic events in childhood, and substance use.
- Family history with an emphasis on psychiatric history and suicide attempts and completed suicides
- Social history with an emphasis on current social support and safety issues in relationships, recent psychosocial stressors, ability to maintain employment, and financial concerns.
- Assessment of safety risk with an emphasis on history of harm to self or others, history of childhood abuse or victimization, plan and intent, and access to firearms and/or weapons.
- Level of functional impairment and need for hospitalization (e.g., ability to work, engage in self-care activities, ability to conduct activities of daily living, and ability to get along with others).

Clinical Presentation: Signs and Symptoms
Hypomanic Episode
- Affect/moods:
  - Up
  - Expansive
  - Irritable
  - Moody
- Behaviors:
  - Busy
  - Active
  - Overinvolved
  - Increased energy
  - Increase in planning and doing things
  - Social warmth
  - Increased creativity and productivity
  - Can be hypersexual

- Others notice their increase in activity but the patient often denies anything about them has changed.
- Thoughts:
  - Optimistic
  - Future-focused
  - Positive attitude
- Perceptions
  - Patients with hypomania typically do not experience perceptual changes.

Dysthymia
- Vegetative symptoms usually seen in MDEs are not as common.
- Affect/moods:
  - Continuously feeling sad
  - Gloomy
  - Irritable
  - Excessive anger
- Behavior:
  - Poor appetite
  - Sleep disturbance
  - Apathy
  - Lack of motivation
  - Introversion
  - Social withdrawal
  - Quiet and less talkative
  - Generalized loss of interest or pleasure and incapable of fun
  - Passive
  - Somatization (e.g., increase in physical or somatic complaints without objective, identified able cause).
  - Conscientious and self-disciplining
- Thoughts:
  - Self-critical, self-reproaching, self-derogatory
  - Pessimistic
  - Poor concentration and indecisiveness
  - Worry and rumination (brooding)
  - Preoccupied with their inadequacy, failures, or negative life events
  - Hopelessness
  - Helplessness
- Perceptions:
  - Patients with dysthymia typically do not experience perceptual changes

Biphasic Characteristics of Cyclothymic Disorder
- Lethargy alternates with good moods
- Unexplained tearfulness alternates with excessive wit and humor.
- Introversion and self-absorption alternate with uninhibited seeking of people.
- Mental confusion alternates with sharpened thinking.
- Shaky self-esteem alternates between low self-confidence and overconfidence.

DSM-IV-TR Diagnostic Guidelines

Cyclothymic Disorder
- For at least 2 years the patient has had multiple periods in which hypomanic symptoms have been present, and multiple periods of low mood that have not fulfilled the criteria for a major depressive episode.
- The longest period in which the patient has been free of mood swings is 2 months.
- During the first 2 years of the disorder the patient had not had periods of mood disturbance in which the criteria for a manic episode, a mixed episode, or a major depressive episode were also met.
- The symptoms are not more easily ascribed to other medical diagnoses, other medical conditions, substance use, or drug withdrawal.
- The disturbances in mood engender significant distress for the individual and/or a reduction in social or other important areas of functioning.

Hypomanic Episode
- For at least 4 days the patient manifests a mood that is elevated, expansive, or irritable, and representing a distinct departure from the patient's nondepressed baseline mood.
- During this period the patient has three or more of the following:
  - Grandiose thoughts, inflated self-esteem
  - Diminished sleep
  - Volubility
  - Racing thoughts
  - Increased levels of distractibility
  - Psychomotor agitation
  - A focus on goal-directed activities

- Poor judgment; activities that have potential for adverse outcomes (e.g., spending sprees)
- Psychotic features are absent.
- Appropriate social and occupational functioning is maintained.
- Hospitalization is not required.
- The symptoms are not more easily ascribed to other medical diagnoses, other medical conditions, substance use, or withdrawal from prescription medication.

Treatment

Acute Treatment
- The primary goal of the acute phase is to manage acute hypomania episodes and subclinical depression and associated safety risk issues.
- Specific treatment studies for cyclothymic disorder separate from other bipolar spectrum disorders are minimal.
- Diagnostic tests should be performed to rule out potential medical etiologies for mood symptoms, especially if this is the first episode of mania, hypomania, mixed mood symptoms, or depression.
- How to handle suicidal ideation:
  - With suicidal ideation with plan and intent patient should be hospitalized (voluntarily or involuntarily) due to acute safety risk.
  - With suicidal ideation with plan but no intent patients may be treated on an outpatient basis with close follow-up if they do not have access to the means to carry out their plan and adequate social support.
  - With suicidal ideation without plan and no intent, patient requires careful assessment of current psychosocial stressors, access to weapons, and other lethal means, substance use, and impulse control issues. Any lethal means should be removed.
- How to handle aggression and potential harm to others:
  - If patients have access to firearms and or weapons, they should be removed.
  - Those with thoughts of harming others with plan and intent should be hospitalized (voluntarily or involuntarily).

- Those with thoughts of harming others with plan but no intent can be treated on an outpatient basis, with increased intensity of treatment with an established provider, depending on risk factors.
- Those with thoughts of harming others without plan or intent do require increased intensity of treatment and perhaps increased dosages of medications.
- Acute hypomanic episode
  - Treatment for hypomania, which can lead to either a manic or depressive episode, may decrease symptom progression.
- Medication noncompliance is common because hypomania may be a desired state for many individuals with cyclothymic disorder, and many are reluctant to take medications.
- Because this disorder is considered a chronic and lifelong illness, long-term treatment is needed to manage and control mood symptoms.

Chronic Treatment

- The primary goal of long-term treatment is to prevent cyclothymia from worsening and progressing to full-blown manic episodes.
- Specific treatment studies for cyclothymia as distinct from other bipolar spectrum disorders are minimal.
- Study results from a large-scale National Institute of Mental Health–funded clinical trial found patients treated with both medications and intensive psychotherapy (30 sessions over 9 months of therapy) for bipolar spectrum disorders demonstrated
  - Fewer relapses
  - Lower hospitalization rates
  - Better ability to stick to treatment plans.
  - More likely to get well faster and stay well longer.
- Medications:
  - Long-term management of cyclothymic disorder should be treated with a mood stabilizer.
  - Antidepressant medications have not been shown to be an effective adjunctive therapy,

and as a monotherapy they can precipitate mania, mixed mood symptoms, or hypomania.
- ECT is used only as a last resort if the patient does not adequately respond to medications and/or psychotherapy.
- Psychotherapy:
  - CBT: helps individuals with bipolar disorder learn to change harmful and negative thought patterns and behaviors, as well as learn coping skills such as stress management, identifying triggers for mood symptoms, and relaxation techniques.
  - Family therapy: this therapy includes family members. By doing so, it helps family members enhance coping strategies, such as recognizing new episodes and how to help their loved one. Therapy also focuses on communication skills and problem solving.
  - Interpersonal therapy: helps people with bipolar disorder improve their relationships with others.
  - Social rhythm therapy: this therapy focuses on maintaining and managing their daily routines such as regular sleep/wake cycles, eating patterns, and social routines.
  - Psychoeducation: focuses on teaching individuals with bipolar disorder about the illness and its treatment. This form of treatment helps people realize signs of relapse so that they can access treatment early before a full episode occurs. This is usually in a group format and it may also be helpful for family members and caregivers.
  - Psychodynamic and psychoanalytic therapies do not appear to have an effect in patients with this disorder.
- Follow-up care by a chemical dependence treatment specialist is recommended when indicated.
- Patients with cardiac comorbidity, abnormal findings on cardiac examination, or significant risk factors for heart disease should be referred to a cardiologist.
- Patients with endocrine dysfunction, such as hyperthyroidism or hypothyroidism, should be referred to an endocrinologist.

- Treatment can be complicated or have a poorer course by having another condition at the same time, such as substance abuse, depression, anxiety disorders, or a personality disorder.
- Concomitant substance abuse/dependence is correlated with increased hospitalizations and a worse course of the illness and increases safety risk.

Recurrence Rate

- Approximately, one-third of all patients diagnosed with cyclothymic disorder will develop a major mood disorder during their lifetime, and it is usually Bipolar II Disorder.
- Retrospective studies of patients with cyclothymia, taking lithium over a 2-year period, indicated the following:
  - Only 26–36% were free of depression symptoms as compared to 42–55% for patients with Bipolar II and 31–42% of patients with a unipolar designation.
  - The probability rate for hospitalization due to severity of depression symptoms was 69% for patients with cyclothymia versus 51% for patients with Bipolar II and 64% for patients with a unipolar designation.
- Prospective studies indicate that patients with cyclothymia, who started on valproate (Depakote) at 150 mg and 250 mg with standard up titration, required lower doses and blood levels to achieve mood stabilization as compared with patients with Bipolar II.
- Patient behaviors that can lead to a recurrence of depressive or manic symptoms:
  - Discontinuing or lowering one's dose of medication.
  - An inconsistent sleep schedule can destabilize the illness. Too much sleep can lead to depression, while too little sleep can trigger and sustain hypomania.
  - Inadequate stress management and poor life-style choices.
  - Medication raises the stress threshold somewhat, but too much stress still causes relapse.

- Using drugs or alcohol can either trigger or prolong mood symptoms.

Patient Education

- Advise patients that it is important to deal with mania early in the episode, and thus recognizing the early warning signs is the key so that more intensive treatment can be administered before symptoms escalate.
- Advise patient to stay on all medications and to not decrease or stop any medications without medical supervision. This is especially important when experiencing mania or hypomania.
- Also advise patients that sometimes several medication trials are needed to find ones that will be efficacious in controlling mood symptoms.
- Advise patients that symptoms will improve gradually, not immediately as they begin to remit.
- In general, there is little research about herbal or natural supplements for bipolar spectrum disorders and not much is known about their efficacy; however, St. John's Wort may cause a switch to mania, and can make other medications less effective (e.g., antidepressants and anticonvulsants). Additionally, the effects of Sam-E or omega-3 fatty acids are not known. All herbal and natural remedies for mood symptoms should be discussed with a medical care provider.
- The best approach to treatment is a combination of psychotherapy and medications. This helps prevent relapses, reduces hospitalizations, and helps the patient get well faster and stay well longer.
- If patients plan extensive travel into other time zones, advise them to call their doctor before leaving to determine if any changes in their medicines should be made and what to do if they have mood episode while away
- Women who are pregnant or would like to become pregnant and have been diagnosed with a cyclothymic disorder should speak with their doctor about the risks and benefits of all treatments during pregnancy. Mood-stabilizing medications used today can cause harm to the developing fetus or a nursing infant. Additionally, stopping or reducing medications during

pregnancy can cause a recurrence of mood symptoms.

■ Helping the individual identify and modify stressors provides a critical aspect of patient and family awareness.

■ Changes in sleep patterns can sometimes trigger a manic or depressive episode. Advise patients to keep a regular routine such as eating meals at the same time every day, and going to sleep at the same time nightly and waking up at the same time daily.

■ Patients should be encouraged to keep a chart of daily mood symptoms, treatments, sleep patterns, and life events to help both themselves and their providers treat the illness most effectively. This is often referred to as a "life chart."

■ Advise patients with cyclothymia to avoid nicotine, sympathomimetic or anticholinergic drugs, caffeine, alcohol, illicit drugs.

■ For excellent patient education resources, visit eMedicine's Mental Health and Behavior Center and Bipolar Center. See also eMedicine's patient education articles on bipolar disorder.

Medical/Legal Pitfalls

■ Failure to assess, monitor, and treat safety risk issues

■ Failure to assess for history of manic or hypomanic episodes when patient presents with depressive symptoms.

■ Failure to assess for coexisting substance-use disorders.

■ Failure to monitor for toxicity or metabolic changes associated with prescribed lithium.

■ Prescribing and not properly monitoring valproic acid (Depakote) for women under the age of 20. This medication may increase the levels of testosterone, which can lead to PCOS. Most PCOS symptoms begin after stopping treatment with valproic acid (Depakene).

■ Prescribing an antidepressant for depressive symptoms and not also prescribing a mood-stabilizing agent in patients with known bipolar spectrum disorders. Only taking an antidepressant increased the risk of switching their mood to either mania or hypomania, or developing rapid cycling symptoms.

Dysthymic Disorder

Background Information

Definition of Disorder

- This is a chronic mood disorder characterized by depressed mood more days than not, but not meeting the criteria for MDD.
- It is associated with increased morbidity from physical disease
- Patients often possess negative, gloomy outlook on life with ruminative coping strategies
- Tendency toward self-criticism and a sense of inadequacy
- Tend to spend limited time in leisure activities
  Also called dysthymia, dysthymic disorder is characterized by long-term (2 years or longer) but less severe symptoms that may not disable a person but which prevent normal functioning or feeling well. People with dysthymia may also experience one or more episodes of major depression during their lifetimes.

Etiology

- It is thought to be a result of an interplay between genetic factors, chronic stress, and personality factors.
- Biological factors such as alterations in neurotransmitters, endocrine, and inflammatory mediators are also thought to play a role.
- Cognitive and personality factors, such as how people view their influence, their ability to change, and their interpretation of stressors, play a role.
- Cases are very likely to have family history of mood disorders, particularly dysthymia and MDD.

Demographics

- Data suggest that the disorder affects 3–6% of the U.S. general population and 5–15% of the primary care population. It affects approximately 36% of patients in outpatient mental health treatment centers.
- Women are twice as likely to present with dysthymic disorder than men.

- It often starts at childhood or adolescence with an early sense of unhappiness without clear cause
- One large study showed it to be more common in African Americans and Mexican Americans than in whites (the opposite pattern from MDD).
- One study showed a 77% of lifetime risk of developing MDD and a higher risk of suicide attempts among patients with dysthymic disorder than patients with MDD.
- The prevalence rate of dysthymic disorder is 0.6–1.7% in children and 1.6–8% in adolescents.
- Patients with dysthymic disorder should not be seen as simply having a "mild form of depression." They are at high risk for developing MDD and often have MDD, which is harder to treat.
- Patients with dysthymic disorder should be evaluated for suicide risk.

Risk Factors

Gender

- Like other depressive disorders, dysthymic disorder is approximately two times more common in women than men.

Family History

- Studies have shown an increased incidence of dysthymic disorder when there is a history of depression, bipolar disorder, or dysthymia in first-degree relatives.
- There are learned or genetic personality factors such as poor coping skills, particularly ruminative, rather than problem solving or cognitive restructuring, strategies.

Past Medical History

- Chronic medical illness
- History of MDD

Social History

- Lack of social support
- Multiple relationship losses

Having Another Mental Disorder

- Diagnosis with a personality disorder (antisocial, borderline, dependent, depressive, histrionic, or schizotypal), in particular, places a patient at higher risk for dysthymia.
- DD places patients at much higher risk for the development of treatment-resistant MDD.
- Alcohol abuse or substance abuse places a patient at higher risk of dysthymic disorder. Approximately, 15% of patients with DD have comorbid substance dependence.

Diagnosis

Differential Diagnosis

- Common:
  - MDD
  - Recurrent brief depressive disorder
  - Alcoholism or substance abuse
  - Thyroid disease
  - Anemia
  - Chronic fatigue syndrome
  - If an underlying chronic health condition such as MS or stroke is the physiologic *cause* of the depressed mood, the diagnosis is mood disorder due to a general medical condition
  - Anxiety disorders, such as PTSD or obsessive-compulsive disorder
  - Dementia
  - Drug interactions or adverse effects
  - Sleep apnea
  - Personality disorder
- Less Common:
  - Bipolar disorder
  - Amphetamine or cocaine withdrawal
  - Infectious disease, such as autoimmune disorder, mononucleosis, or hepatitis C
  - Parathyroid disease
  - Adrenal disease
  - Fibromyalgia
  - Cancer
  - Neurologic disease, such as cerebral vascular accident, MS, subdural hematoma, normal pressure hydrocephalus, or Alzheimer's disease
  - Cardiovascular disease such as congestive heart failure or cardiomyopathy

- Nutritional deficiency, such as B vitamin, folate, or iron deficiency
- Pulmonary disease, such as COPD
- Heavy metal poisoning

ICD Code

300.4 Dysthymic Disorder

Diagnostic Work-Up

- Physical and mental evaluation:
  - Thyroid function studies (T3, T4, TSH levels)
  - CMP
  - Complete blood count with differential
  - Vitamin D level
  - Testing for infectious diseases such as hepatitis C or HIV, if applicable

Initial Assessment

- Mental status exam often shows slowed speech, decreased eye contact, diminished range of facial expression with self-doubt, sadness, guilt, hopelessness, and/or negative outlook. Thought will be organized without disruption of intellect, memory, abstraction, or significant abnormalities (such as delusions).
- Use of a standard depression screening tool such as Beck depression inventory, or Zung self-rating scale, to rule out MDD.
- Past medical history: If any MDD in the past 2 years, the patient does not have dysthymic disorder.
- Family medical history, with emphasis on psychiatric history
- Social history, including safety of relationships, family support, recent or ongoing stressors
- Past suicide attempts or past psychiatric hospitalizations
- Any prior manic/hypomanic episodes (*any* history suggests bipolar or cyclothymia diagnosis)
- What effect symptoms have had on ability to function, particularly participation in nonoccupational activities
- Assess for suicide ideation, suicide plan, and suicide intent

Clinical Presentation: Symptoms

- Low self-esteem
- Difficulties with sleep
- Low energy or fatigue

- Pessimistic outlook
- Feelings of guilt
- Tendency to put energy into work with limited energy left for social/family life
- Difficulties in making decisions
- Obsessive rumination about problems with difficulty in problem solving
- Multiple somatic symptoms

Clinical Presentation: Signs
- Decreased facial expression
- Slowed speech or movements
- Decreased eye contact
- Poor concentration

DSM-IV-TR Diagnostic Guidelines
- Persistent, long-term depressed mood and/or anhedonia (2 years or more in adults, 1 year or more in children and adolescents), in combination with at least 2 of the following:
  - Changes in eating habits
  - Changes in sleep habits
  - Fatigue, low energy
  - Lowered self-esteem
  - Distractibility, problems with concentration
  - Hopelessness
- Periods of remission have not been greater than 2 months.
- There has been no major depressive episode during the same period.
- Psychotic features are absent.
- Absence of manic or hypomanic episodes.
- Evidence for cyclothymia is absent.
- The symptoms engender distress in the individual and/or a reduction in social functioning.

Treatment

Therapies
- Studies support the pharmacological approach as the first line treatment for dysthymic disorder. Approximately, 55% of patients with DD will respond to pharmacologic therapy. Doses are the same as for major depression.
- Both psychological and pharmacologic therapies are effective in the treatment of dysthymic disorder and each has its own merits. The combination of antidepressant and psychotherapy

such as talk therapy is recommended for dysthymic disorder patients for long-term treatment.
- Pay careful attention in the first 1–4 weeks of antidepressant treatment to a sudden lift of depression, or to worsening mood as initial response to antidepressant therapy as these could be signs of increased risk for suicide.
- Be aware of the Federal Drug Administration black box warning regarding antidepressant treatment in children and younger adults and use appropriate caution in these patients.
- Patients should receive long-term (2–5 years) pharmacologic therapy with SSRIs, selective norepinephrine reuptake inhibitors, or atypical antidepressants. Assist patients with side effects, which are more likely to occur early in treatment.
- Regular follow-up for medication management, assistance for overcoming treatment resistance through augmentation therapy, etc., tracking patient progress in individual psychotherapy, monitoring for MDD, and reinforcement of patient self-efficacy are all important to care.
- Stress management and life-style changes, such as regular exercise, are essential to ongoing care.
- Studies suggest that augmentation of antidepressant effect occurs with adjunct use of omega-3 fish oil supplements, 1000 mg twice daily. B vitamin supplementation has also been used in some studies, with equivocal results.
- Psychodynamic therapy, addressing an understanding of maladaptive interpersonal responses, CBT, and interpersonal therapy—which involves addressing interpersonal conflicts through improved strategies—have all been found beneficial in the treatment of patients with dysthymic disorder. Group therapy may also be helpful.
- Treatment may be complicated by having another condition at the same time, such as substance abuse, personality disorders, or other anxiety disorders, and these should also be addressed.

Recurrence Rate
- In one study, there was a 53% estimated 5-year recovery rate from dysthymic disorder, but a very high risk of relapse.

Patient Education

- Advise patients with dysthymic disorder to avoid nicotine and to avoid alcohol.
- Thirty minutes of daily exercise have been found beneficial for dysthymic disorder patients and daily exposure to outdoor light may be beneficial.
- For excellent patient education resources, visit eMedicine's Mental Health and Behavior Center and Depression Center. See also eMedicine's patient education articles on Dysthymic Disorder.

Medical/Legal Pitfalls

- Failure to monitor for suicidal thoughts.
- Failure to screen for bipolar disorder (any history of mania/hypomania).
- Pay careful attention, in the first 1–4 weeks of treatment, to a sudden lift of depression, or to worsening mood as initial response to antidepressant therapy as these could be signs of increased risk for suicide.
- It is important that patients with dysthymic disorder be viewed as having a severe and chronic condition, which must be monitored and managed.
- When initiating treatment, see patients on a more frequent basis until response to antidepressant is clear.
- Have a follow-up system to ensure that there are calls to patients who fail to schedule follow-up appointments or fail to show up for scheduled appointments.
- Patients with dysthymic disorder are more likely than the general population to use alternative therapies. Use of dietary supplements (e.g., herbs) should be discussed to avoid drug interactions.

Other Resources

Evidence-Based References

Akiskal, H. S. (2001). Dysthymia and cyclothymia in psychiatric practice a century after Kraeplin. *Journal of Affective Disorders, 62,* 17–31.

Bauer, M., Beaulieu, S., Dunner, D. L., Lafer, B., & Kupka, R. (2008). Rapid cycling bipolar disorder—diagnostic concepts. *Bipolar Disorders, 10,* 153–162.

Ghaemi, S. N., Hsu, D. J., Thase, M. E., Wisniewski, S. R., Nierenberg, A. A., Miyahara, S., et al. (2006). Pharmacological treatment patterns at study entry for the first 500 STEP-BD participants. *Psychiatric Services, 57*(5), 660–665.

Goldberg, J. F., Allen, M. H., Miklowitz, D. A., Bowden, C. L., Endick, C. J., Chessick, C. A., et al. (2005). Suicidal ideation and pharmacology among STEP-BD patients. *Psychiatric Services, 56*(12), 1534–1540.

Goldberg. J. F., Perlis, R. H., Ghaemi, S. N., Calabrese, J. R., Bowden, C. L., Wisniewski, S. R., et al. (2007). Adjunctive use and symptomatic recovery among bipolar depressed patients with concomitant manic symptoms: findings from the STEP-BD. *American Journal of Psychiatry, 164*(9), 1348–1355.

Harel, E. V., & Levkovitz, Y. (2008). Effectiveness and safety of adjunctive antidepressants in the treatment of bipolar depression: A review. *Israeli Journal of Psychiatry and Related Sciences, 45*(2), 121–128.

Hirshfeld, R. M. (2002). The mood disorder questionnaire: A simple, patient-related screening instrument for bipolar disorder. *Primary Care Companion for the Journal of Psychiatry, 4*(1), 9–11.

Manning, J. S., Saeeduddin, A., McGuire, H. C., & Hay, D. P. (2002). Mood disorders in family practice: beyond unipolarity to bipolarity. *Primary Care Companion for the Journal of Clinical Psychiatry, 4*(4), 142–150.

Martinez, J. M., Marangell, L. B., Simon, N. M., Miyahara, S, Wisniewski, S. R., Harrington, J., et al. (2005). Baseline predictors of serious adverse events at one year at one month among patients with bipolar disorder in STEP-BD. *Psychiatric Services, 56*(12), 1541–1548.

Miklowitz, D. J., Otto, M. W., Frank, E., Reilly-Harington, N. A., Kogan, J. N., Sachs, G. S., et al. (2007). Intensive psychosocial intervention enhances functioning in patients with bipolar depression: results from a 9-month randomized controlled trial. *American Journal of Psychiatry, 164*(9), 1340–1347.

Miklowitz, D. J., Otto, M. W., Wisniewski, S. R., Araga, M., Frank, E., Reilly-Harrington, N. A., et al. (2006). Psychotherapy, symptoms outcomes, and role functioning over one year among patients with bipolar disorder. *Psychiatric Services, 57*(7), 959–965.

National Mental Health. A Report of the Surgeon General. http://www.surgeongeneral.gov/library/mentalhealth/home.html.

Perlis, R. H., Ostacher, M. J, Patel, J. K, Marangell, L. B., Zhange, H., Wisniewski, S. R., et al. (2006). Predictors of recurrence in bipolar disorder: Primary outcomes from the Systematic Enhancement Program for Bipolar Disorder (STEP-BD). *American Journal of Psychiatry, 163*(2), 217–224.

President's New Freedom Commission on Mental Health. (2003). Retrieved from http://www.mentalhealthcommission.gov/reports/Finalreport/toc_exec.html.

Schneck, C. D., Miklowitz, D. J., Miyahara, S., Araga, M., Wisniewski, S. R., Allen, M. H., et al. (2008). The prospective course of rapid-cycling bipolar disorder: Findings from the STEP-BD. *American Journal of Psychiatry, 163*(3), 370–377.

Web Resources

- American Psychiatric Association: http://www.psych.org/.
- American Psychological Association: www.apa.org.
- Depression and Bipolar Support Alliance (DBSA): www.dbsalliance.org.
- MacArthur Initiative on Depression and Primary Care: http://www.depression-primarycare.org/.
- National Alliance of the Mentally Ill (NAMI): http://www.nami.org.
- National Institute of Mental Health: www.nimh.gov/.
- National Suicide Prevention Lifeline: http://www.suicidepreventionlifeline.org/.
- Systematic Enhancement Program for Bipolar Disorder (STEP-BD): http://www.stepbd.org/.

9. ANXIETY DISORDERS
Acute Stress Disorder

Background Information

Definition of Disorder
- Person experienced a traumatic event where death seemed actual or threatened, experienced serious injury or physical threat to the person or others, and the person's response included fear, hopelessness, or horror
- Anxiety, dissociative, and other symptoms occur within 1 month after extreme traumatic stressor and last for at least 2 days
- Types of stressors are the same as posttraumatic stress disorder (PTSD)
- Traumatic event is persistently reexperienced
- Person has at least three dissociative symptoms during or after the experience:
  - Sense of numbing, detachment, or absence of emotional response
  - Reduced awareness of surroundings
  - Derealization, depersonalization, or dissociative amnesia
- Marked avoidance of stimuli may arouse recollections of the trauma
- Marked symptoms of anxiety or increased arousal
- Symptoms cause clinically significant distress, significantly interfere with normal functioning, or impair individual's ability to pursue necessary tasks
- The disturbance lasts for at least 2 days but not more than 4 weeks
- If the disturbance lasts longer than 4 weeks, PTSD may be diagnosed
- Symptoms are not due to the direct physiological effect of a substance, a general medical condition, brief psychotic disorder, or another mental disorder

Etiology
- Severe trauma or traumatic experiences may cause this disorder
- The more extreme the stressor, the more likely a person will develop this disorder
- Severity, duration, and proximity to the stressor will also determine if this disorder develops
- Social support, family history, childhood experiences, personality, and preexisting mental disorders also influence development of this disorder

Demographics
- Prevalence is not known for the general population
- Estimates of prevalence in those exposed to trauma/traumatic experiences range from 14% to 33%

Risk Factors
Age
- Can occur at any age

Gender
- Affects both genders

Family History
- Family history may contribute to development of acute stress disorder

Stressful Events in Susceptible People
- Acute stress disorder is caused by a traumatic experience

Having Another Mental Disorder
- Major depressive episode may occur in conjunction with this disorder
- Eighty percent of those with this acute stress disorder will be diagnosed with PTSD

Diagnosis

Differential Diagnosis
- Mental disorder is due to a general medical condition
- Substance-induced disorder
- Brief psychotic disorder
- Major depressive disorder
- Exacerbation of preexisting mental disorder
- PTSD
- Adjustment disorder
- Malingering

ICD Code
308.3 Posttraumatic Stress Disorder

Diagnostic Work-Up
- Physical and mental evaluation
- Serum and urine drug screen

Initial Assessment
- Full history and physical examination
- Past medical history including psychiatric history
- Traumatic or past event/stressor
- Symptoms experienced (emotional or physical symptoms)
- Labs as needed to evaluate physical complaints:
  - Thyroid function studies (triiodothyronine [T3], thyroxine [T4], thyroid-stimulating hormone [TSH])
  - CMP (complete metabolic panel), including glucose, calcium, albumin; total protein count; levels of sodium, potassium, CO_2 (carbon dioxide and bicarbonate), chloride, blood urea nitrogen (BUN), creatinine, alkaline phosphatase (ALP), alanine amino transferase (ALT, also called serum glutamic pyruvic transaminase [SGPT]), aspartate amino transferase (AST, also called serum glutamic oxaloacetic transaminase [SGOT]), and bilirubin
  - CBC (complete blood count) with differentials: hemoglobin, hematocrit, red blood cell (RBC) count, white blood cell (WBC) count, WBC differential count, and platelet count

Clinical Presentation: Symptoms
- Dissociative, avoidance, numbing, and/or hyperarousal
- Reexperiencing the event
- Anxiety and/or fear
- Avoidance of anything reminding them of the event
- Symptoms interfering with daily functioning
- Recurring depression
- Alcohol/drug abuse

DSM-IV-TR Diagnostic Guidelines
- The affected individual manifests anxiety and dissociative symptoms within 1 month after exposure to a traumatic stressor.

- During or after the traumatic experience, the presence of at least 3 of the following dissociative symptoms: sense of numbing, absence of emotional responsiveness, reduction in awareness of surroundings, derealization, depersonalization, dissociative amnesia.
- The traumatic event is reexperienced and the individual shows marked avoidance of stimuli that may provoke recollection of the trauma.
- The individual demonstrates notable anxiety or increased arousal.
- The symptoms engender significant distress in the individual and/or reductions in social functioning and the ability to carry out necessary tasks.
- Disturbances last at least 2 days but not longer than 4 weeks after the traumatic event. [Note: Posttraumatic stress disorder should be considered if symptoms last longer than 4 weeks.]
- The symptoms are not more easily ascribed to other medical diagnoses, other medical conditions, other psychiatric diagnoses, drug use, or drug withdrawal.

Treatment

Acute Treatment
- The initial meeting with the patient may only be for information gathering if recalling the traumatic event increases distress
- Stabilize the patient medically and give psychological reassurance
- Give supportive psychiatric assessment
- Discuss active coping for psychosocial effects of traumatic event
- Offer supportive and psychoeducational interventions
- Give pharmacotherapy for some patients
- Information regarding resources for locating family, friends, food, and shelter, if needed
- Psychotherapy may be offered

Chronic Treatment
- Psychotherapy
  - Cognitive-behavioral therapy
  - Exposure-based therapy
  - Stress inoculation
  - Imagery rehearsal

- Pharmacotherapy
  - Selective serotonin reuptake inhibitors (SSRIs), tricyclic antidepressants (TCAs), monoamine oxidase inhibitors (MAOIs)
  - Benzodiazepines are for sleep and reducing anxiety only
  - Antipsychotics and anticonvulsants may be useful

Recurrence Rate

A person may experience acute stress disorder more than once in a lifetime, depending on traumatic experience and other factors. Acute stress disorder is either a self-limited disorder or will progress to PTSD or another disorder.

Patient Education

Patient education is critical. Teaching ways to cope with a stressful situation, attendance at stress group therapy sessions, Web site information as listed in the end-of-chapter Other Resources section.

Medical/Legal Pitfalls

- Patients should be monitored for depression
- Ask patient about alcohol or drug use, past and present
- Some patients may relapse to self-medicate
- Search for any injury related to the traumatic event or sequelae of trauma

Generalized Anxiety Disorder

Background Information

Definition of Disorder

- The most common anxiety disorder is seen by primary care physicians.
- Patients have chronic anxiety, worry, and tension, which is without, or out of proportion to, any provocation or stimulus.
- Symptoms are not situational or limited to certain events.
- Patients are unable to assure themselves that their anxiety is greatly exaggerated in comparison to the situation.

Etiology

- Exact cause of generalized anxiety disorder (GAD) is unknown.
- Some research suggests that environmental and genetic factors may play a role.
- GAD may be caused by an imbalance between dopamine and serotonin.

Demographics

- GAD affects between 4 million and 6.8 million adult Americans

Risk Factors

Age
- Patients report symptoms throughout their lives, with no particular age of onset recorded.
  - Onset: childhood
- In some people, GAD has been noted to begin in a person's 20s.

Gender
- GAD affects about twice as many women as men.
  - Women: 55–60% of patients with GAD

Family History
- There is some evidence that anxiety disorders, including GAD, tend to run in families.
- Studies of twins suggest that there may be a genetic factor.

Stressful Events in Susceptible People
- Stressful events can exacerbate symptoms in patients with GAD.

Having Another Mental Disorder
- The comorbidities that accompany GAD include: other anxiety disorders (panic disorder, social phobia), substance-abuse and mood disorders (dysthymic disorder, major depressive disorder). These comorbidities should be treated along with GAD.

Diagnosis

Differential Diagnosis

- Substance-induced anxiety disorder
- Obsessive-compulsive disorder
- Thyroid disorders
- PTSD
- Social phobia
- Panic disorder
- Hypochondriasis
- Somatization disorder
- Separation anxiety disorder
- Adjustment disorder
- Mood disorder

ICD Code

300.02 Generalized Anxiety Disorder

Diagnostic Work-Up

- There are no particular laboratory tests that diagnose GAD, but tests can be done to rule out other organic causes (e.g., thyroid function test, CBCs, basic metabolic panels, urinalysis).
- Diagnosis of panic disorder can be difficult because several other physical and mental disorders may be confused with GAD.
- Physical and mental evaluation is done.
- Two scales are used to evaluate for GAD (GAD 2 and GAD 7 scales).

Initial Assessment

- Medical history
- Symptoms:

- How long has patient been having symptoms?
- When did the symptoms start?
- How often do they occur?
- When and where do they tend to occur?
- How long do they last?
- What effect do they have on your ability to function?

Clinical Presentation: Symptoms
- Patients are unable to relax
- Patient is easily startled
- Difficulty in concentrating
- Difficulty in falling or staying asleep (insomnia)
- Anxiety
- Fatigue
- Diarrhea
- Nausea
- Headaches
- Muscle aches and tension
- Difficulty swallowing
- Trembling
- Twitching
- Irritability
- Sweating
- Nausea
- Lightheadedness
- Shortness of breath
- Hot flashes
- Tachycardia
- Restlessness

DSM-IV-TR Diagnostic Guidelines
- Excessive anxiety and worry about events or activities occur more days than not for a period of at least 6 months.
- The individual is unable to control the worry.
- The anxiety and worry are accompanied by at least 3 of the following: restlessness, fatigue, problems with concentration, irritability, increased muscle tension, changes in sleep habits. (Note: only 1 additional symptom is required in children).
- The anxiety and worry are not a feature of panic attack (as in panic attack disorder); fear of being embarrassed in public (as in social phobia); fear of becoming contaminated (as in obsessive-compulsive disorder); fear of being away from home or close relatives (as in separation anxiety disorder); or fear of being seriously ill (as in hypochondriasis).
- The anxiety and worry are not a part of posttraumatic stress disorder.
- Although affected individuals may not identify their worries as excessive, they report subjective distress (that is owing to the worry), an inability to control worry, or reductions in social or occupational functioning.
- The disturbances in personality and functioning are not the direct physiological effects of exposure to a substance (including medication) or a general medical condition, and do not occur concurrently with a mood disorder, a psychotic disorder, or a pervasive developmental disorder.

Treatment

Acute Treatment
- Psychotherapy
- Medication:
  - Benzodiazepines (first line but do not use in patients with a past history of addiction and drug abuse).
  - Buspirone (BuSpar) (now becoming first-line treatment after benzodiazepines).
  - TCA (imipramine [Tofranil], desipramine [Norpramin], nortriptyline [Aventyl]).
  - Second-generation antidepressants (trazodone [Desyrel], nefazodone [Dutonin]).
  - SSRIs.
  - Serotonin–norepinephrine reuptake inhibitors (SNRIs) Selective norepinephrine reuptake inhibitor (Selective NRI).
  - Complementary and alternative medicine (CAM):
    - Acupuncture
    - Aromatherapy
- Inpatient treatment is necessary in patients with a suicidal ideation and plan, serious alcohol or sedative withdrawal symptoms, or when the differential includes other medical disorders that warrant admission (e.g., unstable angina, acute myocardial ischemia).

Chronic Treatment

- Follow-up care by a chemical dependence treatment specialist is recommended when indicated.
- Psychiatric referral should be considered in patients who do not improve with medical treatment or those with suicidal ideations.

Patient Education

- Patients should continue to take all medications as prescribed and never stop any medicines before discussing this with their physician.
- For excellent patient education resources, visit eMedicine's Mental Health and Behavior Center and Anxiety Center.

Medical/Legal Pitfalls

- Persons with GAD are more likely to have other anxiety disorders (e.g., panic disorder).
- Anxiety disorders are more frequently seen in patients with chronic medical illness (chronic obstructive pulmonary disease [COPD], irritable bowel syndrome [IBS], hypertension) than in the general population.
- Patients are more likely to present to their PCPs frequently with multiple complaints over time.
- Patients with GAD tend to smoke cigarettes and abuse other substances (alcohol, prescription or illicit drugs).

Phobias (Including Social Phobia)

Other Names
- Simple phobia
- Specific phobia
- Social phobia
- Social anxiety disorder

Background Information

Definition of Disorder
- There are two types of phobias: specific and social
- To be diagnosed with a phobia, the person must have a marked, persistent fear of specific objects or situations, social situations, or performance situations
- The fear may be manifested in a panic attack or resemble a panic attack
- The phobic stimulus is avoided or dreaded
- An immediate anxiety response is provoked by exposure to the phobic object or situation
- Adults recognize the fear is unreasonable or excessive
- The avoidance, fear, and panic attacks must significantly interfere with the person's daily routine, occupation, or social life, or else the phobia causes marked distress to the person
- The anxiety, panic attacks, and avoidance must not be caused by another mental condition, a general medical condition, or a drug

Etiology
- Specific phobia
  - Phobias are usually objects or situations that may be threatening or have been threatening in the past
  - Persons may be predisposed to phobia onset by:
    - Personal traumatic experiences or viewing others' traumatic experiences
    - Being attacked by an animal or viewing another being attacked by an animal
    - Observing others fearing an object or situation
    - Informational transmission of things to be feared
    - Unexpected panic attacks in a to-be-feared situation
  - Phobias secondary to trauma or unexpected panic attacks tend to be acute and have no characteristic age of onset
  - Phobias continuing into adulthood remit in about 20% of cases
- Social phobia
  - May emerge in a child with social inhibition and shyness
  - Onset may be abrupt or secondary to stressful or humiliating experience
  - Onset may be insidious
  - Duration is frequently lifelong with remission or attenuation in adulthood
  - Social phobia severity may wax and wane depending on stressors and life events

Demographics
- Prevalence for specific phobia in the community is 4–8.8%
- Lifetime prevalence for specific phobia is 7.2–11.3%, with a decline in the elderly
- Prevalence estimates for social phobias vary depending on the threshold used to determine distress and impairment in each study
- Prevalence estimates have been as high as 20% in those with anxiety disorders but as low as 2% in the general population
- Lifetime prevalence for social phobia is 3–13%

Risk Factors
Age
- Specific phobia
  - Onset depends on type of phobia
  - Usually occurs in childhood/early adolescence
- Social phobia
  - Usually occurs in mid-teens
  - Childhood onset may occur if a child has social inhibition and shyness

Gender
- Specific phobia
  - Women are affected more than men (2:1)
  - 90% of animal and natural environment phobias and situational phobias affect women
- Social phobia
  - Women are affected more than men in the general population
  - Men are affected more than women or are equal in the clinical setting

Family History
- Family members of those with a specific phobia have increased risk for a specific phobia, especially if the phobia is animal-type, situational-type, or fear of blood or injury.
- Especially in the generalized type of social phobia, first-degree biological relatives are more likely to have this phobia than the general population.

Stressful Events in Susceptible People
- Specific phobia:
  - Traumatic events may trigger phobias
  - Stressful events may cause reemergence of a phobia
- Social phobia:
  - May be caused by stressful experience
  - Stress may cause resurgence of a phobia after remission or attenuation

Having Another Mental Disorder
- Having one specific phobia does not predispose a person to having another phobia unless the phobia developed in adolescence
- Having any specific phobia does not predispose or increase risk for another mental disorder
- Those with a social phobia are more likely to also have anxiety disorders, depression, substance abuse, and dependence

Diagnosis

Differential Diagnosis
- Specific phobia:
  - Social phobia
  - Panic disorder with agoraphobia
  - Panic disorder without agoraphobia
  - Posttraumatic stress symptoms
  - Separation anxiety disorder
  - Obsessive-compulsive disorder

- Hypochondriasis
- Anorexia nervosa
- Bulimia nervosa
- Schizophrenia or another psychotic disorder
- Social phobia:
  - Specific phobia
  - Panic disorder without agoraphobia
  - Agoraphobia without history of panic disorder
  - Separation anxiety disorder
  - Generalized anxiety disorder
  - Pervasive development disorder
  - Schizoid personality disorder
  - Avoidant personality disorder

ICD Codes
300.29 Specific Phobia
300.23 Social Phobia

Diagnostic Work-Up
- Physical and mental evaluation is done

Initial Assessment
- Full history and physical exam are included
- Past medical history including psychiatric history
- Traumatic or past event/stressor is determined
- Symptoms you experience (emotional or physical symptoms)
- Physical and mental evaluation is included
- Thyroid function studies (TSH, T3, T4) are done
- CMP includes glucose, calcium, albumin, total protein count, levels of sodium, potassium, CO_2 (carbon dioxide and bicarbonate), chloride, BUN, creatinine, ALP, ALT, AST, and bilirubin
- CBC with differentials: hemoglobin, hematocrit, RBC count, WBC count, WBC differential count, and platelet count

Clinical Presentation: Symptoms
- Panic (or panic-like) attacks
- Extreme anxiety and/or fear
- Extreme avoidance of the phobia

DSM-IV-TR Diagnostic Guidelines
Specific Phobia
- Defined as a marked fear of clearly identifiable objects or situations.
- Exposure to the phobic stimulus almost invariably causes an immediate anxiety response.

- Adults and adolescents are apt to recognize that their fears are excessive or unreasonable, but children are apt not to.
- The phobic stimulus is either avoided or endured with dread.
- The avoidance of, fear of, or anxious anticipation of encounters with the phobic stimulus interferes significantly with the individual's daily routine or social functioning.
- The anxiety, panic attacks, or phobic avoidance are not more easily ascribed to another psychiatric disorder.

Social Phobia

- Defined as marked fear of social or performance situations (in which embarrassment is likely to occur).
- Exposure to the social or performance situation almost invariably provokes an immediate anxiety response. Although adolescents and adults are likely to recognize that their fears are excessive, children are likely not to.
- The individual avoids the social or performance situation, or endures it with dread.
- The avoidance of, fear of, or anxious anticipation of encounters with the phobic stimulus interferes with the individual's daily routine, occupational functioning, or social life.
- The fear or avoidance is not the direct physiological effect of a substance or a general medical condition, and is not better accounted for by the presence of another psychiatric disorder.

Treatment

Acute Treatment
Specific Phobia

- Cognitive-behavioral interventions are the most studied and most efficacious for this disorder
- Multiple exposure treatments, in vivo or virtual reality, work very well in extinguishing the phobia
- Applied relaxation and tension treatments have shown promise but need more studies to show efficacy
- Cognitive restructuring treatments and psychodynamic psychotherapy may also be useful but need more studies to be done

Social Phobia
- Cognitive-behavioral therapies
  - These therapies work on the belief that dysfunctional beliefs and biased information processing strategies are responsible for the social phobia
  - The therapies focus on the patients' beliefs and avoidance
  - Therapies used include exposure treatments alone, exposure treatments plus cognitive restructuring treatments (either in a group session or an individual session), social skills training, and relaxation strategies
  - Exposure treatments with cognitive restructuring treatments are most effective
  - Social skills training and relaxation strategies are less effective alone but have increased efficacy when either is combined with exposure treatments and cognitive restructuring treatments in a group setting
- Medications
  - Various medications have been used to improve patients with a social phobia, including phenelzine (Nardil) and sertraline (Sercerin)
  - Medication use alone was associated with a high relapse rate despite an earlier initial benefit
  - Relapse rate was decreased when medication use was combined with cognitive-behavioral group therapy
  - More studies need to be done to determine better treatment guidelines
- Psychodynamic therapy, interpersonal psychotherapy, and acceptance and commitment therapy are used clinically but should be studied more to determine efficacy as compared to cognitive-behavioral therapies and medication use

Chronic Treatment
Specific Phobia

- Long-term therapy may be needed if exposure therapy does not work
- More research needs to be done on therapy for the specific phobia

Social Phobia

- Long-term therapy may be needed if the patient is refractory to acute treatment

- Therapy may include cognitive-behavioral, medication, or another type of therapy

Recurrence Rate

Rate of recurrence is variable. It depends on life stressors, attenuation, and remission of phobia.

Patient Education

- Both MD Consult and eMedicine have patient education articles on phobias

- Many support groups can be found online, including www.dailystrength.org
- Advise patients to avoid self-medication with alcohol or other drugs

Medical/Legal Pitfalls

- Patients with some phobias may abuse alcohol or illicit drugs as a coping mechanism. Health care workers should screen for this during the H&P.

Posttraumatic Stress Disorder

Other Names
- Shell shock
- Battle fatigue

Background Information

Definition of Disorder
- There are complex somatic, cognitive, affective, and behavioral effects of psychosocial trauma.
- It is seen after patients have undergone a major traumatic or life-threatening event (e.g., war, assault, natural disasters, abuse).
- Patients may have persistent, pervasive thoughts of the traumatic event.
- They may have flashbacks or feel like they're reliving the incident.

  It is important to discern patients with posttraumatic stress symptoms after the occurrence of an acute stressor versus PTSD. Posttraumatic stress symptoms are transient, and will likely resolve within a few weeks. Prophylactive counseling in patients with acute stress has not been shown to prevent the development of PTSD.

Etiology
- Etiology and pathophysiology of PTSD is unclear, but is currently undergoing research.
- According to one study that used MRIs to evaluate the brain, a decreased hippocampal volume was noted in patients with PTSD as compared to controls.

Demographics
- The lifetime prevalence of PTSD ranges from 6.8 to 12.3%.
- It is seen in approximately 2.5% of primary care patients.
- Incidence in the general population is 4–60%.

Risk Factors
Age
- There is no age predilection for PTSD.

Gender
- There is no gender preference for PTSD.

Family History
- There is no family propensity noted for PTSD.

Stressful Events in Susceptible People
- Stressful or traumatic events in people who have undergone prior trauma increase their susceptibility in developing PTSD.

Having Another Mental Disorder
- Psychiatric comorbidity is high in patients with PTSD.
- Screen these patients closely following traumatic stressors.

Diagnosis

Differential Diagnosis
- Posttraumatic stress symptoms
- Acute stress disorder
- Obsessive-compulsive disorder
- Night terrors
- Nightmares
- Anxiety disorder
- Phobia
- Panic disorder
- Personality disorder
- Insomnia
- Depression
- Substance abuse

ICD Code
309.81 Posttraumatic Stress Disorder

Diagnostic Work-Up
- Goal is to rule out other causes of posttraumatic stress symptoms
- Physical and mental evaluation
- Thyroid function studies (T3, T4, TSH)
- CMP, including glucose, calcium, albumin; total protein count; levels of sodium, potassium, CO_2 (carbon dioxide and bicarbonate), chloride, BUN, creatinine, ALP, ALT, AST, and bilirubin
- CBC with differentials: hemoglobin, hematocrit, RBC count, WBC count, WBC differential count, and platelet count

Initial Assessment

- Full history and physical exam are included
- Past medical history includes psychiatric history
- Discern traumatic or past event/stressor
- Symptoms you experience (emotional or physical symptoms)
- Laboratory test is done

There are several questionnaires that are available to primary care physicians to screen for PTSD in patients with exposure to traumatic or stressful events. These questionnaires are based on the level of exposure to the stressor and the associated acute reactions.

Clinical Presentation: Symptoms

- Flashbacks or "reliving" traumatic events
- Nightmares
- Avoidance of reminders of the trauma
- Severe anxiety attacks
- Anhedonia
- Poor appetite
- Irritability
- Depressed mood
- Anger
- Startled reactions
- Sleep disturbances/insomnia
- Guilt
- Other somatic symptoms (fatigue, chronic pain, chest pain, dyspepsia) Symptoms occur most frequently closer to the traumatic event and lessen with time

DSM-IV-TR Diagnostic Guidelines

- The individual has been exposed to a traumatic event.
- The individual experienced or witnessed an event that included actual or threatened death or actual or threatened serious injury (toward the integrity of self or others).
- The individual's response included fear, helplessness, or horror.
- The traumatic event is persistently reexperienced in one or more of the following ways:
  - Recurrent and intrusive recollections of the event
  - Recurrent distressing dreams of the event
  - Acting or feeling as if the event were recurring

- A sense of reliving the experience
- Intense psychological distress at exposure to stimuli that resemble or symbolize the traumatic event
- Physiological reactivity at exposure to stimuli that resemble or symbolize the traumatic event.
- Persistent avoidance of stimuli, associated with the trauma and numbing of general responsiveness, as indicated by 3 or more of the following:
  - Efforts to avoid thoughts or feelings associated with the trauma
  - Efforts to avoid activities, persons, or places that arouse recollections of the trauma
  - Inability to recall some aspects of the trauma
  - Pronouncedly diminished interest or participation in some activities
  - Feelings of detachment or estrangement from others
  - Narrowing of affect
  - Sense of a foreshortened future
- Persistent symptoms of increased arousal (which were not present prior to the trauma), as indicated by two or more of the following:
  - Difficulty falling or staying asleep
  - Irritability, outbursts of anger
  - Problems with concentration
  - Hypervigilance
  - Exaggerated startled responses
- Symptoms are present for more than 1 month. (In the acute disorder, symptoms are present for less than 3 months; in the chronic disorder, symptoms are present for 3 months or more.)
- The overall disturbances cause subjective distress or impairment in social functioning.

Treatment

Acute Treatment

- Inpatient treatment is necessary in patients with a suicidal ideation and plan, serious alcohol or sedative withdrawal symptoms, or when the differential includes other medical disorders that warrant admission (e.g., unstable angina, acute myocardial ischemia).
- Patients should be referred to psychotherapists who are trained in caring for patients with PTSD.

- Some patients are started on medication in the SSRI class. These medications are often started in low doses, and titrated up.
- Antidepressants in other classes are also useful (TCAs, SNRIs, MAOIs), as well as benzodiazepines, mood stabilizers, and sympatholytic agents (alpha-adrenergic inhibitors).

Chronic Treatment

- Long-term psychotherapy may be helpful in monitoring the patient's symptoms and treatment progress, and to evaluate the patient for any signs of drug abuse as a coping mechanism.
- In patients with suspected drug abuse, a consultation with a chemical dependence treatment specialist is recommended.
- Treatment can be complicated by having another condition at the same time, such as substance abuse, depression, or other anxiety disorders.

Recurrence Rate

Rate of recurrence is 50% unless patient is involved in cognitive-behavioral therapy.

Patient Education

- For excellent patient education resources, visit eMedicine's Mental Health and Behavior Center.
- Advise patients with PTSD to avoid using alcohol or other drugs of abuse as coping mechanisms.

Medical/Legal Pitfalls

- Patients with PTSD may abuse alcohol or illicit drugs as a coping mechanism. Health care workers should screen for this during the H&P, and through urine and serum tests when necessary. Alternative coping techniques should be suggested.

Other Resources

Evidence-Based References

American Psychiatric Association-Medical Specialty Association. (2004). *Practice guideline for the treatment of patients with acute stress disorder and posttraumatic stress disorder*. Washington, DC: American Psychiatric Association.

Beckham, J. C., Moore, S. D., Feldman, M. E., Hertzberg, M. A., Kirby, A. C., & Fairbank, J. A. (1998). Health status, somatization, and severity of posttraumatic stress disorder in Vietnam combat veterans with posttraumatic stress disorder. *American Journal of Psychiatry, 155*, 1565–1569.

Bremner, J. D., Randall, P., Scott, T. M., Bronen, R. A., Seibyl, J. P., Southwick, S. M., et al. (1995). MRI-based measurement of hippocampal volume in patients with combat-related posttraumatic stress disorder. *American Journal of Psychiatry, 152*(7), 973–981.

Breslau, N., Davis, G. C., Andreski, P., Peterson, E. (1991). Traumatic events and posttraumatic stress disorder in an urban population of young adults. *Archives of General Psychiatry, 48*(3), 216–222.

Kavan, M. G., Elsasser, G. N., Barone, E. J. (2009). Generalized anxiety disorder: Practical assessment and management. *American Family Physician, 79*(9).

Kessler, R. C., Sonnega, A., Bromet, E., Hughes, M., Nelson, C. B. (1995). Posttraumatic stress disorder in the National Comorbidity Survey. *Archives of General Psychiatry, 52*(12), 1048–1060.

Magee, L., Erwin, B. A., & Heimberg, R. G. (2008). Psychological treatment of social anxiety disorder and specific phobia. In M. A. Antony, M. B. Stein (Eds.), *Oxford handbook of anxiety and related disorders*. New York: Oxford University Press.

Resnick, H. S., Kilpatrick, D. G., Dansky, B. S., Saunders, B. E., Best, C. L. (1993). Prevalence of civilian trauma and posttraumatic stress disorder in a representative national sample of women. *Journal of Consulting and Clinical Psychology, 61*(6), 984–991.

Web Resources

- Anxiety Disorders Association of America (ADAA): www.adaa.org/.
- National Center for Post Traumatic Stress Disorder, sponsored by the US Department of Veterans Affairs: http://www.ncptsd.va.gov/ncmain/index.jsp.
- National Institutes of Mental Health: http://nimh.nih.gov/.

Obsessive-Compulsive Disorder

Background Information

Definition of Disorder

- This anxiety disorder is characterized by obsessions and compulsions
- Obsessions: disturbing thoughts that are seen as excessive
- Compulsions: repetitive behaviors or mental acts that neutralize distress
- Symptoms are egodystonic

Etiology

- Neurobiological disorder
- Multiple sources are implicated
- Frontal–subcortical neuronal circuit
- Subcortical frontal gyrus
- Caudate nucleus
- Thalamus
- Genetics: specific markers have been identified
- Cognitive and behavioral factors

Demographics

- There is a 2.5% lifetime prevalence
- Males/females are equally affected
- Bimodal age of onset is 6–15 years of age for males and 20–29 years for females
- Similar prevalence rates appear around the world
- No difference across socioeconomic backgrounds
- Ranked by the World Health Organization as one of 10 most disabling disorders

Risk Factors

- Males 6–15 years of age are at risk; females, 20–29 years of age
- Family members with an anxiety disorder
- Precipitating factors
- Head injury
- Infection
- Approximately, 39% of women with obsessive-compulsive disorder (OCD) developed it during pregnancy

Comorbidity

- Fifty to sixty percent have at least one additional Axis 1 diagnosis
- Anxiety disorder
- Mood disorder including depression
- Substance abuse
- Two to three times more likely to have Cluster C diagnosis on Axis II

Diagnosis

ICD Code

300.3 Obsessive-Compulsive Disorder

Diagnostic Work-Up

- Interview is based on *DSM-IV-TR* criteria
- Neuropsychological/psychological testing may be helpful for a differential diagnosis
- Yale-Brown obsessive compulsive scale (Y-BOCS) is used to determine severity
- Assess symptoms against Y-BOCS symptom checklist
- Children's version of Y-BOCS (CY-BOCS) is available for pediatric population
- Vancouver Obsessional Compulsive Inventory assesses symptoms
- Padua Inventory—Washington State University Revision assesses symptoms
- Scales above are available online or through authors (for free)
- Assess medical needs due to lack of medical care in severe cases

Initial Assessment

- Family psychiatric history
- Onset of symptoms
- Severity of symptoms
- Functioning at home and school
- Egodystonic/egosyntonic
- Impact on patient/family
- How much time is the patient spending ritualizing/obsessing?
- How much time is family spending accommodating (feeding into OCD symptoms)?

Clinical Presentation

- Severe anxiety, worry, or distress
- Avoidant behavior
- Excessive time spent on parts of daily routine, that is, showering, cleaning
- Obsessions and compulsions

- Odd or excessive behaviors, that is, wearing protective barriers, repeating
- Significant impairment (i.e., patient is unable to work/attend school, or participate in social activities)

DSM-IV-TR Diagnostic Guidelines
- Either obsessions or compulsions.
- Obsessions are defined by the following:
  - Recurrent thoughts are experienced as intrusive and inappropriate, and causing marked anxiety.
  - The thoughts and images cannot be ascribed to undue worry about real-life problems.
  - The individual makes attempts to ignore or suppress the offending thoughts, or to neutralize them with other thoughts and/or activities.
  - The individual recognizes that the obsessional thoughts are products of his or her own mind (not imposed by or from an external source).
- Compulsions defined by:
  - Repetitive behaviors (e.g., hand washing) or repetitive mental activities (e.g., counting items, repeating words silently).
  - The individual feels driven to perform these repetitive behaviors or mental activities (often according to rules that, he or she believes, must be stringently adhered to).
  - The neutralizing behaviors are aimed at reducing stress or preventing some dreaded event. However, these behaviors are not connected in any realistic way with what they are intended to neutralize.
- At some point during the course of the disorder, the individual recognizes that the obsessions or compulsions are excessive or unreasonable. Children are not likely to make this recognition.
- The obsessions or compulsions cause distress for the individual, are time-consuming, or significantly interfere with daily routine.
- If another psychiatric disorder is present, the content of the obsessions or compulsions does not center on that disorder (e.g., preoccupation with food in the presence of an eating disorder).
- The disturbance is not the direct physiological effect of substance use or another medical condition.

Pharmacological Treatment
- Antidepressants: sertraline (Zoloft), fluoxetine (Prozac), fluvoxamine (Luvox), citalopram (Celexa), escitalopram (Lexapro), paroxetine (Paxil), clomipramine (Anafranil) are effective in RCTs (doses for adults)
- Clomipramine (Anafranil): 100–225 mg/day, divided; initiate at 25 mg BID
- Fluvoxamine (Luvox), fluoxetine (Prozac), sertraline (Zoloft), and clomipramine (Anafranil) have FDA approval for use in pediatric population for OCD; start low and go slow
- Fluvoxamine (Luvox) (>8 y/o), initiate 25 mg/day
- Fluoxetine (Prozac) (>7 y/o), initiate 10 mg/day
- Sertraline (Zoloft) (>6 y/o), initiate 25 mg/day
- Clomipramine (Anafranil) (>10 y/o), initiate 25 mg/day
- Selective-serotonin reuptake inhibitors (SSRIs) have black box warning for potential to increase suicidal thoughts in children; similar warnings for adults but not black box.
- Monitor antidepressants for nausea, agitation, sleep disturbance, suicidal thoughts, changes in appetite, and drowsiness; in paroxetine (Paxil) and clomipramine (Anafranil), also monitor for seizures. Medication should not be abruptly stopped. Paroxetine (Paxil) can cause particular problems as discontinued
- Augmentation with an atypical antipsychotic, such as risperidone (Risperdal), quetiapine (Seroquel), aripiprazole (Abilify), may be warranted after weighing the risk/benefits
- Cognitive-behavioral therapy (CBT) is equally as effective as medication
- Refer to clinician trained in CBT using exposure and response prevention

Patient Education
- About diagnosis/prognosis—treatable, but with no cure
- Available treatment is discussed, with side effects carefully explained

Medical/Legal Pitfalls
- Patient may present with life-threatening medical conditions but refuse treatment
- Physician may have to determine if patient needs commitment, based on symptoms

Other Resources

Evidence-Based References

Abramowitz, J. S. (1997). Effectiveness of psychological and pharmacological treatments for obsessive-compulsive disorder: A quantitative review. *Journal of Consulting and Clinical Psychology, 65,* 44–52.

American Psychiatric Association. (2000). *Diagnostic and statistical manual of mental disorders* (4th ed., text revision). Washington, DC: American Psychiatric Association.

American Psychiatric Association. (2007). *Practice guideline for the treatment of patients with obsessive-compulsive disorder.* Arlington, VA: American Psychiatric Association.

Antony, M. M., Downie, F., & Swinson, R. P. (1998). Diagnostic issues and epidemiology in obsessive-compulsive disorder. In R. P. Swinson, M. M. Antony, S. Rachman, et al. (Eds.), *Obsessive-compulsive disorder: Theory, research, and treatment* (pp. 3–32). New York. Guilford Press.

Bjorgvinsson, T., Hart, J., & Heffelfinger, S. (2007). Obsessive-compulsive disorder: Update on assessment and treatment. *Journal of Psychiatric Practice, 13,* 362–372.

Burns, G. L., Keortge, S. G., Formea, G. M., et al. (1996). Revision of the Padua inventory of obsessive compulsive disorder symptoms: Distinctions between worry, obsessions, and compulsions. *Behavior Research and Therapy, 24,* 163–173.

Clomipramine Collaborative Study Group. (1991). Clomipramine in the treatment of patient with obsessive-compulsive disorder. *Archives of General Psychiatry, 48,* 730–738.

Dougherty, D. D., Rauch, S. L., & Jenike, M. A. (2004). Pharmacotherapy for obsessive-compulsive disorder. *Journal of Clinical Psychology, 60,* 1195–1202.

Goodman, W. K., Price, L. H., Rasmussen, S. A., et al. (1989).The Yale-Brown obsessive compulsive scale: Pt. I. Development, use, and reliability. *Archives of General Psychiatry, 46,* 1006–1011.

Jenike, M. A. (1998). Theories of etiology. In M. A. Jenike, L. Baer, & W. E. Minichiello (Eds.), *Obsessive-compulsive disorder: Practical management* (3rd cd., pp. 203–221). St.Louis, MO: Mosby.

March, J. S., Franklin, M. E., Leonard, H. L., & Foa, E. B. (2004). Obsessive-compulsive disorder. In T. L. Morris & J. S. March (Eds.), *Anxiety disorders in children and adolescents* (2nd ed., pp. 212–240). New York: Guilford Press.

Steketee, G. (1997). Disability and family burden in obsessive-compulsive disorder. *Canadian Journal of Psychiatry, 42,* 919–928.

Thordarson, D. S., Radomsky, A. S., Rachman, S., et al. (2004). The Vancouver obsessional compulsive inventory (VOCI). *Behavior Research and Therapy, 42,* 1289 1314.

Weissman, M. M., Bland, R. C., Canino, G. J., et al. (1994). The cross national epidemiology of obsessive compulsive disorder (The Cross National Collaborative Group). *Journal of Clinical Psychiatry, 55,* 5–10.

World Health Organization. (2001). *The world health report 2001—Mental health: New understanding, new hope.* Geneva, Switzerland: World Health Organization.

Web Resources

- American Anxiety Disorders Association: http://www.adaa.org.
- Obsessive Compulsive Foundation: http://www.ocfoundation.org.
- Peace of Mind Foundation: http://www.peaceofmind.com.

11. SOMATOFORM DISORDERS
Somatoform Disorders

Somatoform disorders are presented as one disorder with many components.

Background Information

Definition of Disorder

- Individuals who present to a health care provider with either one symptom or multiple symptoms that through testing and laboratory findings are "unfounded." These symptoms are reported to cause distress, discomfort, and often disability whereby the individual continues to seek help and/or treatment.
- People with a somatoform disorder are not feigning their symptoms (as in factitious disorders). They sincerely believe that they have a serious physical problem, and they do experience the discomfort and distress.
- Historically, this has been linked to terms such as "psychosomatic" disorders, "Briquet's syndrome," and/or "hysteria."
- The somatoform disorders include body dysmorphic disorder, conversion disorder, hypochondriasis, somatization disorder, and pain disorder.

Etiology

- It is no longer viewed as something that is "all in their heads," "not real," "just imagining their symptoms," and/or purely psychological in nature.
- The cause or origin of somatoform symptoms is currently linked to the notion of a mind/body dualism and the fact that these patients do experience their symptoms.
- It is important to acknowledge that, indeed, all symptoms are "in the mind," since the brain is the center of awareness for all physical processes of human beings.
- Somatoform symptoms are etiologically different from symptoms more usually understood as "medical" in origin.

- May be influenced by the patients' sociocultural heritage, their personality, their level of anxiety, and perceived locus of control.
- Recent research has linked the symptoms of somatoform disorders to a past history of abuse and/or trauma, parental neglect, maltreatment, and/or abandonment.

Demographics

- Historically, it has been labeled as being an illness of women (hysteria), but it is equally distributed and frequently misdiagnosed in men.
- It has been estimated that between 4 and 11% of the population experience the disorder, although due to its elusive nature, the incidence is probably much higher.

Risk Factors

- Children or adolescents who have been adopted are at risk
- Children and/or adolescents who lived in foster homes or group homes, due to being orphaned or experiencing parental neglect, maltreatment, and/or abuse are at risk
- Past history of trauma, abuse, neglect, or maltreatment
- Childhood sexual abuse
- Cult membership or experience
- Rigid and unrelenting religious beliefs and/or upbringing
- History of domestic violence
- There is no known genetic heritability among somatoform disorders
- Some studies have suggested that somatic symptoms can be learned within the family of origin or through the learning of behaviors observed during childhood and adolescence. Again, this often links back to the notion of trauma and illness that may have been experienced by the patients during their formative years

Diagnosis

Differential Diagnosis

- Somatoform symptoms, medical symptoms, and amplification of medical symptoms can all coexist in the same patient. This complicates the assessment and treatment but, most importantly, the real possibility of a medical illness.
- There is no definitive medical test to "prove" that a symptom or symptom cluster is caused by a somatoform condition as opposed to a medical illness, so a thorough diagnostic work-up is absolutely necessary and *does not* provide any secondary gain for the patient as previously believed. In actuality, it is useful and therapeutic for patients to trust that you *believe* them and will work toward an end to their suffering.

ICD Codes

300.81 Somatization disorder
- Briquet's disorder
- Severe somatoform disorder
    300.82 Undifferentiated somatoform disorder
- Atypical somatoform disorder
- Somatoform disorder not otherwise specified (NOS)
    300.89 Other somatoform disorders
- Occupational neurosis, including writer's cramp
- Psychasthenia
- Psychasthenic neurosis

Diagnostic Work-Up

- Complete history and physical exam with consideration of previous neurological trauma; past illnesses, surgeries, and health care, seeking for their symptoms.
- Psychiatric evaluation should specifically include a thorough focus on personal and social history to illuminate any past abuse, trauma, conflicted relationships, unstable living situations, and/or parental neglect, or absence in their childhood and adolescence.
- Patients with histories of abuse are unlikely to report this unless specifically asked about abuse in the medical or psychiatric history.
- Patients may fail to report important information because of shame and embarrassment over abuse or maltreatment. However, repeated medical work-ups, multiple invasive procedures, and an extensive search for "unfounded" medical explanations for their symptoms should be carefully weighed against the possible risks such as iatrogenic illness.
- Lab as needed to evaluate physical complaints.
- Thyroid function studies (triiodothyronine [T3], thyroxine [T4], thyroid-stimulating hormone [TSH]).
- CMP (complete metabolic panel), including glucose, calcium, albumin; total protein count; levels of sodium, potassium, CO_2 (carbon dioxide and bicarbonate), chloride, blood urea nitrogen (BUN), creatinine, alkaline phosphatase (ALP), alanine amino transferase (ALT, also called serum glutamic pyruvic transaminase [SGPT]), aspartate amino transferase (AST, also called serum glutamic oxaloacetic transaminase [SGOT]), and bilirubin.
- CBC (complete blood count) with differentials: hemoglobin, hematocrit, red blood cell (RBC) count, white blood cell (WBC) count, WBC differential count, and platelet count.

Clinical Presentation: Symptoms

Note: It is important to recognize that some patients will avoid medical care altogether, just as others compulsively seek a medical work-up.
- Patient may present with one symptom or multiple symptoms crossing over multiple systems within the body
- Each diagnostic category has specifiers to assist in determining the diagnosis

DSM-IV-TR Diagnostic Guidelines

Body Dysmorphic Disorder
- Preoccupation with a slight or an imagined defect in one's appearance.
- The preoccupation engenders personal distress and/or impaired social functioning.
- The preoccupation is not better accounted for by another psychiatric disorder.

Conversion Disorder
- Presence of one or more neurologic symptoms or neurologic deficits (affecting voluntary motor or sensory functioning) that suggest a neurological condition. (Note: psychological factors are

believed to be associated with the symptom or deficit when the symptom or deficit occurs concurrently with, or is preceded by, other conflicts or stressors.)

- The symptom or deficit is not feigned (as in factitious disorder or malingering).
- A neurological explanation does not exist.
- The symptom or deficit is not better accounted for by another medical condition or substance use.
- The symptom or deficit does not comprise or represent a culturally sanctioned behavior.
- The symptom or deficit engenders distress for the individual and/or impedes daily functioning.
- The symptom or deficit is not better accounted for by another psychiatric disorder.

Hypochondriasis

- This is preoccupation with the fear of having, or the idea that one does have, a serious illness.
- The preoccupation persists despite the presence of medical or other counterevidence.
- The preoccupation is not of delusional intensity and is not restricted to a circumscribed concern about appearance (as in body dysmorphic disorder).
- The preoccupation engenders distress in the individual and/or impaired daily functioning.
- The duration of the disorder is 6 months or greater.
- The preoccupation is not more readily ascribed to obsessive-compulsive disorder, panic disorder, separation anxiety, another somatoform disorder, or a major depressive episode.

Pain Disorder

- This is pain at one or more anatomical sites. (Psychological factors are usually believed to play a role in the onset, severity, exacerbation, or maintenance of the pain.)
- The pain is of sufficient severity to warrant medical attention.
- The pain engenders distress for the individual and/or impaired social functioning.
- The pain is not intentionally produced or feigned (as in factitious disorder or malingering).
- The pain is not more readily ascribed to a mood disorder, anxiety, or psychosis, and does not meet criteria for dyspareunia.

Somatization Disorder

- It involves a history of many physical complaints across a period of several years, occurring prior to age 30, resulting in the seeking of treatment and/or impairment of social or occupational functioning.
- The physical complaints cannot be fully explained by a general medical condition or substance use.
- When a medical condition is present, the physical complaints or the subsequent social or occupational impairment are in excess of what would be expected on the basis of the individual's medical history, physical examination, or laboratory findings.
- The physical complaints are not feigned (as in factitious disorder or malingering).

Treatment

Acute Treatment

- The clinician's most important initial task is to develop a relationship with the patients and to help clarify the biopsychosocial components of their symptoms.
- The clinician may also act as an intermediary for the patient vis-à-vis the medical care system. In essence, they clinician becomes the advocate and joins with the patient in a therapeutic relationship.
- This relationship, grounded in psychotherapy, can begin to form an alliance where, with the patient, the clinician endeavors to educate the patient about the pitfalls, challenges, and problems of evaluating and managing the symptoms of somatization. (The clinician, therefore, becomes the "translator" of the medical and health care system.)
- Symptoms must be understood and conveyed to the patient as (a) real; (b) the cause of suffering in the patient; and (c) frequently disabling.
- *Pharmacological management* needs to focus on symptom relief from antidepressants (selective serotonin reuptake inhibitors [SSRIs] and serotonin-norepinephrine reuptake inhibitors [SNRIs]) for mood instability and anxiety, dual-acting antidepressants for bodily pain relief, and atypical antipsychotics for bizarre, mood

congruent symptoms, such as dissociation, psychosis, or severe anxiety.

Chronic Treatment

- It is essential that the clinician, who manages the patient with this disorder, work in tandem with a primary care team, a psychiatric and mental health nurse practitioner (PMHNP), a psychiatrist, and/or all other members involved in the treatment. Without this collaboration, ongoing treatment will most certainly fail, as the patient needs the communication to be maintained among all members of the health care team.
- Psychotherapy for patients with chronic somatic symptoms is usually more successful if the patient is encouraged to be an active participant in the treatment. For some patients, cognitive-behavioral therapy (CBT) has been found to be useful and for others, psychodynamic psychotherapy is indicated for the patient who is insightful and willing to understand how the past influences the current experience of life, living, and interacting with others.
- It is essential that the patients be offered the opportunity to enter into psychotherapy with a clinician that they trust and also are able to see on a regular basis. Referral to a skilled therapist/clinician is also essential.
- *Pharmacological management* needs to be monitored and titrated to manage the symptoms, which may intensify over time.

Recurrence Rate

- This is often defined as a severe and persistent psychiatric and medical illness that requires ongoing assessment, treatment, management, and communication among the entire treatment team. Recurrence is often attributed to a failure or lack of communication between health care systems and providers.

Patient Education

- *Psychoeducation* in the form of individual therapy or group work can assist the patient to understand the cognitive patterns, behaviors, and how they interrelate with the way the body feels and responds.
- For example, if a patient has been neglected by the medical system or by caretakers, it will be important for the patient to learn new ways of interacting and trusting those who will now assist the patient and manage the care.
- The patients also can be guided to utilize alternative ways to relate to the health care system on the basis of the actual current medical needs. They may need to learn how to separate the "past from the present" so that they can seek health care and participate in the examination and workup rather than being a "casualty" of the health care system where they experience more distress because of not being understood or believed.

Medical/Legal Pitfalls

- Medical neglect and/or abandonment, whether perceived or a reality, are certainly litigious and can be a major pitfall for the clinician.
- It is essential that, if a clinician agrees to manage a patient with a somatoform disorder, the clinician be prepared to be working with the patient over a long period of time. If this is outside of the clinician's scope of practice, it is best that the patient be referred to a more skilled and able clinician.
- Often patients are not solely suffering from somatoform disorders, and comorbidity of other illnesses such as mood and anxiety disorders are prevalent as well as personality disorders. This complexity often leads to a complex treatment plan, which must be adhered to and maintained by all members of the treatment team.
- These patients do develop significant medical problems either iatrogenically or through medical neglect. Therefore, it is essential to provide ongoing assessment, diagnosis, and management in the form of a team-based treatment plan.

Other Resources

Evidence-Based References

American Psychiatric Association. (2000). *Diagnostic and statistical manual of mental disorders* (4th ed., text revised). Washington, DC: American Psychiatric Association.

De Gucht, V. & Fischler, B. (2002). Somatization: A critical review of conceptual and methodological issues. *Psychosomatics, 43*, 1–9.

Fallon, B. (2004). Pharmacotherapy of somatoform disorders. *Journal of Psychosomatic Research, 56*, 455–460.

Ford, C. V. (1983). *The somatizing disorders: Illness as a way of life*. New York: Elsevier Biomedical.

Konijnenberg, A. Y., de Graeff-Meeder, E. R., van der Hoeven, J., Kimpen, J. L., Buitelaar, J. K., Uiterwaal, C. (2006). Psychiatric morbidity in children with medically unexplained chronic pain: Diagnosis from the pediatrician's perspective. *Pediatrics, 117*(3), 889–897.

Loewenstein, R. J. (1990). Somatoform disorders in victims of incest and child abuse. In R. P. Kluft (Ed.), *Incest-related disorders of adult psychopathology* (pp. 75–113). Washington DC: American Psychiatric Press.

Sadock, B. J., & Sadock, V. A. (2008). *Synopsis of psychiatry* (10th ed.). Philadelphia: Lippincott, Williams & Williams.

Sar, V., Akyüz, G., Kundakçı, T., Kızıltan, E., Döğan, O. (2004). Childhood trauma, dissociation, and psychiatric comorbidity in patients with conversion disorder. *American Journal of Psychiatry, 161*, 2271–2276.

Soltis-Jarrett, V. (1997). The facilitator in participatory action research: Les raisons d'être. *Advances in Nursing Science, 20*(2), 45–54.

Soltis-Jarrett, V. (2003). *Finding the health in illness: Challenging the concept of somatization*. Flinders University of South Australia: Unpublished doctoral dissertation.

Soltis-Jarrett, V. (2004). Interactionality: Willfully extending the boundaries of participatory research in psychiatric-mental health nursing. *Advances in Nursing Science, 27*(4), 316–329.

Tylee, A., & Gandhi, P. (2005). The importance of somatic symptoms in depression in primary care. *Journal of Clinical Psychiatry, 7*, 167–176.

van der Kolk, B., Pelcovitz, D., Roth, S., Mandel, E. S., McFarlane, A., & Herman, J. L. (1996). Dissociation, somatization, and affect dysregulation: The complexity of adaptation to trauma. *American Journal of Psychiatry, Festschrift Supplement, 153*, 83–93.

Web Resources

- http://emedicine.medscape. com/article/294908-overview.
- http://psyweb. com/Mdisord/jsp/somatd.jsp.
- http://familydoctor.org/online/famdocen/home/common/pain/disorders/162.html.

Adjustment Disorder with Anxiety

Background Information

Definition of Disorder

- There are excessive emotional or behavioral symptoms due to a psychosocial stressor.
- The symptoms occur within 3 months of the onset of the stressor.
- The emotional reaction is more than what would normally be expected for the situation or cause social or occupational impairment.
- This subtype of adjustment disorder (AD) would have primary symptoms of nervousness, fears, and/or worry.

Etiology

- AD classifications provide a way of classifying mental health symptoms that are significant enough to require treatment, but insufficient to meet the specific criteria for another Axis I disorder.
- ADs have no specific symptoms.
- Any combination of maladaptive responses may qualify if they cause distress, impairment in functioning, are a result of a stressor, and develop within three months of the stressor.
- Frequently occurs in patients with physical diagnoses (e.g., MI, cerebrovascular accident [CVA], human immunodeficiency virus [HIV], DM, cancer, head and neck surgery).
- May be a maladaptive response to multiple, relatively minor stressors, not just one large stressor.
- Stressors more likely to be chronic in adolescents than adults.
- Conclusions from a twin study suggest a genetic link.
- The development of AD is partially determined by the meaning of the stressor to the individual, the strength of the person's "sense of self," history of successfully dealing with stressors, and support network.

Demographics

- Equally affects both men and women
- Can occur in any age group
- Consider the patient's cultural context in the clinical judgment of maladaptive behavior

Risk Factors

- There is a history of poor adaptive behaviors
- In children, there is the lack of a warm and supporting primary caregiver
- Medical illness
- Existing Axis I diagnosis
- Disadvantaged life circumstances

Diagnosis

Differential Diagnosis

- Axis I disorders of depression, anxiety, posttraumatic stress disorder (PTSD), acute stress disorder
- Bereavement
- Other subtypes of AD
- Medication noncompliance
- Psychosocial stressors (V codes)

ICD Code

309.24 Adjustment Disorder with Anxiety

Diagnostic Work-Up

- Physical exam
- Medical and psychiatric history
- Lab as needed to evaluate physical complaints
  - Thyroid function studies (triiodothyronine [T3], thyroxine [T4], thyroid-stimulating hormone [TSH])
  - CMP (complete metabolic panel), including glucose, calcium, albumin; total protein count; levels of sodium, potassium, CO_2 (carbon dioxide and bicarbonate), chloride, blood urea nitrogen (BUN), creatinine, alkaline phosphatase (ALP), alanine amino transferase (ALT, also called SGPT), aspartate amino transferase (AST, also called SGOT), and bilirubin

- CBC (complete blood count) with differentials: hemoglobin, hematocrit, red blood cell (RBC) count, white blood cell (WBC) count, WBC differential count, and platelet count

Initial Assessment

- When did symptoms begin?
- What was going on in your life?
- Any recent major health concerns?
- Have you ever had anything like this before?
- How have these symptoms interfered in your life?
- Any thoughts of harm to yourself or another?

Clinical Presentation Symptoms

- Physical complaints, may be vague
- Avoidance of work or school
- Avoidance of social life
- Emotional distress, feeling overwhelmed, restless, fearful
- In children, fear may be of separation from parents or major attachment figure
- Symptoms developed after an identifiable stressor or multiple stressors
- Eleven percent may have a suicidal ideation

DSM-IV-TR Diagnostic Guidelines

- A psychological response to an identifiable psychosocial stressor that includes the development of clinically significant emotional or behavioral symptoms.
- The symptoms develop within 3 months of the onset of the stressor.
- The individual's distress is in excess of what would be expected on the basis of the level or magnitude of the stressor.
- The symptoms cannot be better accounted for by another psychiatric disorder or the exacerbation of a preexisting psychiatric disorder.
- Diagnosis does not apply in the case of bereavement.
- The maladaptive reactions are not better ascribed to adjustment disorder with depressed mood, adjustment disorder with mixed anxiety and depressed mood, adjustment disorder with disturbance of conduct, adjustment disorder with mixed disturbance of emotions and conduct.

- Symptoms are likely to include jitteriness, worry, nervousness, or fear.
- Duration is as follows: Acute—lasting for less than 6 months. Chronic—lasting for more than 6 months.

Treatment

Acute Treatment

- Identify, limit, or reduce the stressor if possible. ADs secondary to a physical illness often remit after the patient becomes well or learns how to adapt to a chronic illness.
  - Psychotherapy is first-line treatment
    - Cognitive-behavioral, interpersonal or psychodynamic
    - Some areas of therapy: identification of the meaning of the stressor, putting feelings into words, understanding existing strengths and capacities, and developing a support network
  - Psychopharmacology is used when psychotherapy has not been effective. Most often, selective serotonin reuptake inhibitors (SSRIs) or anxiolytics are used judiciously

Chronic Treatment

- Short-term therapy is often sufficient. Ongoing therapy is used if there were preexisting symptoms or to help the individual identify reasons for poor stress tolerance.
- Group therapy can be helpful for individuals with similar stressors (e.g., postmastectomy groups).

Recurrence Rate

- A study looking at hospital readmission rates among patients with ADs and major depressive disorder concluded that the readmission rates are fewer for ADs.

Patient Education

- Encourage basic self-care: healthy diet, exercise, plenty of sleep.
- Avoid alcohol, drugs, caffeine, and any stimulating herbal preparation.
- Keep in contact with friends and family. Enlist their support.

- Learn ways to relax with breathing and muscle relaxation techniques.

Medical/Legal Pitfalls

- Suicide attempts and completions occur with ADs as well as other psychiatric disorders.
- The interval from the start of symptoms to the suicide attempt is shorter in ADs as compared to major depressive disorder.
- Suicide attempts tend to be more impulsive with ADs than other mood disorders.
- There is more deliberate self-harm than with other disorders.

Adjustment Disorder with Depressed Mood

Background Information

Definition of Disorder

There are excessive emotional or behavioral symptoms due to a psychosocial stressor. The symptoms occur within 3 months of the onset of the stressor. The emotional reaction is excessive as compared to what would be normally expected for the situation or cause social or occupational impairment. This subtype of AD would have primary symptoms of depressed mood, frequent tearfulness, and/or a loss of interest in activities.

Etiology

- AD classifications provide a way of classifying mental health symptoms that are significant enough to require treatment, but insufficient to meet the specific criteria for another Axis I disorder.
- ADs have no specific symptoms. Any combination of maladaptive responses may qualify if they cause distress, impairment in functioning, are a result of a stressor, and develop within 3 months of the stressor.
- Frequently occurs in patients with physical diagnoses (e.g., MI, CVA, HIV, DM, cancer, head and neck surgery).
- May be a maladaptive response to multiple, relatively minor stressors, not just one large stressor.
- Stressors are more likely to be chronic in adolescents than adults.
- Conclusions from a twin study suggest a genetic link.
- The development of AD is partially determined by the meaning of the stressor to the individual, the strength of the person's "sense of self," the history of successfully dealing with stressors, and the support network.

Demographics

- Equally affects both men and women
- Can occur in any age group
- Consider the patient's cultural context in the clinical judgment of maladaptive behavior

Risk Factors

- There is a history of poor adaptive behaviors
- In children, there is the lack of a warm and supporting primary caregiver
- Medical illness
- Existing Axis I diagnosis
- Disadvantaged life circumstances

Diagnosis

Differential Diagnosis

- Axis I disorders of depression, anxiety, PTSD, acute stress disorder
- Bereavement
- Other subtypes of AD
- Medication noncompliance
- Psychosocial stressors (V codes)

ICD Code

309.0 Adjustment Reaction with Adjustment Disorder with Depressed Mood

Diagnostic Work-Up

- Physical exam
- Medical and psychiatric history
- Lab as needed to evaluate physical complaints
  - CBC with differentials
  - Chemistry panel
  - Thyroid studies

Initial Assessment

- When did symptoms begin?
- What was going on in your life?
- Any recent major health concerns?
- Have you ever had anything like this before?

- How have these symptoms interfered in your life?
- Any thoughts of harm to yourself or another?

Clinical Presentation
- Physical complaints, patient may be vague.
- Avoidance of work or school
- Avoidance of social life
- Emotional distress, sadness, lack of enjoyment in previously enjoyed activities
- Symptoms developed after an identifiable stressor or multiple stressors.
- Eleven percent may have a suicidal ideation.

DSM-IV-TR Diagnostic Guidelines
- A psychological response to an identifiable psychosocial stressor that includes the development of clinically significant emotional or behavioral symptoms.
- The symptoms develop within 3 months of the onset of the stressor.
- The individual's distress is in excess of what would be expected on the basis of the level of magnitude of the stressor.
- The symptoms cannot be more easily ascribed to another psychiatric disorder or the exacerbation of a preexisting psychiatric disorder.
- Diagnosis does not apply in the case of bereavement.
- The maladaptive reactions are not better classified as adjustment disorder with anxiety, adjustment disorder with disturbance of conduct, or adjustment disorder with mixed disturbance of emotions and conduct.
- Primary symptoms are depressed mood, tearfulness, and/or hopelessness.
- The acute illness lasts less than 6 months. The chronic illness lasts more than 6 months.

Treatment

Acute Treatment
- Identify, limit, or reduce the stressor if possible. ADs secondary to a physical illness often remit after the patient becomes well or learns how to adapt to a chronic illness.
- Psychotherapy is first-line treatment.
- Cognitive-behavioral, interpersonal or psychodynamic therapy.
- Some areas of therapy: identification of the meaning of the stressor, putting feelings into words, understanding existing strengths and capacities, and developing a support network.
- Psychopharmacology is used when psychotherapy has not been effective. Most often, SSRIs or anxiolytics are used judiciously.

Chronic Treatment
- Short-term therapy is often sufficient. Ongoing therapy is used if there were preexisting symptoms or to help the individual identify reasons for poor stress tolerance.
- Group therapy can be helpful for individuals with similar stressors (e.g., postmastectomy groups).

Recurrence Rate
- A study looking at hospital readmission rates among patients with ADs and major depressive disorder concluded the readmission rates are fewer for ADs.

Patient Education
- Encourage the basics. Have patient eat a healthy diet, get moderate exercise, and plenty of sleep.
- Avoid alcohol, drugs, and caffeine.
- Keep in contact with family and friends. Ask for their support.

Medical/Legal Pitfalls
- Suicide attempts and completions occur with ADs as well as other psychiatric disorders.
- The interval from the start of symptoms to the suicide attempt is shorter with ADs as compared to major depressive disorder.
- Suicide attempts tend to be more impulsive with ADs than other mood disorders.
- There is more deliberate self-harm than with other disorders.

Adjustment Disorder, Unspecified

Background Information

Definition of Disorder
There are excessive emotional or behavioral symptoms due to a psychosocial stressor. The symptoms occur within 3 months of the onset of the stressor. The emotional reaction is excessive as compared to what would be normally expected for the situation or cause social or occupational impairment. This subtype of AD would not have *primary* symptoms of depressed mood, anxiety, or disturbance in conduct. It would be possible to see physical complaints, social withdrawal, or avoidance of work or school.

Etiology
- AD classifications provide a way of classifying mental health symptoms that are significant enough to require treatment, but insufficient to meet the specific criteria for another Axis I disorder.
- ADs have no specific symptoms. Any combination of maladaptive responses may qualify if they cause distress, impairment in functioning, are a result of a stressor, and develop within 3 months of the stressor.
- Frequently occurs in patients with physical diagnoses (e.g., MI, CVA, HIV, DM, cancer, head and neck surgery).
- May be a maladaptive response to multiple, relatively minor stressors, not just one large stressor.
- Stressors are more likely to be chronic in adolescents than adults.
- Conclusions from a twin study suggest a genetic link.
- The development of AD is partially determined by the meaning of the stressor to the individual, the strength of the person's "sense of self," the history of successfully dealing with stressors, and the support network.

Demographics
- Equally affects both men and women

- Can occur in any age group
- Consider the patient's cultural context in the clinical judgment of maladaptive behavior

Risk Factors
- There is a history of poor adaptive behaviors
- In children, there is the lack of a warm and supporting primary caregiver
- Medical illness
- Existing Axis I diagnosis
- Disadvantaged life circumstances

Diagnosis

Differential Diagnosis
- Axis I disorders of depression, anxiety, PTSD, acute stress disorder
- Bereavement
- Other subtypes of AD
- Medication noncompliance
- Psychosocial stressors (V codes)

ICD Code
309.9 Unspecified Adjustment Reaction

Diagnostic Work-Up
- Physical exam
- Medical and psychiatric history
- Lab as needed to evaluate physical complaints
  - Thyroid function studies (T3, T4, TSH)
  - CMP, including glucose, calcium, albumin; total protein count; levels of sodium, potassium, CO_2 (carbon dioxide and bicarbonate), chloride, BUN, creatinine, ALP, ALT, AST), and bilirubin
  - CBC with differentials: hemoglobin, hematocrit, RBC count, WBC count, WBC differential count, and platelet count

Initial Assessment
- When did symptoms begin?
- What was going on in your life?
- Any recent major health concerns?
- Have you ever had anything like this before?
- How have these symptoms interfered in your life?
- Any thoughts of harm to yourself or another?

Clinical Presentation

- Physical complaints, patient may be vague
- Avoidance of work or school
- Avoidance of social life
- Emotional distress
- Symptoms developed after an identifiable stressor or multiple stressors
- Eleven percent may have a suicidal ideation

DSM-IV-TR Diagnostic Guidelines

- There is a psychological response to an identifiable psychosocial stressor that includes the development of clinically significant emotional or behavioral symptoms.
- The symptoms develop within 3 months of the onset of the stressor.
- The individual's distress is in excess of what would be expected on the basis of the level of magnitude of the stressor.
- The symptoms cannot be more easily ascribed to another psychiatric disorder or the exacerbation of a preexisting psychiatric disorder.
- Diagnosis does not apply in the case of bereavement.
- The maladaptive reactions are not better classified as adjustment disorder with anxiety, adjustment disorder with mixed anxiety and depressed mood, adjustment disorder with disturbance of conduct, or adjustment disorder with mixed disturbance of emotions and conduct.
- Symptoms for the unspecified subtype are likely to include physical complaints, social withdrawal, and impairment in work or academic performance.

Treatment

Acute Treatment

- Identify, limit, or reduce the stressor if possible. ADs secondary to a physical illness often remit after the patient becomes well or learns how to adapt to a chronic illness.
  - Psychotherapy is first-line treatment.

- Cognitive-behavioral, interpersonal, or psychodynamic.
- Some areas of therapy: identification of the meaning of the stressor, putting feelings into words, understanding existing strengths and capacities, and developing a support network.
- Psychopharmacology is used when psychotherapy has not been effective. Most often, SSRIs or anxiolytics are used judiciously.

Chronic Treatment

- Short-term therapy is often sufficient. Ongoing therapy is used if there were preexisting symptoms or to help the individual identify reasons for poor stress tolerance.
- Group therapy can be helpful for individuals with similar stressors (e.g., postmastectomy groups).

Recurrence Rate

- A study looking at hospital readmission rates among patients with ADs and major depressive disorder concluded that the readmission rates are fewer for ADs.

Patient Education

- Encourage the basics: healthy diet, exercise, plenty of sleep.
- Have patient avoid alcohol, drugs, and caffeine.
- Ask friends and family for support. Keep in contact.
- Stress the importance of following up with mental health treatment.

Medical/Legal Pitfalls

- Suicide attempts and completions occur with ADs as well as other psychiatric disorders.
- The interval from the start of symptoms to the suicide attempt is shorter with ADs as compared to major depressive disorder.
- Suicide attempts tend to be more impulsive with ADs than other mood disorders.
- There is more deliberate self harm than with other disorders.

Dissociative Amnesia

Background Information

Definition of Disorder
- Inability to remember personal information
- Information lost is important and too extensive to be caused by forgetfulness
- Gaps in recall occur usually about traumatic or stressful information
- Is not caused by illness, substance use, or injury to the brain
- Memories are stored in the brain and not retrievable, but lack of recall is reversible

Etiology
- Can occur at any age
- Onset can be gradual or sudden
- Time frame lost can be from minutes to years. Most commonly one episode of lost time, but may be multiple time periods
- Different types of memory loss may occur
- Localized amnesia—inability to remember specific events like an earthquake
- Systematized amnesia—inability to remember categories of information, such as friends
- General amnesia—patients inability to remember anything of their life including their own identity
- Continuous amnesia—inability to remember events in the past and up to the current time
- Frequency increases during wartime or natural disasters

Demographics
- Occurs more frequently in women than men.
- Can occur at any age past infancy.
- Occurs most frequently at ages 30–50.
- Approximately, 2–7% of population is affected.
- Controversial as a scientific diagnosis. Difference in how American and Canadian psychiatrists view dissociative amnesia. Only 13% of Canadian psychiatrists think there is strong scientific validity to include it as a mental health diagnosis.

Risk Factors
- Victims of sexual abuse, domestic violence, trauma, combat.

- Difficult to diagnose prior to puberty because inability to remember events prior to age 4 is normal.
- Appears to occur also in other family members, suggesting a possible genetic link.
- Comorbidities: conversion disorders, bulimia nervosa, alcohol abuse, depression, personality disorders (borderline, dependent, histrionic).

Diagnosis

Differential Diagnosis
- Seizure disorder
- Head injury
- Alcohol or substance intoxication
- Korsakoff's disease
- Medication side effect
- Sleep deprivation
- Brain disease
- Delirium or dementia
- Other dissociative disorders
- Malingering factitious disorder

ICD Code
300.12 Dissociative Amnesia

Diagnostic Work-Up
- Diagnosis of exclusion
- Medical and psychiatric history
- Labs as needed to evaluate physical complaints:
  - Thyroid function studies (T3, T4, TSH)
  - CMP, including glucose, calcium, albumin; total protein count; levels of sodium, potassium, CO_2 (carbon dioxide and bicarbonate), chloride, BUN, creatinine, ALP, ALT, AST, and bilirubin
  - CBC with differentials: hemoglobin, hematocrit, RBC count, WBC count, WBC differential count, and platelet count
- Psychological exam to include possible screening:
  - The dissociative experiences scale (DES): this is a self-report screen
  - The Structured Clinical Interview for *DSM-IV* Dissociative Disorders (SCID-D): this is a

guided interview; it is the "gold standard" in diagnosis of dissociative disorders, but time consuming

Initial Assessment

- Is the amnesia transient or persistent?
- Has there been a recent blow to the head?
- Is there fever?
- Is recent memory intact?
- Any recent medication or substance?
- Functional limitations?

Clinical Presentation

- Loss of memory of important life events is usually retrograde (traumatic event is prior to amnesia).
- The unconscious memories influence the conscious state.
  - A rape victim may not remember being raped, but may act like a victim of a violent crime
  - Demoralization and detachment
  - Mild depression and/or anxiety
  - Agitation at stimuli related to the unrecalled traumatic event

DSM-IV-TR Diagnostic Guidelines

- One or more episodes of the inability to recall important personal information (often though not necessarily of stressful or threatening import).
- The deficit is too extensive to be ascribed to ordinary forgetfulness.
- The disturbance does not occur concurrently with dissociative identity disorder, dissociative fugue, somatization disorder, or posttraumatic stress disorder.
- The disturbance is not the direct physiological effect of substance use or a neurological or other condition.
- The symptoms engender distress in the individual and impairment of social functioning.

Treatment

Acute Treatment

- Initially supportive therapy and creating a safe environment may restore past memories.

- Hypnosis
  - Age regression may help patients access previously unavailable memories.
  - Screen technique—recalling the traumatic event on an imaginary movie screen, allowing the patient to separate the psychological from the somatic aspects of the memory to make it more bearable. Assists with the cognitive restructuring of the trauma. Patients who are not highly hypnotizable may benefit from this technique.
- Medication if there is depression and/or anxiety:
  - Usually SSRIs, SNRIs, anxiolytics, or atypical antipsychotics for severe symptoms.

Chronic Treatment

- Psychotherapy is used to strengthen the ego, find new ways to cope, improve relationships, and optimize functioning.

Recurrence Rate

- Rarely recurs

Patient Education

- Advise patients to avoid alcohol and drugs.
- Encourage healthy lifestyle and treatment follow-up.
- Online resources: Cleveland Clinic, National Alliance on Mental Health (NAMI), Psychcentral.org (also support group information).

Medical/Legal Pitfalls

- Criminal cases have involved the recall of previously "repressed" memories of abuse. It is not completely accepted that recovery of repressed memories exists. Some argue that false memories can occur through the power of suggestion during therapy. The position of the American Psychological Association is that a recovered memory cannot be distinguished from a false memory without corroborating information.

Other Resources

Evidence-Based References

American Psychiatric Association. (2000). *Diagnostic and statistical manual of mental disorders* (4th ed.). Washington, DC: American Psychiatric Association.

Collins, R. D. (2003). *Algorithmic diagnosis of symptoms and signs.* Philadelphia: Lippincott, Williams & Wilkins.

Jones, R. (2002). Readmission rates for adjustment disorders: Comparison with other mood disorders. *Journal of Affective Disorders, 71*(1), 199–203.

Kay, J., & Tasman, A. (2006). *Essentials of psychiatry.* West Sussex, England: John Wiley & Sons.

Sadock, B., & Sadock, V. (2000). *Kaplan & Sadock's comprehensive textbook of psychiatry* (7th ed.). Philadelphia: Lippincott, Williams & Wilkins.

Steinberg, M., Barr, D., Sholomskas, D., & Hall, P. (2005). SCL-90 symptom patterns: Indicators of dissociative disorders. *Bulletin of the Menninger Clinic, 69*(3), 237–249.

Web Resources

- http://www.psychcentral.com.
- Freedom from Fear: http://www.freedomfromfear.org. Information on anxiety and mental health treatment, not specifically adjustment disorders.
- International Society for the Study of Dissociation: http://www.issd.org.
- National Institute of Mental Health: http://www.nimh.nih.gov.
- WebMD: http://www.webmd. com.

13. SEXUAL DYSFUNCTION
Female Sexual Arousal Disorder

Background Information

Definition of Disorder
- There is a persistent or recurrent inability to attain or maintain the arousal response of sexual excitement
- Marked distress or interpersonal difficulty
- Dysfunction cannot be better accounted for by another Axis I disorder except another sexual dysfunction
- It cannot exclusively be the result of a substance, medication, or general medical disorder
- The normal sexual arousal response consists of vasocongestion of the pelvis, vaginal lubrication and expansion, and swelling of the external genitalia

Etiology
- May be due to psychologic cause, organic cause, or a combination of both
- Psychologic causes include relationship issues, cognitive and affective factors, and cultural and societal factors
- Relationship issues can stem from communication difficulties inside and outside the bedroom and can be the sole issue behind arousal dysfunction
- Depression and anxiety affect arousal
- Anxiety (an emotional response, not just having the trait for anxiety) which is produced just before erotic stimuli will decrease subjective arousal in women
- Stress, worry, obsessive thoughts and behaviors, history of sexual abuse, and panic attacks also affect arousal
- Women who are unhappy with their physical bodies can have problems with arousal
- Organic causes include endocrine dysfunction, autonomic nervous system (ANS) dysfunction, and cardiovascular/medicine issues
- Most often, the causes are combined
- For sexual arousal to occur in women, normal amounts of estrogens and androgens must be present along with a normal, functioning sympathetic nervous system
- Women with decreased or absent estrogen production have reduced tissue sensitivity of the vagina and vulva and decreased or absent vaginal lubrication
- ANS dysfunction includes spinal cord lesions
- Cardiovascular issues include vascular disease and hypertension
- Female sexual arousal disorder may be lifelong or acquired and situational or generalized

Demographics
- Arousal difficulties are present in 64% women seeking sex therapy.
- Prevalence statistics differ depending on the instruments in the study.
- Literature reports vary on prevalence statistics due to unstandardized approaches in studying female sexual disorders.
- It is fairly uncommon for a premenopausal woman to have an arousal problem without a decreased libido.
- Antidepressants and antipsychotics are two common classes of drugs that may interfere with orgasm.

Risk Factors
- Age: can develop at any age
- Family history: there is no evidence that this disorder is familial
- Stressful events in susceptible people: stressful events in one's life and stressful situations between couples may be the sole cause of this disorder
- Having another mental disorder
- More likely to have another sexual function disorder
- Also likely to have a mood or anxiety disorder

Diagnosis

Differential Diagnosis
- Sexual dysfunction due to a general medical disorder
- Substance-induced sexual disorder

- Another Axis I disorder (major depressive disorder, etc.)
- Occasional problems with sexual arousal
- History of rape, physical, and/or sexual abuse
- Current rape, physical, and/or sexual abuse
- Relationship conflict
- Significant stress
- Menopause

ICD Codes
302.72 Psychosexual Dysfunction, Sexual Excitement

Diagnostic Work-Up
- Complete history, physical exam, and mental evaluation
- Labs as needed to evaluate physical complaints:
  - Thyroid function studies (triiodothyronine [T3], thyroxine [T4], thyroid-stimulating hormone [TSH])
  - CMP (complete metabolic panel), including glucose, calcium, albumin; total protein count; levels of sodium, potassium, CO_2 (carbon dioxide and bicarbonate), chloride, blood urea nitrogen (BUN), creatinine, alkaline phosphatase (ALP), alanine amino transferase (ALT, also called SGPT), aspartate amino transferase (AST, also called SGOT), and bilirubin
  - CBC (complete blood count) with differentials: hemoglobin, hematocrit, red blood cell (RBC) count, white blood cell (WBC) count, WBC differential count, and platelet count

Initial Assessment
- Medical history with detailed social history
- Psychiatric history
- Traumatic history (including any form of abuse)
- Sexual history
- Current medication use
- Any recent changes in medication?
- Have you ever had problems with attaining arousal? If so, for how long?
- Have you ever had a problem with lubrication? If so, for how long?
- Does this problem occur only in a certain situation or with a certain partner?

- Do you have difficulty with arousal only while masturbating or using a vibrator?
- How long does it take to become aroused now, compared with the past?
- What effect is this having in your relationship?
- Did any emotional or other life stress occur when the problems with arousal began?
- When did you undergo menopause?
- Have you ever had your ovaries removed?
- Have you ever taken hormone replacement therapy?
- What brought you to seek treatment now?
- What effect is this problem having on your daily functioning?
- Do you feel safe with your partner?
- Have you ever been threatened or harmed by him in any way?

Treatment

Acute Treatment
- Interventions include psychologic and biologic interventions.
- Psychologic therapy consists of marital therapy, explorations of emotions from abuse, psychotherapy for trust and intimacy issues, and cognitive-behavioral therapy (CBT).
  - There is limited evidence of effectiveness in CBT therapy for this disorder.
  - CBT consists of identifying and correcting dysfunctional attitudes toward sexual pleasure, masturbation, and sensate focus.
  - Emphasis is also on couple communication.
- Biologic therapy includes:
  - For decreased lubrication, there are lubricants, and estrogen-related products
    - In postmenopausal patients, be cautious using estrogen-related products
    - These products may increase risk of breast cancer
  - Eros
    - Clitoral vacuum device approved by FDA
  - Zestra
    - Botanical massage, oil is applied to vulva
    - Investigation for efficacy is ongoing
  - Phosphodiesterase inhibitors and alprostadil

- ◆ Only one study with unreplicated results showed any promise of these medications helping women with sexual arousal disorder and normal libido.
- ◆ Sildenafil and nitric oxide do increase the physical arousal stage but do not affect the subjective arousal feelings in women with this disorder.

Chronic Treatment
- Continue psychologic therapy to completion
- Continue medication with regular follow-up
- Patients should be aware that this condition may recur and treatment may not be permanent

Recurrence Rate
More research needs to be done on this subject with more studies using standardized instruments.

Clinical Presentation
- No specific physical symptoms.
- Patients may be in distress if treatment has not worked or if this disorder recurs after treatment.

Patient Education
- Information regarding this disorder can be found at the Merck Web site under the subject of sexual dysfunction in women.
- For more patient education resources, visit eMedicine's Web site under the topic of female sexual problems and visit familydoctor.org under "sexual dysfunction in women."

Medical/Legal Pitfalls
- Patients may become very frustrated if treatments do not work.
- In some cases, therapy will not work unless the patient's partner agrees with therapy.
- Patients may try herbal supplements in attempts to increase arousal.
- Patient should be counseled on side effects and interactions of supplements with other medications.
- Arousal difficulties may be due to cardiovascular issues; patients should be screened for hypertension and vascular disease.

Gender Identity Disorder

Background Information

Definition of Disorder
- Must have evidence of strong and persistent desire to be of the opposite sex or the patients insisting on being the opposite sex.
  - Must not only be a desire to have cultural advantages of the opposite sex.
- Patient has persistent discomfort about the patient's sex or feels the gender role is inappropriate.
- This disorder cannot be diagnosed in a person with an intersex disorder (congenital adrenal hyperplasia, etc.).
- It is essential to the diagnosis that the patient has clinically significant distress or impairment in social, occupational, or other areas of functioning.

Etiology
- Unknown etiology
- One theory involves structure formation of the uncinate nucleus

Demographics
- The most recent statistics show a less than 1% prevalence in the general population
  - 1:12,900 for male-to-female (MtF) transsexualism
  - 1:33,800 for female-to-male (FtM) transsexualism
- MtF transsexualism is 2–3 times more prevalent than FtM transsexualism.
- Age of onset is often in early childhood with one report of onset in a child less than 3 years old.
- FtM transsexuals and the homosexual MtF usually apply for sex reassignment surgery in their 20s.
- Heterosexual MtF usually applies for sex reassignment surgery much later.
- These patients usually have married and fathered children before applying.
- Those with this disorder will either continue to have unresolved issues with gender, will accept their birth gender, will have part-time cross-gender behavior, or will have sex reassignment surgery.

Risk Factors
Age
- Age of development varies.
- Most common ages of onset of gender dysphoria reported are from younger than 3 years old to middle childhood.

Gender
- This disorder is found in both genders.
- Men are affected 2–3 times more often than women.

Family History
- There is no evidence that this disorder runs in families.

Stressful Events in Susceptible People
- Significant crisis or loss may worsen this disorder. Once the crisis or loss is resolved, the patient usually returns to baseline.

Having Another Mental Disorder
- Higher likelihood of having schizophrenia, affective psychosis, or adjustment disorder.
- They are more likely to have substance abuse problems, although statistics vary on prevalence.
- Also more likely to have a personality disorder, have attempted suicide in the past, have engaged in self-harm behavior, have an increased risk for violence (assault, rape, attempted rape), HIV infection, and other sexually transmitted diseases (STDs).

Diagnosis

Differential Diagnosis
- Nonconformity to stereotypical sex-role behavior
- Transvestic fetishism
- Gender identity disorder not otherwise specified (persons with intersex conditions)
- Schizophrenia and other psychotic conditions
- Dissociative identity disorder
- Cluster B personality disorder
- Gender nonconformity

ICD Codes
302.6: if diagnosis is during childhood
302.85: if diagnosis is during adolescence or adulthood

Diagnostic Work-Up
- Complete history, physical exam, and mental evaluation

Initial Assessment
- Complete medical history
- Sexual history
- Psychiatric history
- Psychosexual development
- For how long have you felt you are of the opposite sex?
- What brought you to seek help now?
- What is your sexual orientation?
- How do you feel about your body?
- Are you currently in a relationship?
- Tell me your feelings related to your birth gender.
- How were you raised?
- Did your family raise you in your birth gender?
- Do you have a social support system?
- What is your occupation?
- What outcome are you looking for? (counseling, sex reassignment surgery, etc.)

Laboratory Tests
None are relevant to diagnosis of this disorder.

Treatment

Acute Treatment
- Psychodynamic psychotherapy focused toward acceptance of birth gender has been the accepted therapy for years.
  - Multiple studies have been unable to determine exact efficacy of psychodynamic psychotherapy
  - Patients with any of the following characteristics are most likely to respond to this therapy:
    - Patient treated and controlled comorbid psychological problems
    - Religious beliefs inconsistent with sex reassignment surgery
    - Anatomic features preventing passing as the opposite sex despite sex reassignment surgery (extremely tall stature or very large size)
      - Fear of losing spouse, children, and alienating other family members
  - Individual psychotherapy can also help the patient
    - It provides a safe setting for the patient to discuss feelings and concerns
    - This is recommended but not required during real-life experience
  - Group psychotherapy is also helpful for patients
    - It provides a supporting environment
- Hormone therapy
  - This is used in those who decide to not undergo sex reassignment surgery but still want to be the opposite gender part-time
  - These patients will undergo either masculinizing or feminizing hormonal therapy
  - Episodically they will live as the opposite sex
  - This occurs more often in cross-dressing adult males and less often in adult females with this disorder
- Real-life experience
  - Homosexual MtF transsexuals usually will undergo this "test"
  - Heterosexual MtF transsexuals are least likely to undergo this "test"
  - FtM transsexuals usually have an easier time with this "test" than the other two groups
  - There are irreversible social consequences to living as the opposite sex without surgery
  - This is usually done while taking hormone therapy
- Sex reassignment surgery
  - This is a permanent solution
  - The patient must have a thorough evaluation before being allowed to undergo surgery
  - They must also have either completed at least 1 year of cross-sex hormone therapy or at least 1 year of real-life experience in their gender role
  - The process to completely become the opposite sex takes years to decades

Chronic Treatment
- Psychotherapy
  - About 50% of those undergoing evaluation or psychotherapy for this disorder will stop treatment

- Some, but not all, return to treatment at a later time
- Reasons for not continuing therapy include impatience, seeing the therapist as unempathetic, expensiveness of therapy, or decision not to resolve gender identity problem
- Hormone therapy
- Sex reassignment surgery:
  - This is the most permanent solution
  - The surgery takes place in stages
  - The physical transition may take place over years but the complete emotional, psychological, and identity changes may take decades

Recurrence Rate
Depends on the patient, the outcome decided by the patient, and other factors.

Clinical Presentation
- No specific physical symptoms are related to this disorder
- They may have symptoms related to hormonal therapy or surgical procedures

Patient Education
- Information on gender identity disorder can be found at www.merck. com under the Merck manual of diagnosis and therapy (psychiatric disorders, then sexuality and sexual disorders, then gender identity disorder).

- E-medicine (emedicine.medscape. com) also has a good Web site under the topic of psychiatry and sexual and gender identity disorders.

Medical/Legal Pitfalls
- During acute psychotic episodes, those with bipolar disorder, schizophrenia, and other psychotic disorders may have delusions of becoming the opposite sex.
- Care should be taken to diagnose and treat these conditions before jumping ahead toward treatment.
- Treatment of the psychotic disorders will resolve the desire to become the opposite sex.
- Those with antisocial or borderline personality disorders will also seek sex reassignment surgery for unrelated reasons.
- Sex hormone therapy often leads to permanent sterilization, so patients should be counseled on sperm/egg preservation.
- Estrogen therapy can cause thrombosis, pulmonary embolism, and they should be monitored for insulin resistance.
- Testosterone therapy may predispose the patient for cardiovascular disease; regular screening should be done, including lipid profiles and tests for insulin resistance.
- Patients undergoing sex hormone therapy should be monitored for cancer.
  - Ovarian malignant changes and endometrial hyperplasia with testosterone therapy.

Hypoactive Sexual Desire Disorder

Background Information

Definition of Disorder

- Patient must have persistent or recurrent deficient or absent sexual fantasies and desire for sexual behavior.
- Factors affecting sexual functioning must be taken into account.
- There must be marked distress or interpersonal difficulty due to decreased or absent desire.
- This problem cannot be better attributed to another Axis I disorder.
- This problem cannot be better attributed to a general medical condition.
- Patient usually does not initiate sexual encounters.
- When the partner initiates sexual encounter, the patient is reluctant to engage in activity.
- Patient usually has diminished expression when deprived of sexual expression.
- The patient usually has low frequency of sexual activity, unless patient is pressured by partner or wants nonsexual needs met (physical comfort, intimacy).
- Patient may have a partner with excessive sexual desire.

Etiology

- May be physiological, psychological, situational, or environmental.
- Androgens, which are linked to sexual desire, are produced by the female body and production decreases with age.
- This change occurs independent of menopause.
- Oral contraceptives may increase sex hormone binding globulin, leading to a decrease in free testosterone levels and sexual desire.
- Low sexual desire has been correlated with hyperprolactinemia.
- Not all patients with chronic hyperprolactinemias have low sexual desire.
- Worry, low self-esteem, stress, abuse, negative sexual attitudes, longer relationship duration, low partner attractiveness, and low outcome expectancy can cause decreased sexual desire.
- Having another sexual disorder or having a partner with a sexual disorder may decrease desire.
- Low sexual desire has not been linked with illicit drug or alcohol use.

Demographics

- Present in almost 20% of entire U.S. population.
- Several studies indicate that this disorder is on the rise.
- CBT therapy is not very effective.
- According to data, sexual desire difficulties are the most reported female sexual complaint.
- Increased incidence occurs in those with mood and anxiety disorders.
- In untreated patients, this disorder is more prevalent in those with mood disorders.
- Prevalence of hypoactive sexual desire is higher among those with mood and anxiety disorders than in the general population.
- Prevalence statistics differ depending on the instruments in the study.

Risk Factors

Age
- May develop at any age
- Is more common after menopause

Gender
- Is more common in women

Family History
- There is no evidence that this disorder runs in families

Stressful Events in Susceptible People
- Abuse or a traumatic event may cause this disorder

Having Another Mental Disorder
- Patient is more likely to have another coexisting sexual disorder
- Patient is more likely to have schizophrenia or another psychosis

- Patient is more likely to have a mood or anxiety disorder
- Patient is may be more likely to have premenstrual disorder

Diagnosis

Differential Diagnosis

- This sexual dysfunction may be due to a general medical condition (female androgen insufficiency, chronic renal failure, hyperprolactinemia, pregnancy, and lactation)
- Substance-induced sexual dysfunction
- Another Axis I disorder (major depressive disorder, etc.)
- History of rape, physical, and/or sexual abuse
- Current rape, physical, and/or sexual abuse
- Relationship conflict
- Significant stress
- Menopause

ICD Codes

302.71 Psychosexual Dysfunction with Hypoactive Sexual Desire

Diagnostic Work-Up

- Complete history, physical, and mental exam.
- The patient should complete one of the following to aid in diagnosis and treatment: the sexual interest and desire inventory—female, Hurlbert index of sexual desire, or sexual desire inventory questionnaire.

Initial Assessment

- Medical history with detailed social history
- Psychiatric history
- Traumatic history (including any form of abuse)
- Sexual history
- Current medication use
- Any recent changes in medication?
- Have you ever had problems with low or absent sexual desire?
- For how long have you had low or absent sexual desire?
- Does this problem only occur in a certain situation or with a certain partner?
- Do you have decreased desire to masturbate or use a vibrator?

- What effect is this having in your relationship?
- Did any emotional or other stressful life event occur when you began to have decreased or absent sexual desire?
- When did you undergo menopause?
- Have you ever had your ovaries removed?
- Have you ever taken hormone replacement therapy?
- Do you feel safe with your partner?
- Have you ever been threatened or harmed by him in any way?
- What brought you to seek treatment now?
- What effect is this decreased/absent sexual desire having on your daily functioning?
- Is there anything you do not like or do not feel comfortable with in your sexual encounters?
- Do you feel like your partner pushes you or is upset with your decreased desire?
- Do you ever have problems attaining orgasm?
- Do you have pain during sex?

Laboratory Tests

- Physical exam
- Medical and psychiatric history
- Lab as needed to evaluate physical complaints:
  - Thyroid function studies (T3, T4, TSH)
  - CMP, including glucose, calcium, albumin; total protein count; levels of sodium, potassium, CO_2 (carbon dioxide and bicarbonate), chloride, BUN, creatinine, ALP, ALT, AST), and bilirubin
  - CBC with differentials: hemoglobin, hematocrit, RBC count, WBC count, WBC differential count, and platelet count
  - Hormone level determination: testosterone, dehydroepiandrosterone sulfate (DHEA-S), sex hormone binding globulin levels, and prolactin

Treatment

Acute Treatment

- If hypoactive desire is the only symptom, outcome for this disorder is especially poor
- According to some literature, this disorder is highly resistant to treatment, with low long-term success rates

- Psychologic therapy
  - Marital therapy
  - Sexual therapy
    - May include sex education
    - May include instruction on sexual techniques and orgasm consistency training
    - May encourage increased recognition and perception of pleasurable body sensations
  - Individual and/or couples counseling:
    - In individual counseling, the patient may include exploration of emotions from abuse, therapy for trust and intimacy issues, and understanding of conscious versus unconscious motives in not desiring sex
    - Couples counseling may include sex education but also communication issues
  - Cognitive-behavioral therapy:
    - There is limited evidence of the effectiveness in CBT therapy for this disorder
    - CBT consists of identifying and correcting dysfunctional attitudes toward sexual pleasure, masturbation, and sensate focus
    - Emphasis is also on couples communication
- Biologic therapy
  - Sexual education counseling with patient and partner if necessary
  - Androgens
    - Testosterone patches, gels, and intramuscular (IM) injections have been used since the 1940s
    - Most often used for low sexual desire at post-oophorectomy
    - If using IM injection, monitor serum free-testosterone levels after 3 months and monitor lipids
    - Tibolone has also been used with good results
    - New recommendations include androgen therapy in women with normal estrogen levels or androgen therapy along with estrogen therapy for postmenopausal women (natural and surgical)
  - Dehydroepiandrosterone (DHEA)
    - It is available as nutritional supplement in the United States, therefore not regulated by FDA
      - Some forms are not bioavailable
      - Studies on efficacy have resulted in conflicting data
  - Drugs depleting serotonin or augmenting dopamine:
    - One is apomorphine, used for erectogenic properties in men
    - Clinical trials for women were conducted, but the results were not published.
    - The company is no longer conducting trials for female sexual dysfunction
    - Bupropion (Wellbutrin) may help with sexual arousal in nondepressed, postmenopausal women
    - Compared to other antidepressants, bupropion (Wellbutrin) and nefazodone (Dutonin) seem to have the least effect on female sexual function
  - Flibanserin and other 5-HT$_{1a}$ agonists
    - May reverse selective serotonin reuptake inhibitor (SSRI) sexual side effects without decreasing SSRI efficacy
    - Research is currently being conducted

Chronic Treatment
- Continue care under a psychiatrist until psychologic therapy is complete
- Continue medication with regular follow-up with a physician

Recurrence Rate
- There are varied reports of recurrence
- More studies need to be done with standardized questionnaires

Clinical Presentation
- No physical symptoms, although patient may appear in distress if the problem is still ongoing at follow-up

Patient Education
- Information regarding this disorder can be found at the Merck Web site under the topic of sexual dysfunction in women.
- For more patient education resources, visit eMedicine's Web site under the topic of female

sexual problems and familydoctor.org under the subject of sexual dysfunction in women.

Medical/Legal Pitfalls

- Patients may become very frustrated if treatments do not work.

- In some cases, therapy will not work unless the patient's partner agrees with therapy.
- If a history of sexual abuse, or current sexual abuse, is admitted by the patient, she needs to be screened for posttraumatic stress disorder (PTSD) and depression.

Voyeurism

Background Information

Definition of Disorder
- Observation of an unsuspecting person who is naked, disrobing, or in a sexual act.
- Most of the unsuspecting persons are strangers.
- The act of "peeping" is for the observer to achieve sexual excitement.
- Sexual activity with the unsuspecting person is not usually sought.
- Orgasm may occur during the initial observation or later while reminiscing.
- The voyeur may later have fantasies involving the person observed.
- In reality, sexual acts with the observed person rarely occur.
- The most severe form is the voyeur observing only sexual activity.
- This behavior usually begins before 15 years of age and is a chronic condition.
- In more severe forms, voyeurs will spend a very large amount of time seeking out observation opportunities.

Etiology
- The exact etiology is unknown.
- May be due to an unfortunate learning history secondary to conditioning, modeling, and reinforcement.
- From a psychoanalytical perspective, three key occurrences are present in voyeurs:
  - Hypercathexis (preoccupation with visual function): this is often found in artists and mathematicians, but not solely in these two classes of people.
  - Postnatal experience with the mother: this includes early visual exchanges and fear of loss of her and her breasts.
  - Early trauma in the first or second year of life: this trauma must severely affect the mother and child's relationship. This may lead to pregenital fixation and other problems with the ego and superego.
- From a biologic perspective, in the past, voyeurs have been thought to have high testosterone levels, although most current research shows that testosterone levels in voyeurs are in the normal range.
- It is currently thought that voyeurs have an abnormal androgen receptor, either enhanced or producing an abnormal response to androgens.
- Therapy causing hypoandrogenism has been highly effective in suppressing voyeuristic desires, behaviors, and the relapse of both.

Demographics
- The exact incidence and prevalence are unknown.
- Voyeurism is not included in national mental health questionnaires.

Risk Factors
Age
- Begins to develop in adolescence and early adulthood
- Persists throughout life

Gender
- Men have this disorder at least twice as often as women
- Men are more likely to have risk-taking behaviors associated with this disorder

Family History
- There is no evidence that this disorder is directly related to family history

Stressful Events in Susceptible People
- There is no association between this disorder and stressful events

Having Another Mental Disorder
- Men with a hypersexual disorder are more likely to have voyeurism or another paraphilia or paraphilia-related disorder than the general population.
  - Those diagnosed with voyeurism have a higher likelihood of having another mental disorder than the general population.

- They are also more likely to have another paraphilia than the general population.
- Those with voyeurism have more risk-taking behavior (substance use and sexual behavior).

Diagnosis

Differential Diagnosis
- Other paraphilia disorders
- Obsessive-compulsive disorder

ICD Codes
302.9 Paraphilia Not Otherwise Specified

Diagnostic Work-Up
- The diagnosis is based on the patient's history and honesty.
- Legal records and other medical records can help identify voyeurs.
- Physical and mental evaluation

Initial Assessment
- Medical history
- Family history
- Social history
- Sexual history
- Psychosexual history
- Psychiatric history
- Legal history
- For how long has patient been having voyeuristic desires?
- For how long has patient been acting out on those desires?
- How is the behavior affecting personal relationships?
- Amount of time spent seeking out places to observe people?
- Amount of time spent seeking out people to observe?
- When and where they tend to occur?
- What effect do they have on the patient's ability to function?

Laboratory Tests
- Physical exam
- Medical and psychiatric history
- Lab as needed to evaluate physical complaints:
  - Thyroid function studies (T3, T4, TSH)

- CMP, including glucose, calcium, albumin; total protein count; levels of sodium, potassium, CO_2 (carbon dioxide and bicarbonate), chloride, BUN, creatinine, ALP, ALT, AST), and bilirubin
- CBC with differentials: hemoglobin, hematocrit, RBC count, WBC count, WBC differential count, and platelet count
- Free and total serum testosterone levels
- The following should be done before medical treatment:
  - Pregnancy test

Treatment

Acute Treatment
- The goal of therapy is to decrease or completely extinguish voyeuristic desires and actions without a recurrence of these desires and behaviors.
- Treatment consists of psychotherapy and/or medication.
- Surgical castration has been used in the past but is not commonly used today due to ethical/legal concerns.
- Psychotherapy includes behavior, cognitive, and group therapy.
- Behavioral and cognitive strategies attempt to make the social context of voyeurism unfavorable.
  - Use of aversion therapy:
    - Pair the deviant but pleasurable stimulus with some painful stimulus.
  - Classical conditioning:
    - Patient masturbates to deviant but pleasurable stimulus (fantasy, etc.) and approaches orgasm, but, right before orgasm, changes the stimulus to a nondeviant and pleasurable stimulus.
    - This links orgasm (pleasurable stimulus) with nondeviant and pleasurable stimuli.
- Group therapy works very well but, if used alone, may take 6 months to several years to extinguish behavior.
  - Provides support from other voyeurs.
  - Works well to reverse incorrect beliefs (all disrobing women like to be watched, even if they are unaware of it).
- Improves insight and knowledge base.

- Compared to group therapy for other topics, these groups take longer for members to become completely comfortable with each other.
- Medications commonly used in the United States are antiandrogenic (medroxyprogesterone acetate, nafarelin, leuprolide, flutamide, triptorelin) and psychotropic (fluoxetine, paroxetine [Aropax], fluvoxamine [Favarin]).
- More double-blind controlled studies need to be done on medication use.
- Antiandrogens seem to produce better results than psychotropics.

Chronic Treatment
- Treatment consists of surgical castration or continuation of acute treatment (psychotherapy or medication).
- Surgical castration was used in the past but is now rarely used.
- It has the lowest relapse rate but is permanent as compared to other treatments.
- The effectiveness of chronic treatment with psychological and medical therapy depends on patient compliance.
- Group therapy is considered the best psychological therapy to use, although behavioral and cognitive therapies are good as well.
- Patients with surgical castration or on antiandrogen therapy should be monitored for liver function changes and signs/symptoms related to hypogonadism and hypoandrogenism.
- Hypogonadism and hypoandrogenism caused by long-acting gonadotropin-releasing hormone (GNRH) analogues can be reversed with small doses of testosterone (25–50 mg) monthly.
- This regimen alleviates the side effects with no increase in voyeuristic desires or behaviors.

Recurrence Rate
- Recurrence rate depends on the method of treatment used.
- The highest recurrence rate found after surgical castration was 7.4%.

- Average recurrence rate for medical castration using antiandrogens reaches 6–7%.
- More research needs to be done on recurrence rate when using antidepressants.
- Those medically castrated with a long-acting GNRH inhibitor have the lowest rate of recurrence compared to the other antiandrogen.

Clinical Presentation
- No biologic symptoms or signs help diagnose this disorder.
- If following up for medication use, look for side effects (liver failure, etc.).
- Psychologic symptoms may include mental distress over the patients' behavior.
- May have stress-related symptoms if problem is interfering with important relationships.

Patient Education
- A good support system can help with rehabilitation and prevent relapse.
- Support systems can include spouse, partner, therapist, therapy group, counselor, etc.
- For patient education resources, visit MD Consult's patient education page on voyeurism.
- Contact a mental health specialist for information on treatment.

Medical/Legal Pitfalls
- Voyeurs may be arrested and imprisoned; teens are less likely to be arrested than adults.
- Charges are more likely to be pressed if there are other concurrent legal problems or past legal issues.
- Those with this disorder are more likely to have psychological problems.
- Those with this disorder may have problems with interpersonal relationships, hypersexuality, or other paraphilias.
- Those with one paraphilia are more likely to have a second.
- They also have a higher incidence of risk-taking behaviors, leading to STDs, substance-use-related issues, and other sequelae.

Other Resources

Evidence-Based References

American Psychiatric Association. (1994). *Diagnostic and statistical manual of mental disorders (DSM-IV)* (4th ed.). Washington, DC: American Psychiatric Association.

Bancroft, J. (1989). *Human sexuality and its problems* (2nd ed.). Edinburgh: Churchill Livingstone.

Covington, S. (1991). *Awakening your sexuality*. San Francisco: Harper.

Cranston-Cuebas, M. A., & Barlow, D. H. (1990). Cognitive and affective contributions to sexual functioning. *Annual Review of Sex Research, 1*, 119–162.

Fisher, R., & Brown, S. (1988). *Getting together*. Boston: Houghton Mifflin.

Haas, K., & Haas, A. (1993). *Understanding human sexuality*. St. Louis: Mosby.

Lipsius, S. H. (1987). Prescribing sensate focus without proscribing intercourse. *Journal of Sex and Marital Therapy, 13*(2), 106–116.

Masters, W. H., & Johnson, V. E. (1970). *Human sexual inadequacy*. London: Churchill.

Mathers, N., et al. (1994). Assessment of training in psychosexual medicine. *BMJ, 308*, 969–972.

Pollack, M. H., Reiter, S., & Hammerness, P. (1992). Genitourinary and sexual adverse effects of psychotropic medication. *International Journal of Psychiatry in Medicine, 22*(4), 305–327.

Paraphilias

Background Information

Definition of Disorder
- A paraphilia is an attraction that is outside the normal range of sex.
- The term "paraphilia" has replaced earlier terms, "sexual perversion" and "sexual deviation."
- "Paraphilia" comes from the Greek terms "*para*," meaning along the side, and "*philia*," meaning love.
- Most paraphilias are usually chronic, lasting for many years, unless treated.
- Paraphilias could either be used as a stimulus that is always required for erotic arousal or can be episodic (e.g., during times of stress).
- Some paraphilias are playful and harmless. Others are considered sexual offenses.
- Paraphilias can be a nuisance to partners.
- The compulsive behaviors seen in sexual paraphilias may be related to obsessive-compulsive disorders.

DSM-IV-TR Diagnostic Criteria
- The paraphilias are mental disorders characterized by recurrent sexual fantasies, urges, or behaviors that center on: nonhuman objects (e.g., fetishism, transvestic fetishism); children or other nonconsenting partners (e.g., pedophilia, voyeurism); or the humiliation or hurting of one's sexual partner (e.g., sexual sadism).

Etiology
- There is no single answer as to the etiology of paraphilias, but there are a few theories.
- One prevalent theory includes a manifestation of real or fantasy experiences, desires, and/or conflicts that stems from the individual's early psychosexual development. This is called "lovemap." The person is then fixated at that stage, depending on the lovemap, and the nature of the paraphilia is determined by this.
- Another theory is that a paraphilia is seen as coming from a sudden emergence of an association with a previously neutral object and a sexually arousing object/experience.
- There are several factors involved with the development of paraphilias, such as anxiety, skill, and relationship deficits.

Diagnosis

Differential Diagnosis
- Developmental disability
- Dementia
- Personality changes due to general medical conditions
- Substance intoxication
- Manic episodes
- Schizophrenia

Initial Assessment
- Whether there is a problem in arousal in relation to a normal stimuli
- Anxiety about normal sexual activity
- Anxiety about social interactions with adults
- Skills deficits in social interactions
- Skills deficits in normal sexual activity
- Whether the individual has an underlying gender role identity problem

Clinical Presentation
- Individuals present to the clinic due to referrals by law-enforcing agents.
- Individuals who are distressed by their paraphilias.
- Individuals whose partners are distressed by their paraphilias.
- Individuals who report erectile disorders or other dysfunctions, which are secondary to the person's paraphilia.
- Individuals who report sexually transmitted diseases, unwanted pregnancy, or car accidents while being sexual.

Treatment

Clinical Management
- A general strategy is for the combination of different types of treatments.

Behavioral/Psychotherapy

- Psychotherapy can be divided between group and individual therapy.
- With individual therapy, the focus is on insight-oriented, cognitive-behavioral, and supportive psychotherapies.
- This is the most common form of treatment used.

Medical

- The majority of medical treatments are used for sexual offenders.
- Medroxyprogesterone acetate inhibits gonadotropin secretion, which inhibits sexual behavior.
  - Onset of action: 3 weeks, and the effects are reversible
  - Indicated to reduce recidivism in sexual offenders
- Antidepressants appear to reduce sexual behavior.
  - This is usually prescribed at the depression-dose level
- Long-acting gonadotropin-releasing hormone (GnRH) agonists are the most potent of the antiandrogen agents.

- The use of GnRH agonists and psychotherapy is extremely effective in controlling selected paraphilias (pedophilia, exhibitionism, and voyeurism).
- Luteinizing hormone-releasing agents produce complete "chemical castration" with hypoandrogenism.
- Cyproterone acetate, a testosterone antagonist, is approved for reduction of sex drive and hot flashes after orchiectomy.

Surgical

- Surgical castration (orchiectomy) involves removal of testes.
- Until the early decades of this century, surgical castration had been widely used in several countries, but it is practiced rarely these days because of ethical and legal issues.
- It is still done in Germany and certain states in the United States (California, Florida, Iowa, Louisiana, and Texas) as one condition of parole or probation.

Exhibitionism

Definition of Disorder

- Exposure of genitals to unsuspecting strangers.
- Most offenses occur in the daylight.
- The onset of exhibitionism occurs before 18 years of age.
- Most individuals who have conducted exhibitionism are between the ages of 20 and 35 years.
- Can be classified into two types: Rooth type I and Rooth type II.
- Rooth type I: individual with no criminal or dissocial personality, who struggles with the urge to expose, finally performing the act with anxiety. If this person is a male, he exposes a flaccid penis, gaining little sexual pleasure. Afterward, they have feelings of guilt.
- Rooth type II: individuals who have a lot less inhibition in exposing themselves. Tend to be more sociopathic. Tend to expose themselves in a state of excitement (for men, he would have an erect penis). The person tends not to have any guilt. They may masturbate during the act or afterward. They may also have a criminal record for nonsexual offenses.
- In some cases, frontal lobe dysfunction is believed to contribute to this sexual behavior.

ICD Code

302.4 Exhibitionism

Legal Ramifications

- There are concerns that in an uninhibited individual, progression from exhibitionism to other, more serious sexual assault can occur. In cases with individuals who expose flaccid penis, the progression is less likely than individuals with erect penis.

Fetishism

Definition of Disorder

- The use of nonliving objects as a repeatedly preferred method of achieving sexual stimulation.
- Fetish may involve a certain setting or scenario where role-play is engaged.
- People may possess more than one type of fetish.
- The mean age of onset is 16 years.
- Bancroft divided fetishism into three levels: partialism, extension of the body via an inanimate object, and tactile stimulation.
- Partialism occurs when there is a part of the body that has been the primary love object. An example would be a man's sexual obsession for the large breast of women.
- The second level occurs when an individual's sexual urges comes about because of an inanimate object. An example of that is when an individual has a fetish for an article of clothing, like a woman's underwear.
- The third level involves an individual's having a sexual desire for stimulation by touch. A particular fetish that would be incorporated in this level would be the sexual attraction with feeling leather.
- There are several postulates as to how this paraphilia may be developed. Some suggest that these individuals may have an underlying anxiety or inability for normal sexual acts, which causes an episode or series of episodes in which the individual becomes sensitized to fetish objects.

ICD-9 Code

302.81 Fetishism

Legal Ramifications

- About 25% of people with a fetish steal their objects (i.e., women's underwear).
- Majority of the individuals try to avoid being caught by the law.

Transvestic Fetishism

Definition of Disorder
- Behavior involves the individual who gains sexual pleasure from cross-dressing.
- The mean age of onset is 13.6 years.
- Bancroft describes four types of transvestites: transsexual, transvestite, double-role transvestite, and homosexual transvestite.
- The transsexuals retain their primary sex identity. For example, if the transsexual is a male, he may dress like a female, but in his mind, he is still a male.
- "Transsexual" should not be confused with the term "transvestite"; the latter is defined as individuals who feel that their sexual identity is of the opposite sex. For instance, a female transvestite would identify with a male sexual identity.
- Double-role transvestites: they genuinely do not want sex reassignment surgery, but rather opt for the double life. This involves the individual spending part of their time as a man and part as a woman.
- Homosexual transvestite: an individual who dresses up as the opposite sex to attract individuals of their sex. An example would be a woman dressing up as a man to attract females.
- This paraphilia has been a factor for the dissolution of marriages, although a few spouses do tolerate it.

ICD-9 Code
302.3 Transvestic Fetishism

Legal Ramifications
- Individuals rarely seek treatment for this paraphilia unless forced by circumstances, such as stealing opposite sex clothes to cross-dress or when their spouse seeks a divorce.

Pedophilia

Definition of Disorder

- An individual is usually sexually attracted either exclusively, or in part, toward prepubescent children.
- Not all individuals who have this sexual attraction actually abuse children.
- The mean age of onset for nonincestuous homosexual pedophilia is 18.2 years and for nonincestuous heterosexual pedophilia is 21.1 years.
- According to Fitch, there are five different types of pedophiles: immature, frustrated, sociopathic, pathologic, and miscellaneous.
- Immature types of pedophilia occur when the individual exhibits a childish personality with no identification with the adult sex role.
- A frustrated type of pedophile would often be an individual who conducts pedophilic activities due to a reaction against a sexual and emotional frustration.
- A sociopathic pedophile is an individual who is regarded as part of a group of people who lack social conformity.
- A pathologic pedophile is an individual who has a psychiatric disorder that may be a factor in the choice of pedophilia.
- Miscellaneous pedophiles are individuals who act on an impulse and don't usually match a pattern.

ICD Code

302.2 Pedophilia

Legal Ramifications

- Note that terms that describe sex with a minor involve criminal actions, while pedophilia is a sexual attraction toward children. Without the actual act being done, this paraphilia would only be considered a psychiatric disorder. Hence an individual with pedophilia is not a sexual offender unless the person commits the act.
- This paraphilia, when enacted on a child, infringes on the child's right to physical and psychological integrity because children do not have the ability to give consent to this sexual relationship.
- Sex with a minor inhibits the child's sense of security and control of personal boundaries with daily relationships.
- Studies show that many pedophiles have themselves been victims of sexual abuse in their childhood.
- Behavioral problems, suicidal ideation, and drug abuse appear to be the aftermath for people who have had childhood abuse.
- There is also an increased risk of childhood sexual-abuse victims being rape victims in their adolescence and adult life.

Sexual Masochism

Definition of Disorder
- Individuals enjoy receiving humiliation/ suffering.
- This can include acts that can even lead to death, such as a subtype of sexual masochism called "hypoxyphilia" (sexual arousal during hypoxia).

ICD Code
302.83 Voyeurism

Legal Ramifications
- This type of paraphilia can be dangerous because the rights of others can be disregarded, which breeds a criminal activity such as rape and death.

Sexual Sadism

Definition of Disorder

- It is defined as the pairing of sexual arousal with the infliction of physical or emotional pain and dominance and control over another person.
- Krafft-Ebing coined the term "sadism" to show the relations between cruelty, violence, and lust.
- It is named after a Frenchman Marquis de Sade who was known for his stories of women being hurt by men for sexual pleasure.
- Generally, severity increases over time.
- Studies show that the visual stimuli in sexual arousal stems from the activation within the temporal lobe. Hence, it is believed that individuals who are sexual sadists have a high frequency of neurological abnormalities that affect the temporal lobe.
- It is often a comorbidity with past and present Axis II disorders, like narcissistic, schizoid, antisocial, sadistic personality disorders.

- These individuals usually exhibit a number of other paraphilias.
- There is also an association between these individuals and drug and alcohol abusers' obsessional traits, collecting pornography, a history of impaired social relationships, physical and sexual abuse in childhood, and extensive fantasy lives incorporating detailed sadistic fantasies.

ICD Code

302.84 Sexual Sadism

Legal Ramifications

- This type of paraphilia can be dangerous because the rights of others can be disregarded, which breeds criminal activity such as rape and death.

Other Resources

Evidence-Based References

American Psychiatric Association. (2006). *Diagnostic and statistical manual of mental disorders* (4th ed.). Washington, DC: American Psychiatric Association.

Bossini, L., Fagiolini, A., Valdagno, M., Polizzotto, N. R., & Castrogiovanni, P. (2007). Sexual disorders in subjects treated for mood and anxiety diseases. *Journal of Clinical Psychopharmacology, 27*(3), 310–312.

Briken, P., & Kafka, M. (2007). Pharmacological treatments for paraphilic patients and sexual offenders. *Current Opinion in Psychiatry, 20*, 609–613.

Brown, G. R. (2006). Sexuality and sexual disorders. In M. H. Beers, R. S. Porter, T. V. Jones, J. V. Kaplan, & M. Berkwitz (Eds.), *The Merck manual of diagnosis and therapy* (18th ed.). Whitehouse Station, NJ: Merck Research Laboratories.

Faden, B. (2005). Psychological therapies. *BRS: Behavioral science* (4th ed., pp. 163–164). Baltimore, MD: Lippincott, Williams & Wilkins.

Fedoroff, J. (2008). Sadism, sadomasochism, sex, and violence. *The Canadian Journal of Psychiatry, 53*(10), 637–646.

Garcia-Falgueras, A., & Swaab, D. F. (2008). A sex difference in the hypothalamic uncinate nucleus: Relationship to gender identity. *Brain: A Journal of Neurology, 131*(12), 3132–3146.

Guay, D. (2008). Drug treatment of paraphilic and nonparaphilic sexual disorders. *Clinical Therapeutics, 31*(1), 1–31.

Hayes, R. D., Bennet, C. M., Fairley, C. K., & Dennerstein, L. (2006). What can prevalence studies tell us about female sexual difficulty and dysfunction? *Journal of Sexual Medicine, 3*(4), 589–595.

Hayes, R. D., Dennerstein, L., Bennet, C. M., & Fairley, C. K. (2008). What is the "true" prevalence of female sexual dysfunctions and does the way we assess these conditions have an impact? *Journal of Sexual Medicine, 5*(4), 777–787.

Kirsch, L., & Becker, J. (2007). Emotional deficits in psychopathy and sexual sadism: Implications for violent and sadistic behavior. *Clinical Psychology Review, 27*, 904–922.

Kreuger, R., & Kaplan, M. (1997). Voyeurism: Psychopathology and theory. In R. Laws & W. O'Donohue (Eds.), *Sexual deviance: Theory, assessment, and treatment* (pp. 305–319). New York: Guilford Press.

Långström, N., & Hanson, R. K. (2006). High rates of sexual behavior in the general population: Correlates and predictors. *Archives of Sexual Behavior, 35*, 37–52.

Långström, N, & Seto, M. (2006). Exhibitionistic and voyeuristic behavior in a Swedish national population survey. *Archives of Sexual Behavior, 35*, 427–435.

Rowland, D. L., & Incrocci, L. (2008). *Handbook on sexual and gender identity disorders* (pp. 188–213). Hoboken, NJ: John Wiley & Sons.

Saleh, F. M., & Guidry, L. L. (2003). Psychosocial and biological treatment considerations for the paraphilic and nonparaphilic sex offender. *Journal of the American Academy of Psychiatry and the Law, 31*, 486–93.

Seagraves, R. (2007). Female sexual dysfunction. *Primary Psychiatry, 14*(2), 37–41.

Sharma, B. (2003). Disorders of sexual preference and medicolegal issues thereof. *The American Journal of Forensic Medicine and Pathology, 24*(3), 277–282.

Thyer, B., & Wodarski, J. (2007). *Social work in mental health: An evidence-based approach.* Hoboken, NJ: John Wiley & Sons.

Web Resources

- American Psychiatric Association: http://www.psych.org.
- http://behavenet.com.

15. EATING DISORDERS
Anorexia Nervosa

Background Information

Definition of Disorder

- Anorexia nervosa (AN) is defined in the *Diagnostic and Statistical Manual of Mental Disorders 1994 (DSM-IV)* as a persistent and severe restriction of energy intake (especially fat), in combination with compulsive exercising in pursuit of thinness (APA, 1994). According to the *DSM-IV* (307.1), anorexia nervosa is defined as constituting the following (adapted from *DSM-IV*):
  - Refusal to maintain body weight at or above a minimal normal weight for age and height, leading to a body weight <85% of the expected weight or failure to make an expected weight gain during a period of growing up which leads to a body weight of <85%.
  - Body mass index is <17.5 kg/m² for older adolescents.
  - Intense fear of gaining weight or being fat, even when underweight.
  - Disturbance in the way in which one's body weight, shape, or size is experienced, undue influence of body weight or shape on self-evaluation, or denial of seriousness of body weight.
  - In postmenarcheal females, amenorrhea for at least three consecutive menstrual cycles.

DSM-PC Classification

[Note: The *Diagnostic and Statistical Manual for Primary Care—Child and Adolescent Version (DSM-PC)*, a supplement to the *DSM*, the APA classification of mental illness was intended to encompass children and younger adolescents who may exhibit some behaviors of mental illness but not the entire sets of criteria for those illnesses. It distinguishes between variations and problems. A *variation* is a concern for a parent or clinician. A *problem* constitutes evidence of pathology. Most clinicians refer to the presenting symptoms when considering treatments, rather than relying heavily on labeling.]

Dieting/Body Image Variation V65.49: This classification, according to the *DSM-PC*, is concerned primarily with the individual who has restricted his or her food consumption and who prefers thinness, but nevertheless has a realistic image of himself or herself.

Dieting/Body Image Problem V69.1: This classification, according to the *DSM-PC*, is concerned primarily with the individual who has acquired a distorted body image, and has begun to deny that weight loss or dieting is a problem.

- Anorexia nervosa is not just a desire to be thin, but an overwhelming desire to be thin and to reduce weight to lower and lower weight targets. The individual, in lowering his or her weight, may thereby reduce stress and improve his or her sense of empowerment.
- The individual may be clinically depressed.
- The individual denies his or her weight problem, and feels better as a result of continued weight loss.
- Younger individuals (pre-adolescent) may not lose weight, but may fail to gain weight and to achieve their ideal weights. Younger children very often have a poor ability to express inner turmoil, and may refuse to eat certain foods or to increase exercise activity.
- The anorexic individual may also engage in binging/purging (as seen in bulimia nervosa).
- Approximately half of individuals with anorexia nervosa have experienced a phase of binging/purging. During binging, the amounts of food ingested may not be large, and the foods themselves are often "forbidden foods," high in calories or fat.

Etiology

- The pathogenesis for AN, BN, and binge eating disorder (BED) is complex and is postulated to be associated with a combination of biological, psychological, and societal factors.
- More recent studies have indicated the interplay of an imbalance of neurotransmitters such as serotonin (5-HT) as a factor (K).

- The role of neurotransmitters and BED is not well understood.
  - BN and BED are associated with self-esteem and conflict in family dynamics. Psychosocial factors in association with eating disorders are related with difficulty in achieving the developmental task of transitioning to adulthood; these include poor acceptance of physical changes of puberty, peer group pressure, and issues related to nonacquisition of a stable self-identity. Adolescent girls may receive conflicting messages about acceptable body images and conflicting messages from society and the media on the role of women.
- Other psychosocial factors may include family conflict or ineffective coping during stressful times, such as when entering high school or college. Conversely an individual feels "power or control" while participating with weight control behaviors, especially if there is secondary acceptance, such as compliments or acceptance by peers. The studies suggest that females in late childhood and adolescence who feel a need to diet or lose weight are at a risk of adopting harmful eating disorders.
- Any individual who participates in restrictive diets can trigger obsessive focus on food and feelings of loss of control, often seen with repeated weight loss and weight gains, "yo-yo dieting." Modern Western culture cultivates and reinforces a desire for thinness, compounded by the influence of the media of very thin models and actors. Individuals in this society may view thinness as "successful." AN, however, did exist prior to the sociocultural values of the modern Western culture.
- Although social, economic, and cultural factors may be influencing factors, eating disorders have not been found among the majority of society.
- Anorexics have low self-worth and often an obsessive-compulsive personality trait for perfectionism; therefore these individuals never consider themselves to be at a "perfect weight."
- AN can be influenced by transitions in life experiences, requirements of sports, work, or artistic activity, and the media and society.

Demographics

- Eating disorders are found more in the female patients, 90%; Caucasians, 95%; and first develop among adolescents in 75%.
- Although most patients are from middle class or upper-socioeconomic-status families, the disorders can be found among any gender, race, age, or socioeconomic group. In fact, recent studies suggested that the disorder among minority females and adolescents of color is higher than suspected.
- Approximately, 0.5–1% of teenage females develop AN.

Complications

- Death: AN has the highest incidence of death related to starvation than any other mental illness.
- Anemia
- Cardiac problems, such as mitral valve prolapse, arrhythmias, and heart failure
- Osteoporosis
- Respiratory problems resembling emphysema
- Renal insufficiency and/or renal failure

Risk Factors

Age

- It first occur in middle school and then throughout adolescence.
  - Young girls starting at middle school who have a body image distortion and often diet to control weight.
  - Children who refuse to eat.
  - Young children who do not gain weight as expected.
  - Desire to target oneself to continuously lose more weight (control factor).
  - Individuals who eat small amounts of food, often fewer than 1000 kcal/day. Individuals who skip meals, or make excuses for not eating, as well as eating only certain "safe foods" low in fat and calories, such as popcorn, lettuce, diet drinks, etc.
  - Use of diet pills along with diets to manage weight, especially diet pills that contain ephedrine, caffeine, or phenylpropanolamine.
  - Individuals who plan and cook elaborate meals but eat little of it, as well as rituals related to

food preparation and eating. Cutting food into very small portions, or chewing and then spitting out food.

- Repeated weighing of self and complaining about being fat.
- Unintentional weight loss that provides secondary rewards will trigger individuals to continue to lose weight.

Gender

- Young girls of the Caucasian race, with most being adolescents.
- Pregnancy is often hindered due to changes in menstrual cycles or amenorrhea.

Family History

- In a study on risky eating disorders of mothers and sisters who had AN, there was an incidence of occurrence 8 times more often.
- Genetic studies also have indicated an underlying biologic influence on eating disorders, especially in twins. AN and other anxiety disorders tend to run in families.
- Perfectionism with compulsive behaviors.

Stressful Events in Susceptible People

- Females in late childhood and adolescence who feel a need to diet or lose weight are at risk for harmful weight-loss habits.
- Transitioning time in childhood or adolescence, such as times of entering high school or college.

Having Another Mental Disorder

- Those with other mental disorders, such as depression or substance abuse (alcoholism or drug abuse), have an increased risk for suicide or suicidal tendency. It is estimated that 30% of individuals seeking medical care are depressed or have depressive episodes such as sadness or depressed mood, lack of interest or enjoyment, or reduced energy or fatigability (WHO, 2000, p. 6).

Diagnosis

Differential Diagnosis

- Hypothyroidism
- Cardiac insufficiency or arrhythmias
- Inflammatory bowel disease

- Malignancy, CNS neoplasm
- Pregnancy
- AIDS/acute onset
- Systemic lupus erythematosum
- Depression
- Substance abuse

ICD Code

307.1 Anorexia Nervosa

Diagnostic Work-Up

- Assessment of vital signs, especially for hypothermia and for presence of orthostatic hypotension.
- Assessment for hypovolemia.
- Dental assessment for presence of dental enamel erosion.
- Assessment for Russell sign—abrasion or callus of metacarpophalangeal joint of the index of middle finger of dominant hand.
- Assessment for alopecia.
- Assessment for edema, especially peripheral, indicative of poor capillary integrity due to malnutrition.
- Assessment of weight and height is done by using standard growth charts for children or for those younger than 10 years of age; calculate body mass index (BMI). Children, especially boys, have an increase of BMI with age. It is best to use standard growth charts.
- BMI = (weight in kg)/(height in m^2).
- Physical and mental, and psychosocial evaluation; use of screening tools for depression, mood.
- Nutritional intake history and assessments for weight loss or weight cycling.
- Low white blood cell count, increased margination of the leukocytes not related to an infection.
- Blood plasma protein levels and pre-albumin (determine malnourishment).
- Erythrocyte sedimentation rate is usually normal and may be elevated with organic illness such as inflammatory bowel disease.
- Thyroid function studies—may be depressed.
- CMP-14—biochemical profiles, especially for presence of electrolyte imbalance such as hypoglycemia, hypomagnesia, hypokalemia.

- Liver function studies, may be elevated with severe dehydration as much as 2× the normal.
- Cholesterol levels may be elevated, with starvation due to depressed triiodothyronine (T3); cholesterol binding with globulin is low and possible fatty infiltration and leakage of cholesterol into hepatic system.
- Complete blood count (CBC) with differential; elevated hemoglobulin levels may be related to dehydration.
- Electrocardiogram may reveal presence of bradycardia, prolong QT interval.
- Transferritin and iron levels may be low.
- X-rays to rule out fracture, pneumonia, respiratory or infectious process.

Initial Assessment
- Medical history
- Symptoms experienced
- Diet recall:
  - How does patient feel about weight?
  - Is the patient satisfied with eating patterns?
  - Has the patient tried to control or lose weight by vomiting, diet pills, laxative, or starving?
  - Exercise practices of the patient
- Family history or sibling eating disorder patterns
- History of mental illness/affective disorders, inpatient, and/or of family members

Clinical Presentation
- Physical symptoms:
  - Amenorrhea
  - Cold hands and feet
  - Constipation
  - Dry skin and hair
  - Headaches
  - Fainting or dizziness
  - Lethargy or lack of energy
  - Anorexia
  - Lanugo (body's attempt to maintain body heat)
  - Low blood pressure for the age
- Emotional and behavioral symptoms:
  - Refusal to eat
  - Denial of hunger
  - Excessive exercise
  - Flat mood, or lack of emotion
  - Difficulty concentrating

- Preoccupation with food
- Black-and-white thinking (resistant to change)

DSM-IV-TR Diagnostic Guidelines
- The individual's refusal to maintain body weight at or above a minimal normal weight (for her or his age and height), leading to a body weight of less than 85% of the expected weight, or failure to make an expected weight gain, which leads to a body weight of less than 85% of the expected weight.
- BMI is less than 17.5 kg/mg^2 for older adolescents.
- There is an intense fear of gaining weight or of becoming fat, even in one who is noticeably underweight.
- There is an aberration in the way the individual experiences his body weight, shape, and size.
- There is an undue emphasis on body weight in the individual's self-evaluation.
- In postmenarcheal females: amenorrhea for three consecutive menstrual cycles.

Treatment

American Psychiatric Association Practice Guidelines
- The psychiatrist may assume the leadership role within a program or team that includes other physicians, psychologists, registered dietitians, and social workers or may work collaboratively on a team led by others. Additionally, these same practice guidelines require that communication among all disciplines is essential (Recommendation I).
- A team approach is recommended by the APA Practice Guidelines (Recommendation III) as well using various resources for treatment, inpatient, outpatient, psychological therapy, and pharmacotherapy including patient education (Recommendation I).
- Obtain a history, and a physical that is comprehensive with a review of the patient's height and weight history, restrictive and binge eating and exercise patterns and their changes, purging and other compensatory behaviors, core attitudes regarding weight, shape, and eating,

and associated psychiatric conditions (Recommendation I).

- Obtain a family history of eating disorders or other psychiatric disorders, including alcohol and other substance-use disorders, a family history of obesity, the family's reactions or interactions in relation to the eating disorder, and family attitudes toward eating, exercise, and appearance (Recommendation I).
- It is important to determine stressors that may trigger the eating disorders in order to facilitate amelioration of the eating disorder.
- When assessing children and adolescents, it is essential to involve parents, significant others, and, when appropriate, school personnel and health professionals who routinely work with the patient (Recommendation I).
- With older adults, while spouses and significant others should be part of the treatment program, the clinician should consider whether others should be involved (Recommendations II and III).

Acute Treatment

- Treatment is multifaceted and interdisciplinary.
- Goal is to stop weight loss and gain weight. The ultimate goal is to establish a structured pattern of three meals and one to three snacks daily.
- Breakfast is essential as this is the meal most often to be missed with dieters, anorexics, and adolescents. Patients who eat breakfast often have less chance of binge eating later in the day (are less hungry and thus may avoid binging). Adolescents will perform better in school or with hospital-based classes.
- In severe situations, acute treatment may be indicative for life-threatening conditions such as cardiac arrhythmias, severe dehydration, or electrolyte imbalance. Intensive care has been instituted for life-threatening situations.
  - Total parenteral nutrition may be indicated along with intravenous replacement of electrolytes.
  - Albumin may be given to prevent sudden *refeeding syndrome*—a potentially fatal condition resulting from rapid changes in fluids and electrolytes in malnourished

individuals given oral, enteral, or parenteral feeding. Monitor for hypophosphatemia occurring as a result of glycolysis.
  - Hypophosphatemia can result in impairment of myocardial contractility.
  - Heart failure can occur in the presence of fluid retention with an inadequate cardiac status.
  - Hypokalemia may result as well from insulin secretion in response to an increase in calories, which shifts the potassium into the cells.
  - A daily multivitamin with thiamine should be used to prevent Wernicke's encephalopathy.
  - Nasogastric feeding may be necessary to replenish caloric requirements once the acute phase for refeeding occurs.
- Supervise and monitor weight daily; some patients with AN have learned how to increase weight by drinking fluids.
- Monitor vital signs for hypothermia and fluid and electrolytes, especially urine-specific gravity. Patients may try to falsify weight by wearing increased underclothing garments; however, urine-specific gravity can indicate dehydration or starvation.
- A dietitian should be an integral part of the inpatient treatment to evaluate and treat specific deficiencies or excesses.
- Food should be balanced with a flexible exchange system to allow for variety. All food consumption should be monitored. Diet must be balanced, and limit "fat-free foods" and emphasize healthy foods. Adolescents may perceive "fat-free foods" as "good" food, not realizing the increase in sugar and calories. Educate the patient on a balanced diet and nutritional concepts.
- The patient can maintain a journal of eating patterns and identify dysfunctional eating patterns (purging) that occur during the inpatient episode. Provide feedback and encouragement for adherence to health; try not to stress the increase in food intake.
- The individuals with AN may not think that they have a problem but rather that they have chosen a life style.
- Inpatient treatment in a mental health setting is necessary in patients with a suicidal ideation and plan, serious alcohol or sedative withdrawal

symptoms, or when the differential includes other medical disorders that warrant admission (e.g., unstable angina, acute myocardial ischemia).

- Cognitive-behavioral therapy (CBT) allows patients to monitor progress and identify triggers for dieting, binge eating, and purging as well as refusal to eat. CBT focuses on restructuring thoughts that lead to distorted eating.
- Psychotherapy that establishes trust is essential, as individuals with AN may not be willing to relinquish their coping mechanism or eating patterns. AN must be explained in terms of the patient's stage of psychosocial development. Reassure the patient that others need to be incorporated in care to assist with improving health and that the clinician is not abandoning the patient.
- Family therapy can help resolve family conflicts or elicit support from concerned family members; this is especially important for children who live at home.
- Group therapy can help persons with AN to connect with others facing similar complications, stressors, and coping behaviors. Group therapy must be carefully monitored as persons with AN may use it as a means to compete as to who is thinnest.

Chronic Treatment

- A multidisciplinary approach with a psychologist, primary care providers, and a dietitian is essential. Any therapy can last for over 1 year while the individual attempts to gain insight into triggers that can induce the eating disorder behavior.
- Interpersonal therapy and family therapy have proven to be more effective than CBT, with or without pharmacotherapy, for AN.
- A meta-analysis study revealed that intervention was more successful if it was interactive and had multisessions.
- Measurement of bone density should be evaluated initially and every 6 months. Findings demonstrate that depressive symptoms and anxiety are associated with low bone density.
- Menses resumption occurs with return to at least 86% of ideal body weight; therefore, the goal should be to assist adolescents to acquire a healthy habit of eating nourishing foods and exercise.

- Use screening tools to determine the presence of depression, child abuse, or sexual abuse in older adolescents and use the SCOFF questionnaire:
  - S—Do you make yourself *Sick* because you feel uncomfortably full?
  - C—Do you worry you have lost *Control* over how much you eat?
  - O—Have you recently lost more than *One* stone (14 lb or 7.7 kg) in a 3-month period?
  - F—Do you believe yourself to be *Fat* when others say you are too thin?
  - F—Would you say that *Food* dominates your life?

Pharmacotherapy

- Selective serotonin reuptake inhibitors (SSRIs) may be useful with AN to maintain weight gain and prevent relapse, such as fluoxetine (Prozac, Fontex, Ladose, Sarafem, Solax), with the initial dose of 20 mg once daily increased to 40–60 mg for maintenance.
- SSRIs are not useful in AN when patients are at low weights.
- Appropriate pharmacological therapy and CBT, individually or in combination, are effective in more than 85% of cases.
- Although tricyclics antidepressants, such as clomipramine (Anafranil) and amitriptyline (Elavil), have been prescribed to anorexics, these medicines produce sedation, tachycardia, constipations, dry mouth, and confusion.
- Cyproheptadine (Periactin), an antihistamine, and serotonin antagonists have proven beneficial in increasing food intake. Serotonin in the hypothalamus is responsible for decreased food consumption; therefore, it is hypothesized that a serotonin antagonist would have the opposite effects. Cyproheptadine has been successful in treatment of patients with inappropriate caloric intake such as patients with HIV, cancer, and other chronic illnesses.
- Dronabinol (Marinol), a cannabinoid, has been used with patients to increase appetite (see Web Resources).
- In some patients with AN, anxiolytic agents such as olanzapine (Zyprexa, Zyprexa Zydis, Zalasta, Zolafren, Olzapin), prior to eating, have been effective.

- Because gastric motility is impaired with AN, drugs such as metoclopramide (Reglan), and cisapride (Propulsid) help to accelerate gastric emptying and enhance gastric motor activity. Osmotic agents such as Gl-Lytely or Glycolax can help with constipation and bloating.
- Zinc supplementation, alone or along with a multivitamin, has been associated with weight gain.
- Treatment of osteopenia may be initiated with estrogen/progesterone combinations such as birth control pills if the chance of recovery from anorexia appears lengthy.
- Rate, growth factors (IGF-1), and dehydroepiandrosterone (DHEA), a naturally occurring adrenal hormone, may be of some benefit in patients with severe bone loss.
- The Society for Adolescent Medicine has suggested 1200–1500 mg of elemental calcium, a multivitamin with 400 units of Vitamin D, along with *dual emission X-ray absorpiometry* (DEXA) scans on baseline and to monitor bone regrowth.
- Natural herbs may improve appetite and have a placebo effect on weight gain, Kiddie Florish™ has been used by some parents with younger school age children to improve appetite.
  - The ingredients consist of the following:
    - *Emblica officinalis* (amalki) is thought to improve protein synthesis
    - *Withania somnifera* (ashwagandha), Indian ginseng, is thought to improve energy and stamina
    - *Trigonella foenumgraecum* (fenugreek) is thought to support a natural steroid production
    - *Scutellaria lateriflora* (skullcap) is used as a calmative
    - *Zingiber officinale* (ginger) is used for digestive purposes
    - *Borago officinalis* (borage) is used as a digestive aid. Borage contains gamma linolenic acid (GLA), a fatty acid that converts to prostaglandin E1

Note: The FDA has not approved natural remedies as pharmacological treatments for eating disorders.

Recurrence Rate

Rate of recurrence is approximately 15–25% as individuals with AN who are hospitalized have a 75–85% chance of full recovery.

Patient Education

- Information regarding AN and support groups can be obtained from the NIMH (see Internet support).
- Advise patients with AN to avoid nicotine, sympathomimetic or anticholinergic drugs, caffeine, and alcohol.
- Avoid weighing self, resist urge to isolate self from caring individuals.
- Provide information on healthy life styles such as supplements and vitamins.
- Avoid pro-anorexia Web sites, chat rooms, or media that emphasize thinness.
- Avoid contact with anorexic friends. Stick to your *healthy* life style plan, use of cognitive-behavioral intervention such as student bodies, an Internet program.

Medical/Legal Pitfalls

- A common finding in those who commit suicide is the presence of more than one mental disorder such as mood disorder (i.e., depression), and personality disorder and other psychiatric disorders (WHO, 2000, p. 6). Individuals with AN are at risk for depression due to their distorted body image and perfectionist psychological profile (Wattula, 2008).
- As of May 2, 2007, the National Clearing House has labeled antidepressant drugs, with a black box warning on the prescribing information to include warnings about the increased risks of suicidal thinking and behavior in young adults aged 18–24 years during the first 1–2 months of treatment.
- As of May 12, 2006, the National Clearing House has given paroxetine (Paxil) and Paxil CR, a *Clinical Worsening and Suicide Risk* label in the prescribing information related to adult patients, especially younger adults.
- Individuals with an eating disorder display symptoms as a result of psychological problems; failure to recognize the relationship may result in inappropriate care.

Bulimia Nervosa

Background Information

Definition of Disorder

- BN and BED occur when a large amount of food is eaten in a short time period.
- With BN, there is often no weight loss and there may be episodes of weight gain.
- Individuals may not have a body image distortion or may actually see themselves as not as heavy as they actually are.
- BED was formally known as "compulsive eating disorder."

DSM-PC Classification

[Note: The *Diagnostic and Statistical Manual for Primary Care—Child and Adolescent Version (DSM-PC)*, a supplement to the *DSM*, the APA classification of mental illness, was intended to encompass children and younger adolescents who may exhibit some behaviors of mental illness but not the entire sets of criteria for those illnesses. It distinguishes between variations and problems. A *variation* is a concern for a parent or clinician. A *problem* constitutes evidence of pathology. Most clinicians refer to the presenting symptoms when considering treatments, rather than rely heavily on labeling.]

Binging/Purging Eating Variation V69.19: This classification, according to *DSM-PC*, is concerned with the individual for whom there is intermittent concern about body image and getting fat. Typically, normal weight is maintained.

- Occurs as part of experimentation with induced vomiting, use of laxatives, fasting, or rigorous exercise to prevent weight gain.
- Perceptions of body shape and body size have become distorted.
- The behaviors are not sufficiently pronounced or advanced to qualify as bulimia nervosa or eating disorder, not otherwise specified.
- Purging is the compensatory behavior most often used to avoid weight gain. Binge eating, however, is the defining element of the diagnosis.

- In adolescents, purging includes: self-stimulation of the upper pharynx, pressure put on the abdomen, and the use of ipecac and laxatives.
- Adolescents may also use rigorous exercise and fasting to prevent weight gain.
- The individual with bulimia nervosa may exhibit attitudes of self-deprecation or have depressed mood after becoming aware of his or her anomalous eating patterns.
- In contrast, those individuals with binge eating disorder may use compensatory methods to avoid weight gain when other attempts to avoid weight gain have failed.
- Individuals with binge eating disorder often eat alone, as they are embarrassed about binging.
- BED can be distinguished from BN in that, in BED, there is a recurring compensatory weight control habit, such as dieting, when overeating occurs.
- BED has been associated with male athletes' attempts to control weight during sports events.

Etiology

- The pathogenesis believed to occur with an imbalance of serotonin is that at the hypothalamus, higher levels of 5-HT tend to decrease appetite and food intake while lower levels are associated with decreased satiety. The central nervous system precursor to serotonin, 5-hyroxyindolacetic acid (5-HIAA), is lower in patients with AN when they are ill but returns to a higher level during recovery from AN (Kaye). A similar process occurs with BN.
- Two other factors associated with BN and BED are sexual trauma and depression. Patients with BN and BED have histories of depression. There is a higher incidence of sexual trauma among adolescents who have BN than the general population. Depression is difficult to determine if it precedes BN or is associated with affective disorder.

- BN has been associated with dissatisfaction with body after sexual abuse, poor attachment to others, and insecurity.
- Athletes of any gender, especially gymnasts and runners who have low self-esteem, are predisposed to eating disorders.
- Male patients with eating disorders who constitute a much lower incidence have either BN or BED. Male athletes with BED avoid weight gain or maintain a certain weight for sports activities. Male athletes will often engage in binge eating and vomiting.
- Increased incidence or prevalence of BN may account for the increase in eating disorders.
- Increased media attention, better screening of patients for eating disorders, and less stringent diagnostic criteria may also be responsible for the apparent increase in eating disorders.
- Binge eating and purging allow patients to be *in control* when engaged in weight control behaviors, especially if secondary gains occurs.

Demographics
- Eating disorders are found more in the female patients 90%; Caucasians, 95%; and as first developed among adolescents, 75%.
- Five percent of older adolescents affected are female.
- BN and BED are more common in high school and college students with a peak incidence occurring around 18 years of age. BN affects approximately 3% of young women.
- Although there are no reliable data available for the incidence of BED, clinical experience with obesity in adults suggests that it is common. Ten to fifty percent of adolescent girls and boys frequently engage in eating disorders.
- Many children do not meet stringent diagnostic criteria for BN but may exhibit partial symptoms.
- BN is found across racial and socioeconomic groups, with boys representing one-fifth of adolescents and about one-tenth of adult males. Recent data suggest that binging and/or purging may occur when the individual perceives an increase in food intake and not on a regular basis.
- The peak incidence for BN is around 18 years of age.

- Twenty-five percent of adolescents regularly engage in self-induced purging as a means to control weight.
- Five to ten percent of mild variants of eating disorders do not meet the full diagnostic criteria for the *DSM-IV* but represent a threat to growth and development of the adolescent according to the variations or problems in the *DSM-PC* classification.
- There is an increase in prevalence for eating disorders primarily due to media attention, improved detection, and less stringent diagnostic criteria such as the *DSM-PC*.
- BN is thought to be a learned behavior, acquired from modeling of peer groups.

Risk Factors
- Age: adolescents in high school and college, young adults.
- Athletes who have specific weight requirements.
- Both genders are equally at risk.
- Patients who binge and/or purge and develop depressed moods and self-deprecating thoughts often seek relief of the thought processes by ridding the body of the excess calories.
- BN and BED patients often have episodes of dieting to lose weight rapidly.
- Patients with BED may recognize their eating patterns as abnormal, but have experienced negative results at losing weight and use compensatory mechanisms to avoid weight gain, such as self-induced vomiting, laxatives, exercise, or fasting.
- Patients who have BED often can be overweight and may have parents who are overweight, as well as maternal control over feeding (restricting or urging).
- Patients may use the excuse of binging as an attempt to bulk up for sports in a repeated frequency and then use purging or vomiting as an attempt to avoid weight gain.
- BN and BED often have compulsive and impulsive behaviors not only in eating but also in use of drugs and alcohol, self-mutilation (cutting), sexual promiscuity, or self-harm, lying, stealing, and other personality disturbances.

- Children over the age of 2 with a BMI of 85% are considered at risk for becoming overweight or children at the 95th percentile are overweight.
- It is hypothesized that resistance to insulin and leptin (hormones related to a feeling of satiety) may lead to obesity. Decreased exercise and diets high in fructose and low in fiber may lead to hyperinsulism.
- Gender
  - Although both genders are at risk, female adolescents are more likely to participate in BN or BED.
  - Postpubertal females constitute 5–10% of cases of mild variants of eating disorders as classified by the *DSM-PC*.
- Family history
  - Individuals with a history of sexual trauma and depression.
  - Genetic studies have indicated an underlying biologic influence on eating disorders, especially in twins. There is an association with BN and being a twin of up to 35–50%.
  - Overweight parents, especially fathers.
- Stressful events and susceptible people
  - BN and BED have been associated with individuals who might have experienced a form of sexual trauma.
  - Difficulty with transitioning through developmental stages such as high school and college may predispose individuals to BN and/or BED.
  - Individuals who participate in sports activities that require weight requirements, such as gymnastics, football, and track, are more likely to become involved in binge eating and purging. BN and BED are used to increase or decrease weight, depending on requirements of the sport.
- Having another mental disorder
  - Individuals with BN and/or BED tend to have compulsive and impulsive personality behaviors.
  - Those with other mental disorders, such as depression or substance abuse (alcoholism or drug abuse), have an increased risk for suicide or suicidal tendency. It is estimated that 30% of individuals seeking medical care are depressed or have depressive episodes such as sadness—depressed mood, lack of interest or enjoyment, or reduced energy or fatigability.

Diagnosis

Differential Diagnosis
- Esophageal tears
- Cardiac insufficiency or arrhythmias
- Insulin resistance
- Sleep apnea/daytime somnolence
- Pseudotumor cerebri
- Hyperthyroidism
- Inflammatory bowel disease
- Malignancy, CNS neoplasm
- Pregnancy
- AIDS/acute onset
- Systemic lupus erythematosum
- Depression
- Substance abuse

ICD Code
307.51 Bulimia Nervosa

Diagnostic Work-Up
- Assessment of vital signs, especially for hypothermia and for presence of orthostatic hypotension
- Assessment for hypovolemia
- Dental assessment for presence of dental enamel erosion
- Assessment for Russell sign—abrasion or callus of metacarpophalangeal joint of the index of middle finger of dominant hand
- Assessment for alopecia
- Assessment for edema, especially peripheral, indicative of poor capillary integrity due to malnutrition
- Assessment of weight and height is done by using standard growth charts for children or for those younger than 10 years old; calculate body mass index. Children, especially boys, have an increase of BMI with age. It is best to use standard growth charts. BMI = (weight in kg)/(height in m^2).
- Physical and mental and psychosocial evaluation.
- Nutritional intake history and assessments for weight loss or weight cycling.
- Blood plasma protein levels and pre-albumin (determine malnourishment).

- Erythrocyte sedimentation rate is usually normal and may be elevated with organic illness such as inflammatory bowel disease.
- Thyroid function studies—may be depressed.
- Cholesterol levels may be elevated, with starvation due to depressed T3, cholesterol binding with globulin is low, and there is possible fatty infiltration, and leakage of cholesterol into hepatic system.
- CBC with differential, elevated hemoglobulin levels may be related to dehydration and hemoconcentration.
- Transferritin and iron levels: levels may be normal.
- Electrolyte studies often indicate hypokalemia, hypochloremia metabolic alkalosie due to recurrent vomiting. The absence of abnormality in electrolytes does not exclude BN.
- Hypomagnesium may be present with excessive use of laxatives or water-diarrheal stools.
- CMP-14—biochemical profiles, especially for presence of electrolyte imbalance such as hypoglycemia, hypomagnesia, hypokalemia.
- Liver function studies: may be elevated with severe dehydration as much as $2\times$ the normal.
- Electrocardiogram, presence of bradycardia, prolonged QT interval when BN occurs in low weight individuals. U waves may be present secondary to hypokalemia and if cardiomyopathy has occurred due to alkaloid emetine contained in syrup of ipecac.
- Screening with appropriate instruments for depression.

Clinical Presentation
- Binge eating
  - Weight gain or weight fluctuation
  - Bloating
  - Lethargy
  - Salivary gland enlargement (if vomiting)
  - Guilt
  - Depression
  - Anxiety
- Purging
  - Weight loss
  - Electrolyte imbalance: $\downarrow$ potassium, $\uparrow$ CO_2
  - Hypovolemia
  - Guilt

- Depression
- Anxiety/guilt
- Knuckle calluses (vomiting)
- Dental enamel erosion (vomiting)
- Any form of self-mutilation such as cutting
- Frequent overeating used for coping
- Self-induced vomiting, hematemesis
- Excessive exercise

DSM-IV-TR Diagnostic Guidelines
- In bulimia nervosa, recurrent episodes of binge eating are characterized by:
  - Eating amounts of food that are unquestionably larger than what most persons would consume in the same time period and under similar circumstances.
  - Absence of self-control during the episodes.
- Presence of compensatory behaviors to prevent weight gain: induced vomiting, use of laxatives and diuretics, use of enemas, use of other medications, fasting, rigorous exercise.
- Binge eating and the accompanying compensatory behaviors, both occurring at least twice a week for 3 months.
- Self-evaluation is unduly influenced by body shape and weight.
- The episodes of bulimia nervosa do not occur exclusively during episodes of anorexia nervosa.

American Psychiatric Association Practice Guidelines
The psychiatrist may assume the leadership role within a program or team that includes other physicians, psychologists, registered dietitians, and social workers or may work collaboratively on a team led by others. Additionally, these same practice guidelines note that communication among all disciplines is essential (Recommendation I).
- A team approach is recommended by the APA Practice Guidelines (Recommendation III) as well as using various resources for treatment, as inpatient and outpatient, psychological therapy and pharmacotherapy, including patient education (Recommendation I).
- Obtain a history and a physical that are comprehensive with a review of the patient's height and weight history, restrictive and binge eating and exercise patterns and their changes, purging and other compensatory behaviors, core

attitudes regarding weight, shape, and eating, and associated psychiatric conditions (Recommendation I).

- Obtain a family history of eating disorders or other psychiatric disorders, including alcohol and other substance-use disorders, a family history of obesity, the family's reactions or interactions in relation to the eating disorder, and family attitudes toward eating, exercise, and appearance (Recommendation I).

- It is important to determine stressors that may trigger the eating disorders in order to facilitate amelioration of the eating disorder.

- When assessing children and adolescents, it is essential to involve parents, significant others, and, when appropriate, school personnel and health professionals who routinely work with the patient (Recommendation I).

- With older adults, while spouses and significant others should be part of the treatment program, the clinician should consider whether others should be involved (Recommendations II and III).

Acute Treatment

- Treatment is multifaceted and interdisciplinary, including a mental health professional, a primary care provider or medical person, a dietitian, school personnel, and religious persons if indicated.

- The medical personnel work to correct and manage medical issues such as electrolyte imbalances and dental problems.

- The dietitian is essential in providing nutritional education and a rationale for selection of certain foods and a meal plan. In some organizations a dietitian is supplemented by a sports physiologist or trainer to assist individuals with weight management.

- If exercise therapy, caution is provided that excessive exercising could occur along with binge-purge eating with susceptible individuals.

- The nutritional intake for those requiring a weight gain should consist of 2–3 lb (0.9–1.4 kg) per week of controlled weight gain and for outpatients, 0.5–1 lb per week. The intake should start at 3040 kcal/kg (1000–1500 kcal/day) and advance progressively.

- In severe situations, acute inpatient treatment for BN may be indicative of life-threatening conditions. Some of these conditions include cardiac arrhythmias, severe dehydration or electrolyte imbalance, arrested development, failure of outpatient treatment, acute food refusal, suicidal ideation, comorbid diagnosis such as depression, or severe family dysfunction.

- Intensive care has been instituted for life-threatening situations.
  - Total parenteral nutrition may be indicated along with intravenous replacement of electrolytes.
  - Albumin may be given to prevent sudden *refeeding syndrome*—a potentially fatal condition resulting from rapid changes in fluids and electrolytes in malnourished individuals given oral, enteral or parenteral feeding. Monitor for hypophosphatemia occurring as a result of glycolysis.
  - Hypophosphatemia can result in impairment of myocardial contractility.
  - Heart failure can occur in the presence of fluid retention with an inadequate cardiac status.
  - Hypokalemia may result as well from insulin section in response to an increase in calories, which shifts the potassium into the cells.
  - A daily multivitamin with thiamine should be used to prevent Wernicke's encephalopathy.
  - Nasogastric feeding may be necessary to replenish caloric requirements once the acute phase for refeeding occurs.

- Caution should be provided that some patients may gain weight rapidly due to fluid retention, possibly due to low protein levels.

- Treat electrolyte or nutritional deficits first, inpatient treatment may be indicated.
  - CBT emphasizes that thoughts and feelings may lead to distorted eating patterns. CBT has higher efficacy and lower cost, dropout rates, and relapse rates than pharmacological treatments.
  - Psychotherapy and antidepressant medications in combination provide the best chance for remission.
  - Appetite suppressants and psychological treatment have been effective in the treatment

of individuals who are overweight or with bulimia.

- Individuals with BED may need to be treated for other physical problems such as sleep apnea, snoring, diabetes, hyperlipidemia, cardiovascular disease.

Chronic Treatment

- Multidisciplinary approach with a psychologist, primary care providers, and a dietician is essential. Any therapy can last for over 1 year while the individual attempts to gain insight into triggers that can induce the eating disorder behavior.
- Interpersonal therapy and family therapy have proven to be more effective than CBT, with or without pharmacotherapy, for AN.
  - Use screening tools to determine presence of depression, child abuse, or sexual abuse in older adolescents and use the SCOFF questionnaire:
  - S—Do you make yourself *Sick* because you feel uncomfortably full?
  - C—Do you worry you have lost *Control* over how much you eat?
  - O—Have you recently lost more than *One* stone (14 lb or 7.7 kg) in a 3-month period?
  - F—Do you believe yourself to be *Fat* when others say you are too thin?
  - F—Would you say that food *Dominates* your life?
- Use of cognitive-behavioral intervention such as student bodies and an Internet program.

Pharmacotherapy

- SSRIs may be useful with BN and BED to maintain weight gain and prevent relapse, such as fluoxetine (Prozac, Fontex, Ladose, Sarafem, Solax).
- Appropriate pharmacological therapy and CBT, individually or in combination, are effective in more than 85% of cases.
- Antiepileptic agents like topiramate (Topamax) have been useful in individuals with BN. Both of these drugs have demonstrated a reduction in binge-eating behavior and in self-induced vomiting.

- Sibutramine (Meridia), an appetite suppressant, has been used with BED in individuals who are overweight.
- In some patients with AN, anxiolytic agents such as olanzapine (Zyprexa, Zyprexa Zydis, Zalasta, Zolafren, Olzapin), prior to eating, have been effective.
- Because gastric motility is impaired with AN, drugs such as metoclopramide (Reglan), cisapride (Propulsid) help to accelerate gastric emptying and enhance gastric motor activity. Osmotic agents such as Gl-Lytely or Glycolax can help with constipation and bloating.
- Zinc supplementation alone, or along with multivitamin, has been associated with weight gain.

Recurrence Rate

- Poorer outcomes have been associated with later age of onset of eating disorders.
- Low self-esteem can impact the recurrence of binge-purging behaviors. Thirty percent of individuals may continue to engage in binging-purging up to 10 years after follow-up if substance abuse is coupled with the eating behavior.

Medical/Legal Pitfalls

- A common finding in those who commit suicide is the presence of more than one mental disorder.
- Mood disorder (i.e., depression), personality disorder and other psychiatric disorders may be overlooked. As of May 2, 2007, the National Clearing House has labeled antidepressant drugs with a black box warning on the prescribing information to include warnings about the increased risks of suicidal thinking and behavior in young adults aged 18–24 years old during the first 1–2 months of treatment.
- As of May 12, 2006, the National Clearing House has labeled paroxetine (Paxil) and Paxil CR with a *Clinical Worsening and Suicide Risk* in the prescribing information related to adult patients, especially younger adults.

Other Resources

Evidence-Based References

American Psychiatric Association. (2006). *Practice guideline for the treatment of patients with eating disorders* (3rd ed.). Washington DC: Author. Retrieved on January 5, 2009, from http://www.guideline.gov/summary/summary.aspx?doc_id=9318&nbr=004987.

American Psychiatric Association. (2009). Treatment of patients with eating disorders (3rd ed.). *American Journal of Psychiatry, 163*(7 Suppl.) 4–54. Retrieved on January 5, 2009, from http://www.guideline.gov/Compare/comparison.aspx?file=EATING_DISORDERS2.inc#t4 comprehensive PubMed.

Berkman. N. D., Lohr, K. N., & Bulik, C. M. (2007). Outcomes of eating disorders: A systematic review of the literature. *International Journal of Eating Disorders, 40*(4), 293–309. Retrieved on January 5, 2009, from [PubMed].

Burns, C. E., Dunn, A. M., Brady, M. A., Starr, N. B., & Blosser, C. G. (2009). *Pediatric Primary Care* (4th ed.). St. Louis, MO: Saunders, an imprint of Elsevier Inc.

Dorn, L. D., Susman, E. J., Pabst, S., Huan, B., Kalkwarf, H., & Grimes, S. (2008). Association of depressive symptoms and anxiety with bone mass and density in ever-smoking and never smoking adolescent girls. *Archives of Pediatrics and Adolescent Medicine, 162*(12). Retrieved on January 12, 2009, from http://iiiprxy.library.miamie.edu.

Forman, S. F. (2008). Eating disorders: Treatment and outcome. *UpToDate.* Retrieved on January 7, 2009, from www.uptodate.com/online/cotnent/topic.do?topicKey-psychiat//11503&view

Sanci, L., Coffey, C., Olsson, C., Reid, S., Carlin, J. B., & Patton, G. (2008). Childhood sexual abuse and eating disorders in females: Findings from the Victorian Adolescent Health Cohort Study. *Archives of Pediatrics and Adolescent Medicine, 162*(3). Retrieved on January 9, 2009, from http://iiiprxy.library.miami.edu.

Stice, E., & Shaw, H. (2004). Eating disorder prevention programs: A meta-analytic review. *Psychology Bulletin, 130*, 206.

Wattula, A. L. (2008*). Anorexia nervosa: Pharmacologic treatments.* Psychology Department, Vanderbilt University. Retrieved on December 26, 2008, from http://www.vanderbilt.edu/AnS/psychology/health_psychology/anorexia_drugs.htm.

Web Resources

- http://www.guideline.gov/Compare/comparison.aspx?file=EATING_DISORDERS2.inc. This site provides a comprehensive comparison of the American Psychiatric Association (APA), Finnish Medical Society Duodecim (FMSD), and National Collaborating Center for Mental Health/National Institute for Health and Clinical Excellence (NCCMH/NICE) recommendations for the management of eating disorders depicted in tables. Table 2 specifically addresses the guidelines requirements by the NCCMH/NICE for nurse practitioners.

- National Alliance of Mental Illness: http://www.nami.org/template.cfm?section=by_illness&template=/contentmanagement/. This useful site provides information with discussions on diagnosis, treatment, and patient education for individuals with eating disorders.

- National Institute of Mental Health: http://www.nimh.nih.gov/. Available at: 718–351-1717. This site is a primary reference source for identification and classification of major mental health illnesses. Navigating through the site can lead to information on treatment and guidelines.

- http://ssl.search.live.com/health/article.aspx?id=articles. This Web site provides the history of the compilation and development of the *Diagnostic and Statistical Manual of Mental Disorders* (*DSM IV*) published by the American Psychiatric Association and the World Health Organization's classification of diseases found in the *International Statistical Classification of Diseases and Related Health Problems* (*ICD*). The ICD-9-CM is the standard for reporting morbidity with the ICD-10-CM (clinical code) and the ICD-10-PCS (procedure code) used for specific coding purposes. Additionally, a discussion is provided on the revision of the *DSM-IV-TR* (text revision) due for publication in May 2012. The *DSM-IV-TR* and the ICD classification systems both use the same diagnostic codes. The multi-axial system is discussed in relation to the different aspects of disorder or disability. In addition, this site provides a list of external links for WHO official sites and conversion between ICD codes.

- http://www.pharmacy-and-drugs.com/Weight_loss/Anorexia.html
  This concise Internet source provides a review of the diagnosis of eating disorders, symptoms associated with major eating disorders, and the physiological findings of these eating disorders. Provided are the categories of drugs commonly used along with major therapies commonly used.

- http://familydoctor.org/online/famocen/home/common/mentalhealth/eating/063.html. This site provides quick reference for health care providers on the diagnosis, treatment, and risk factors for anorexia nervosa and other eating disorders.

- http://ssl.search.live. com/health/article.aspx. This university-based Web site provides a review of the symptoms, causes, and treatment for eating disorders. A discussion on helpful diagnostic tests, psychological evaluations, and history review is also provided for health care providers.
- Vanderbilt University: http://www.vanderbilt.edu/ AnS/psychology/health_psychology/anorexia_ drugs.htm. This Web site provides a useful review of common classification of drugs used for eating disorders, especially for anorexia nervosa as well as a discussion of drugs used for gastric emptying, and mineral supplementation.
- http://www.drugs.com/condition/anorexia.htmll This useful Web site discusses the common medications used to stimulate appetite as well as patient education on the uses of these drugs.
- Center for Disease Control: http://www.cdc.gov/ nccdphp/dnpa/bmi/00binaries/bmi-tables.pdf, is useful for calculating body mass index (BMI) for individuals from ages 2–20, while http://www.cdc.gov/nccdphp/ dnpa/bmi/00binaries/bmi-adults.pdf is useful for calculating body mass index (BMI) for adults.

Resources for Patients

These sites provide a description of outpatient and inpatient residential services available to individuals with eating disorders, dual diagnosis, and/or additive behaviors.

- http://www.milestonesprogram.org/program.html.
- http://palmpartners3-px.rtrk. com/.
- http://www.raderprograms. com.

PDA Support

- *Treating eating disorders. Quick reference guide.* Arlington, VA: APA, 2006, July. Electronic copies: Available in portable document format (PDF) from the American Psychiatric Association (APA) Web site.
- *American Psychiatric Association practice guideline development process.* Washington, DC: APA, 2006, May. Electronic copies: Available in portable document format (PDF) from the APA Web site.

Antisocial Personality Disorder

Background Information

Definition of Disorder

- Persistent pattern of disregard for and defiance of the rights of others that begins in childhood or early adolescence and remains consistent up to adulthood.
- Deceit and manipulation are central features whereby the individuals also lack empathy as they have a tendency to disregard the feelings, rights, and suffering of others.
- History of pathological lying.
- Inflated sense of self that appears confident and assured but is often to the determent of others, as they tend to be opinionated, coarse, and verbose, rambling about topics to impress others.
- Cannot be diagnosed until the age of 18.

Etiology

- Also known as sociopathic or psychopathic.
- Previous research has debated whether it is due to nature or nurture.
- Biological studies have identified that there are no known genetic risk factors for personality disorders in the cluster A, B, and C classifications.
- Psychosocial studies have identified that the lack of socialization, the increasing incidence of childhood traumas, as well as childhood maltreatment and neglect such as abuse, lack of empathy shown, poverty, family instability, and community violence, may be related to the development of this disorder.

Demographics

- Thirty to seventy percent of childhood psychiatric admissions are for disruptive behavior disorders. A small percentage of antisocial children (about 3% of males and 1% of females) grow up to become adults with antisocial personality disorder (ASPD), while the remainder of those individuals persist with severe problems with authority, maintaining gainful employment, and/or satisfying relationships.

- Higher incidence in correctional and substance-abuse facilities, forensic settings.

Risk Factors

- Usually begins in childhood or adolescence
- Has been linked with head injuries in childhood
- Predominately males
- Low socioeconomic status and living in urban settings
- More common among first-degree biological relatives
- Familial linkage to female relatives is higher than to male relatives
- Children adopted into homes with parents who have ASPD are at increased risk of developing this disorder

Diagnosis

Differential Diagnosis

- Pathological gambling
- Anxiety disorders
- Substance-related disorders
- Malingering
- Somatoform and factitious disorders
- Developmental and pervasive disorders
- Attention-deficit hyperactivity disorder (ADHD)
- Schizophrenia and psychotic disorders
- Bipolar, mania

ICD Code

F60.2 Antisocial Personality Disorder (ASPD)

Diagnostic Work-Up

- Complete history and physical exam with consideration of previous neurological trauma.
- No laboratory tests are indicated for this diagnosis.
- Psychiatric evaluation should specifically include a thorough focus on personal and social history as this area will highlight the individual's lack of empathy, disregard for the feelings, rights, and suffering of others (i.e., multiple marriages, relationships, criminal history, lack of long-term plans or goals).

- Individuals will have underlying beliefs about themselves and this will be manifested in their behaviors. The consideration of these beliefs or cognitive schemas can also be a useful way to validate the diagnosis. Therefore, here are a few examples of beliefs, thoughts, or sentiments that the individual may share with you as part of the diagnostic interview:
  - Force and cunning are the best ways to get things done
  - "People will get at me if I don't get them first"
  - "It is not important to keep promises or honor debts"
  - "What others think of me really does not matter"
  - "I can get away with things so I do not need to worry about bad consequences"
  - "If it wasn't me, it would be someone else (on raping a woman)"

Clinical Presentation

- Failure to conform to rules in society so that often behaviors are in direct violation of the law
- Deceitful, tells lies, and distortions to the pleasure and advantage of the self
- Lack of empathy and disregard for others
- May be initially pleasant and cooperative but then becomes nasty and difficult
- Impulsive, irritable, aggressive physically as well as verbally
- Lacks the ability to plan ahead, lack of goals
- Consistently irresponsible and has lack of remorse for deviant activities and behaviors
- Pathological lying

DSM-IV-TR Diagnostic Guidelines

- Since the age of 15 the individual has demonstrated a disregard for the rights and well-being of others, and a disregard for sociocultural norms.
- At least 3 of the following must be present:
  - A failure to conform to the rules of society, and disrespect or contempt for the law (often leading to actions that are grounds for arrest).
  - Deceitfulness, use of aliases, the manipulation of others for personal profit or pleasure.

- An inability to set goals or to plan ahead.
- Impulsive behaviors.
- A history of antisocial actions and behaviors: assaults, aggressiveness, irritability.
- Recklessness; disregard for the safety of self and others.
- An inability to meet obligations, including financial obligations, or to honor debts.
- Low levels of regret or shame.
- Relative indifference vis-à-vis harm that comes to others (or to self).
- The antisocial behaviors are not concurrent with schizophrenic illness or manic episodes.

Treatment

Acute Treatment

- There is no acute treatment for this disorder, as personality disorders and, in particular, ASPD are persistent and pervasive patterns of maladaptive behaviors that require chronic treatment in the form of psychotherapy.
- The individual with this personality disorder often ends up in the prison system or in a substance-abuse treatment facility where the treatment focuses on detainment (due to criminal activity) or for withdrawal from substances (that they have become addicted to), not for the treatment of their antisocial behaviors.

Chronic Treatment

- Previous studies have suggested that long-term intervention is the only form of treatment for this individual whether it is incarceration or long-term psychotherapy. There is no psychopharmacological treatment indicated specifically for ASPD.
- Cognitive-behavioral therapy (CBT) is one example of a modality of psychotherapy that has been suggested as a method of psychotherapy for individuals who present with antisocial behaviors and ASPD.
- Rather than attempt to change the *moral structure* of the individual as evidence in psychodynamic psychotherapy, CBT instead can be implemented to focus on improving moral and

social *behaviors* through enhancement of cognitive functioning.

- Individuals with ASPD would need to (a) identify and address the possible negative outcomes for their behaviors; and (b) have an increased awareness of their dysfunctional beliefs about themselves, the world, and the future toward making cognitive changes. CBT would focus on assisting the individual with APD to make a transition from their concrete beliefs to a broader spectrum of possibilities and outcomes.
- A small percentage of children who have conduct disorder (about 3% of males and 1% of females) grow up to become adults with ASPD, while the remainder of those individuals persist with severe problems with authority, maintaining gainful employment, and/or satisfying relationships.
- Individuals do not have episodes of a personality disorder; rather, they have these traits as lifelong behavioral patterns.

Patient Education

- Individual would have to make personal life changes to correct deviant behaviors through psychosocial education, CBT, ongoing long-term psychotherapy, and/or incarceration.
- In general, most individuals with this disorder have no interest in changing or understanding their behaviors. Education would most likely occur for family and friends who have been injured, deceived, or in some way manipulated by these individuals.
- Family therapy for those who have been affected by an individual with ASPD would include (a) understanding the diagnosis; (b) identifying the behaviors that are manipulative and deceitful; (c) being able to set limits with the individual with ASPD so as not to be hurt, abused, or deceived in the future.

Medical/Legal Pitfalls

- These individuals are dangerous and often can fool even the most experienced clinician. It is best to consider a forensic evaluation or consultation with a forensic specialist (psychiatrist or psychologist) for further direction.

- Forensic psychiatry is a branch of medicine which focuses on the interface of law and mental health.
- Forensic psychiatrists have additional education, training, and/or experience related to the various interfaces of mental health (or mental illness) with the law and are able to distinguish between a personality disorder or a clinical syndrome (i.e., when violent and hostile/aggressive behaviors are criminal or immoral).
- Forensic psychiatrists often determine whether an individual is "clinically competent" to stand trial for their actions or they provide expert evidence about their actions and behaviors.
- Clinicians can be at risk for violence directed at them from individuals through threats, or physical or emotional abuse or harm.
- Forensic research has identified three *key principles* when confronted with an individual with ASPD who is violent or has a history of violence: (a) in general, ASPDs are rarely ego-dystonic; (b) most patients and violent situations associated with clinical issues involve comorbid conditions; and (c) violence and violence risk are often associated with intoxication. In other words, most individuals with ASPD will not seek treatment for their symptoms of this personality disorder; rather, they will present to health care providers for other symptoms, illnesses, and/or treatment (i.e., related to their violent behaviors). As well, treating or managing the coexisting conditions (which may include illness, substance abuse, or environmental factors such as being arrested and imprisoned) may alleviate some violence potential if they are incarcerated as they are out of the general public community. Finally, their outcome or prognosis for treatment of their substance abuse or dependence is poor.
- Risk assessment includes being aware of a history of violence with the following antisocial behaviors: (a) *purposeful, instrumental violence* (acts in which violence is a means to a conscious, gainful end such as a robbery, as well as violence designed to manipulate or mislead another into some wanted behavior; (b) *purposeful, noninstrumental violence* is exemplified in seeking the pleasure of a stimulating or antisocial

activity, but the actual injuring of others is not integral to the activity's purpose; and (c) *purposeful, targeted, defensive violence* is identified in an individual who fears abandonment or humiliation and strikes out in illogical ways such as murder or injury. Examples are "paranoid stalkers" who follow their "victims" and are threatened by anything getting between their victims and themselves (i.e., police, children, spouse of victim).

- Clinicians need to understand the importance of identifying these signs and symptoms in clinical practice, and how their relationship is defined in terms of the individual with ASPD.
- The key is to recognize and assess risk in order to remain safe.

Borderline Personality Disorder

Background Information

Definition of Disorder

- Persistent pattern of mood instability, intense interpersonal relationships, impulsivity, identity disturbance, recurrent suicidal acts, and/or self-mutilating behaviors, intense anger, and rage as well as the potential for dissociation and psychosis.
- Begins in adolescence and the behaviors vary throughout adulthood.
- Fears of abandonment occur.
- Idealizes and devalues people.
- Sees the world in black and white ("no gray areas").
- Three specific components help to conceptualize the disorder: (a) an unstable self; (b) impulsive thoughts; and (c) sudden shifts of mood.
- Often confused with bipolar disorder due to impulsivity and mood instability.

Etiology

- During the past 20 years, the literature has expanded with multiple reasons for the development of this personality disorder.
- Includes a history of childhood abuse, unstable or otherwise detrimental family environment, and family history of psychopathology.
- Childhood sexual abuse (CSA) is the most significant correlation with severity, chronicity, and age of onset of sexual abuse, and co-occurrence (and severity) of other forms of abuse and neglect taking a second place in the determination.
- Psychoanalytic theories focus on poor parental/caretaker attachment and the individual's difficulty with separation as a consequence.

Demographics

- About 1–2% of the population, with 10–25% of patients presenting in clinical settings, and 20% in hospital settings

- More females than males
- No difference for ethnic origin or socioeconomic status

Risk Factors

- Childhood physical, sexual, and emotional abuse.
- Children who experience CSA are four times more likely to develop borderline personality disorder (BPD) than those who do not.
- Severity, chronicity, and age of onset of sexual abuse (the younger the abuse, the poorer the prognosis), as well as the co-occurrence of other forms of abuse and neglect place individuals at greater risk.
- Family factors such as difficult relationships, poor attachment, poor parental care.
- Social factors such as low socioeconomic status of family, being raised in a single-parent family, welfare support of family, parental death, and social isolation.
- Temperament has been studied and findings suggest that children and adolescents who cope by "internalizing" symptoms such as anxiety and depression and "externalizing" symptoms such as impulsivity, defiance, and oppositional behavior are at greater risk for a poorer prognosis.
- Genetic factors play a role in the potential for individual differences in BPD features in Western society. This finding surmised that the symptoms and presentation of this disorder were consistent across three countries studying twins.
- Poor parenting and lack of attachment are frequently associated with the development of the symptoms of BPD in childhood, adolescence, and into adulthood.

Diagnosis

Differential Diagnosis

- Frequently comorbid with Axis I disorders, especially substance-use disorders in males, eating disorders in females, anxiety disorders, and mood disorders, so it is often missed or misdiagnosed.

- Due to the mood instability, impulsivity, and psychotic symptoms, bipolar disorder is often mistaken for this personality disorder (although individuals can have both).

ICD Code

301.83 Borderline Personality Disorder

Diagnostic Work-Up

- Complete history and physical exam, with consideration of previous neurological trauma and careful assessment of the potential for seizure disorder (i.e., temporal lobe epilepsy).
- Psychiatric evaluation, including a focus on personal and social history including history of abuse, problems with attachment and separation as a child and/or adolescent.
- Physical and mental evaluation
  - Thyroid function studies (triiodothyronine [T3], thyroxine [T4], thyroid-stimulating hormone [TSH]).
  - CMP (complete metabolic panel), including glucose, calcium, albumin; total protein count; levels of sodium, potassium, CO_2 (carbon dioxide and bicarbonate), chloride, blood urea nitrogen (BUN), creatinine, alkaline phosphatase (ALP), alanine amino transferase (ALT, also called SGPT), aspartate amino transferase (AST, also called SGOT), and bilirubin.
  - CBC (complete blood count) with differentials: hemoglobin, hematocrit, red blood cell (RBC) count, white blood cell (WBC) count, WBC differential count, and platelet count.
  - Careful assessment for cuts, bruises, and scars where patient could have caused self-harm through cutting, burning, or self-injury.

Clinical Presentation

- Three specific components help to conceptualize the disorder: (a) an unstable sense of self; (b) impulsive thoughts; and (c) sudden shifts of mood.
- Reports mood instability, intense interpersonal relationships, impulsivity, identity disturbance, recurrent suicidal acts, and/or self-mutilating behaviors, intense anger, and rage as well as the potential for dissociation and psychosis.

- Relates interpersonal issues in terms of extremes (black or white, good or bad, idealized or failed parenting or relationships).

DSM-IV-TR Diagnostic Guidelines

- A pattern of instability of interpersonal relationships.
- A pattern of instability of self-image.
- Marked impulsivity beginning in early childhood and present in a variety of contexts.
- Presence of 5 or more of the following:
  - Urgent efforts to avoid real or imagined abandonment.
  - Interpersonal relationships that are characterized by alternations between extremes of valuation and devaluation.
  - Notably and persistently unstable self-image or sense of self.
  - Impulsivity in two or more areas that carry the possibility of bad outcomes (e.g., spending sprees, reckless driving, binge eating, substance abuse).
  - Suicidal ideation, behavior, gestures, or threats, or self-mutilating behavior.
  - Labile mood, hyperreactivity (e.g., episodes of intense dysphoria, high anxiety).
  - Feelings of emptiness.
  - Inappropriate anger, difficulty in controlling anger.
  - Transient stress-related paranoid ideation.
  - Dissociative symptoms.

Treatment

Acute Treatment

- Establish a trusting interpersonal professional relationship.
- Stabilize symptoms that are the most distressing to the individual (mood instability, psychosis, suicidal thoughts and actions).
- May consider atypical antipsychotics to assist with the transient psychosis and mood instability as well as serotonin reuptake inhibitors (SSRIs) for depression. Stay away from tricyclic and MAO-I antidepressants as they have a higher risk of overdose and lethality.
- Crisis intervention is frequently the most common acute treatment, along with brief

hospitalizations for threats to self (i.e., suicidal ideation, plan, and intent), and others (homicidal ideation, plan, and intent); self-mutilating behaviors; brief psychosis.

- If individual is not in therapy, it is best to consider initiating this or referring to an experienced outpatient therapist as these individuals will present in crisis and need to know that there is a contact person.
- Prescribe medications for short periods of time to avoid the potential for overdose of medications when the individual is in crisis or impulsive.
- If one is not the therapist or prescriber, one should maintain an ongoing collaborative relationship with the therapist or prescriber as individuals with this disorder often split and play one against the other.
- Refer to DBT (dialectical behavioral therapy)— see references and recommended readings.

Chronic Treatment

- Studies have shown that long-term psychodynamic psychotherapy is the most useful, if not the most successful, long-term form of treatment.
- DBT is also very successful but often individuals need to repeat the group and individual sessions on a long-term basis to acquire the necessary skills to learn how to cope with their thoughts and feelings.
- Medications for symptom relief are useful, such as SSRIs and/or mood stabilizers for management of mood instability. Cautiously use benzodiazepines or other addictive substances.
- This is a long-term pervasive personality disorder that does not "go away" and come back. It is frequently "crisis driven" and individuals with this disorder need to learn to live with the symptoms as well as learn to cope appropriately with their internalized emotions as well as the externalized behaviors.
- Some individuals do mature and can move toward a healthier way of living and coping with stresses. This seems to be an outcome of

long-term psychotherapy where the patient has insight and a willingness to change.

Patient Education

- Multiple Web sites and "chat rooms" where individuals and families can learn about the disorder and also obtain support (see sites below).

Medical/Legal Pitfalls

"When you touch the patient, therapy is over" (Gutheil, 1989).

- It is extremely important to understand that patients who suffer from this disorder have difficulty with boundaries (personal, social, and professional) and will "test" the limits in their relationships.
- Hugging and/or touching the patients without some discussion of its meaning can be very dangerous for the clinician. It is best *not* to have physical contact with them and set this boundary early on in treatment.
- Individuals with BPD are, for the most part, likely to provoke various kinds of boundary violations, including sexual acting out and testing your "affection" for them (i.e., they may invite you to an event that they are attending or offer you tickets to a theater production).
- These individuals (sadly) also represent the majority of those patients who falsely accuse therapists of sexual involvement, touching, and inappropriate contact. Many clinicians choose not to work with these patients and also demoralize them because of their own lack of skill. Therefore, be aware of your own scope of practice and if you are not skilled, refer them to someone who is trained and/or skilled.
- In general, therapists can take advantage of developing an awareness of any repeating patterns of behaviors that occur with these individuals and in how they respond (both the patient and the clinician). With this knowledge, clinicians can then steer clear of the highly destructive litigation that can and will ensue.

Narcissistic Personality Disorder

Background Information

Definition of Disorder

- A persistent pattern of grandiosity (in fantasy or behavior), need for admiration, and lack of empathy, beginning by early adulthood and present in a variety of contexts.
- Grandiose sense of self-importance (e.g., exaggerates achievements and talents, expects to be recognized as superior without commensurate achievements).
- Preoccupation with fantasies of unlimited success, power, brilliance, beauty, or ideal love.
- Patient believes that he or she is "special" and unique and can only be understood by, or should associate with, other special or high-status people (or institutions).
- Requires excessive admiration.
- Sense of entitlement, i.e., unreasonable expectations of especially favorable treatment or automatic compliance with his or her expectations.
- Interpersonally exploitative, i.e., takes advantage of others to achieve his or her own ends.
- Lacks empathy, i.e., is unwilling to recognize or identify with the feelings and needs of others.
- Often envious of others or believes that others are envious of him or her.
- Shows arrogant, haughty behaviors or attitudes (DSM-IV-TR, 2000).

Etiology

- As with all personality disorders, early childhood development plays a role in the progression of the pathology that is inherent in each of the maladaptive behaviors listed in the definition of narcissistic personality disorder (NPD).
- Some theories (i.e., psychoanalytic) focus on the lack of paternal availability and the strength (or lack) of the relationship between the mother and father as a determinant in the development of a narcissistic child, adolescent, and adult as well as an outcome of the insufficient gratification of the normal narcissistic needs of infancy and childhood.
- Neoanalytical thinking takes an antithetical view that narcissism is the outcome of narcissistic overgratification during childhood. This view focuses on parents who overindulge their child, protect the child from disappointment and failure, and minimize the criticisms of others about their child. It also presents the child who displays difficulties in self-esteem regulation and a tendency toward massive externalization of emotions.

Demographics

- About 0.7–1% of the general population suffer from NPD; about 2–16% of the clinical population
- Between 50 and 75% are males

Risk Factors

- There have been no known genetic factors contributing to risk.
- An oversensitive temperament as a young child.
- Children who are adopted and therefore struggle to cope with the loss and rejection of their biological parents, especially if there is dysfunction within the current family of origin.
- Various developmental pathways may present a special risk for the formation of NPD: (a) having narcissistic parents; (b) being adopted; (c) being abused; (d) being overindulged; (e) having divorced parents; and/or (f) losing a parent through death.
- Some theorists believe that this is learned behavior and that narcissistic children come from narcissistic parents or caretakers.

Diagnosis

Differential Diagnosis

- Histrionic personality disorder (HPD)
- Antisocial personality disorder (ASPD)

- Obsessive-compulsive personality disorder (OCPD)

ICD Code
F60.8 Narcissistic Personality Disorder

Diagnostic Work-Up
- Complete history and physical exam with consideration of previous neurological trauma
- No laboratory tests are indicated for this diagnosis
- Psychiatric evaluation including a focus on personal and social history

Clinical Presentation
- The essential features are grandiosity, lack of empathy, and need for admiration.
- A sense of superiority, a sense of uniqueness, exaggeration of talents, boastful and pretentious behavior, grandiose fantasies, self-centered and self-referential behavior, need for attention and admiration, arrogant and haughty behavior, and high achievement.
- Individuals with NPD can be at high risk for suicide during periods when they are not suffering from clinical depression.
- The individual learns to use defenses, including projection, and splitting into all good and all bad, and, along with that, idealization.

DSM-IV-TR Diagnostic Guidelines
- Grandiose thoughts, grandiose behavior
- A need for admiration
- Lack of empathy
- Begins at early childhood and is present in a variety of contexts
- The presence of at least 5 of the following:
  - Self-importance (e.g., the individual exaggerates his or her achievements, expects to be recognized as superior in the absence of notable achievements)
  - Preoccupied with notions of unlimited success, power, beauty, brilliance
  - Believes that he or she is exceptional and can only be understood by, or should only associate with, persons of high status
  - Wants or needs excessive admiration

- Possesses a sense of entitlement, has expectations of especially favorable treatment, has expectations of automatic compliance with his or her wishes
- Is exploitive, takes advantage of others in order to achieve his or her own ends
- Lacks empathy, seems unable to recognize or identify with the feelings and needs of others
- Is often envious of others, believes that others are envious of him/her
- Displays haughty or arrogant behaviors, attitudes

Treatment

Acute Treatment
- Currently, with the onset of the twenty-first century, there are no medications that have been developed specifically for the treatment of NPD.
- Patients with NPD who are also depressed or anxious may be given medications for relief of those symptoms.
- However, there are subjective reports in the literature that the SSRIs may reinforce narcissistic grandiosity and lack of empathy with others and thus worsen the disorder.

Chronic Treatment
- Intensive psychoanalytic psychotherapy. Requires referral to a therapist or extensive training to implement this type of treatment.
- The goals of treatment are to work on (a) the grandiose self; (b) the pathologic defense mechanisms that interfered with people's normal development; and (c) their manipulative interactions with their family and friends.
- CBT can be implemented in some cases to assist the individuals to identify their negative behaviors and replace them with more functional ways of interacting with others.
- Most individuals who suffer from NPD cannot form a sufficiently deep bond with a therapist to allow healing of early-childhood injuries, so treatment is usually long-term if the individual can tolerate it.

■ This is a long-term pervasive personality disorder, which originates in childhood and/or adolescence and is retained throughout adulthood.

Patient Education

See Other Resources section at the end of the chapter.

Medical/Legal Pitfalls

■ Significant relationships were found between NPD and incarceration for violent crimes; therefore, obtain a thorough social and legal history.

Other Resources

Evidence-Based References

American Psychiatric Association. (2000). *Diagnostic and statistical manual of mental disorders* (Revised 4th ed.). Washington, DC: American Psychiatric Association.

Beck, A., & Freeman, A. (2003). *Cognitive therapy of personality disorders* (2nd ed.). New York: Guilford Press.

Bradley, R., Jenei, J., & Westen, D. (2005). Etiology of borderline personality disorder: Disentangling the contributions of intercorrelated antecedents. *Journal of Nervous and Mental Disorders, 193*, 24–31.

Cohen, P. (2008). Child development and personality disorder. *The Psychiatric Clinics of North America, 31*(3), 477–493, vii.

Distel, M. A., Trull, T. J., Derom, C. A., Thiery, C. W., Grimmer, M. A., & Martin, N. G. et al. (2008). Heritability of borderline personality disorder features is similar across three countries. *Psychological Medicine, 38*(9), 1219–1229.

Fonagy, P., & Bateman, A. (2008). The development of borderline personality disorder—a mentalizing model. *Journal of Personality Disorders, 22*(1), 4–21.

Gutheil, T. A. (1989). Borderline personality disorder, boundary violations, and patient-therapist sex: Medicolegal pitfalls. *American Journal of Psychiatry, 146*, 597–602.

Kendler, K. S., Aggen, S. H., Czajkowski, N., Røysamb, E., Tambs, K., Torgersen, S., et al. (2008). *Archives of General Psychiatry, 65*(12), 1438–1446.

Paris, J. (2009). The treatment of borderline personality disorder: Implications of research on diagnosis, etiology, and outcome. *Annual Review of Clinical Psychology, 5*, 277–290.

Reid, W. H., & Thorne, S. A. (2007). Personality disorders and violence potential. *Law and Psychiatry: Journal of Psychiatric Practice, 13*(4).

Sadock, B. J., & Sadock, V. A. (2008). *Synopsis of psychiatry* (10th ed.). Philadelphia, PA: Lippincott, Williams & Wilkins.

Smith, C. A., Ireland, T. O., Thornberry, T. P., & Elwyn, L. O. (2008). Childhood maltreatment and antisocial behavior: Comparison of self-reported and substantiated maltreatment. *American Journal of Orthopsychiatry, 78*(2), 173–186.

Torgersen, S., Kringlen, E., & Cramer, V. (2001). The prevalence of personality disorders in a community sample. *Archives of General Psychiatry, 58*, 590–596.

I hate you, don't leave me: Understanding the Borderline Personality (1991)

Skills Training Manual for Treating Borderline Personality Disorder. (There is a whole series of books by Marsha Linehan, PhD, related to assessment and treatment using various psychotherapies including DBT, starting in 1993.)

Stop Walking on Eggshells: Taking Your Life Back When Someone You Care About Has Borderline Personality Disorder (1998)

Surviving a Borderline Parent: How to Heal Your Childhood Wounds & Build Trust, Boundaries, and Self-Esteem (2003)

Understanding the Borderline Mother: Helping Her Children Transcend the Intense, Unpredictable, and Volatile Relationship (2002)

Web Resources

Antisocial Personality Disorder
- http://www.mentalhealth.com/dis/p20-pe04.html.
- http://www.ptypes.com/antisocialpd.html.

Forensic Psychiatry
- http://www.reidpsychiatry.com/index.html.
- http://www.umdnj.edu/psyevnts/forensic.html.

Borderline Personality Disorder
- http://www.bpdcentral.com/index.php.
- http://www.mhsanctuary.com/borderline/bkindex.htm.

Primary Insomnia

Background Information

Definition of Disorder

- It is associated with physical factors and physiological disorder excluding anxiety or depression
- Trouble falling asleep or maintaining sleep for 1 month
- Patient complains of not feeling rested

Epidemiology

- Women are 1.5 times more likely to have insomnia-related office visits
- Predominant between the ages of 18 and 64
- Ten to fourteen percent of adults present in primary care
- Accounts for 16% of all insomnia complaints

Risk Factors

- Acute stress
- Depression
- Anxiety
- Medications (nonprescription and prescription)
- Obesity
- Geriatric considerations:
  - Medications should be used only for short-term management
  - Benzodiazepines or sedative-hypnotics increase risk of confusion, delirium, and/or falls
- Pregnancy considerations:
  - Physiological changes are associated with pregnancy, may disrupt sleep
  - Avoid medications
  - Consider other comfort measures such as a change to a softer bed or a position change

Diagnosis

Differential Diagnosis

- Thyroid disorders
- Anxiety/stress
- Drug interactions
- Substance abuse
- Hypersomnia
- Parasomnia

Diagnostic Work-Up

- Subjective complaints of inability to fall asleep or maintain sleep
- Feeling of not being rested
- Impacts daytime functioning

Initial Assessment

- Sleep hygiene
- Related medical conditions
- Snoring, sleep movements, irregular breathing patterns, length of sleep, changes in mood should be obtained from family
- Length of time with sleep disturbance, difficulty falling asleep, thoughts racing, repeated awakenings or early morning awakening history should be obtained
- New stressors
- New medications, over-the-counter (OTC) meds, or herbal supplements

Laboratory Tests

- Thyroid function studies (triiodothyronine [T3], thyroxine [T4], thyroid-stimulating hormone [TSH])
- CMP (complete metabolic panel), including glucose, calcium, and albumin; total protein analysis; and levels of sodium, potassium, CO_2 (carbon dioxide, bicarbonate), chloride, blood urea nitrogen (BUN), creatinine, alkaline phosphatase (ALP), alanine amino transferase (ALT, also called SGPT), aspartate amino transferase (AST, also called SGOT), and bilirubin
- CBC (complete blood count) with differentials: hemoglobin, hematocrit, red blood cell (RBC) count, white blood cell (WBC) count, WBC differential count, and platelet count

ICD Code

780.50 Sleep Disturbance, Unspecified

DSM-IV-TR Diagnostic Criteria

- Difficulty falling asleep or staying asleep, occurring for at least one month.
- Daily functioning is impaired.

- The insomnia is not caused by anxiety, depression, or other medical conditions related to sleep, such as obstructive sleep apnea.

Treatment

Behavioral Modification

- Eliminate stressors or assist patient in developing coping strategies
- No caffeine after 3 P.M.
- No alcohol intake within 3 hours of bedtime
- Daily exercise (avoid 4 hours prior to sleep)
- Establish sleep routine

Pharmacotherapy

Short-term use of nonbenzodiazepine medications such as eszopiclone (Lunesta), zaleplon (Sonata), zolpidem (Ambien), or ramelteon (Rozerem)

- Adult treatment only:
  - Eszopiclone (Lunesta)
  - Zaleplon (Sonata)
  - Zolpidem (Ambien)
  - Ramelteon (Rozerem)

  Short-term use of benzodiazepine medications such as flurazepam (Dalmane), temazepam (Restoril), or triazolam (Halcion)
- Flurazepam (Dalmane)

- Temazepam (Restoril)
- Triazolam (Halcion)

Follow-Up

- Consider psychiatric evaluation if mental, emotional, or behavioral disorder suspected
- Consider sleep lab evaluation if symptoms persist

Patient Education

- Use bed for sleep or intimacy only
- Encourage patient to establish a routine before sleep
- No caffeine 6 hours before sleep
- No exercise 4 hours before sleep
- Evaluate response to medication within 7 days
- Avoid refills of medications
- Avoid diet high in protein or alcohol 3–6 hours before sleep
- Exercise regularly at least 5–6 hours before bedtime
- Avoid use of OTC antihistamines or alcohol to induce sleepiness
- Create a calm, cool, quiet atmosphere for sleep
- If unable to sleep for 30 minutes, leave bedroom and engage in a quiet activity such as light reading
- Pharmacologic agents are for short-term or intermittent use only

Primary Hypersomnia

Background Information

Definition of Disorder
- Recurring excessive daytime sleepiness or prolonged nighttime sleep, impacting activities of daily living without central origin
- Three categories of hypersomnia include insufficient nighttime sleep, fragmented nighttime sleep, and increased drive to sleep
- May present as monosymptomatic or polysymptomatic
- Monosymptomatic person presents solely excessive daytime sleepiness without abnormal nighttime awakenings
- Polysymptomatic person presents with abnormally long nighttime sleeping and sleep drunkenness upon awakening

Etiology
- Idiopathic
- No genetic, environmental, or other relating factors are identified

Demographics
- Most common onset is during adolescence
- Rarely presents after age of 30
- Affects male and females equally
- Exact prevalence is unknown in the United States
- Five to ten percent of all patients referred to a sleep laboratory for evaluation are diagnosed with primary insomnia

Risk Factors
- Acute stress
- Depression
- Anxiety
- Medications (nonprescription and prescription)
- Physiological changes associated with pregnancy may disrupt sleep
- Poor sleep hygiene

Diagnosis

Differential Diagnosis
- Sleep apnea
- Kleine-Levin syndrome
- Depression
- Head trauma
- Insomnia

ICD Code
9-CM 780.54 Hypersomnia, Unspecified

Diagnostic Work-Up
- Excessive daytime sleepiness requiring frequent naps
- Does not awaken feeling refreshed
- Night sleep longer than 12 hours
- Difficult to awaken, once asleep
- Sleep hygiene
- Related medical conditions
- Snoring, sleep movements, irregular breathing patterns, length of sleep, changes in mood should be obtained from family
- Length of time with sleep disturbance
- New medications, OTC meds, or herbal supplements

Laboratory Tests
- Thyroid function studies (T3, T4, TSH)
- CMP, including glucose, calcium, albumin; total protein count; levels of sodium, potassium, CO_2 (carbon dioxide and bicarbonate), chloride, BUN, creatinine, ALP, ALT, AST, and bilirubin
- CBC with differentials: hemoglobin, hematocrit, RBC count, WBC count, WBC differential count, and platelet count
- Confirmed by multiple sleep latency test (MSLT)
- Mean initial sleep latency of <8 minutes without early onset of rapid eye movement (REM) sleep
- Polysomnography is used to exclude other sleep disorders
- Epworth sleepiness scale is used

Clinical Presentation
- Prolonged sleep patterns
- Sleep drunkenness
- Less common
  - Headache
  - Orthostatic hypotension

- Syncope
- Raynaud's phenomenon

DSM-IV-TR Diagnostic Guidelines

- Consistent sleepiness for greater than one month.
- Engenders personal distress or impaired social functioning.
- Other sleep disorders have been excluded.
- Does not occur concurrently with and exclusively during the course of another mental disorder.
- Is not a direct physiological effect of a substance.

Treatment

Behavioral

- Stimulants at the lowest dose produce optimal alertness and minimize side effects
- Avoidance of sleep deprivation
- Establish regular sleep and wake times
- Work in a stimulating environment
- Avoid shift work

Pharmacotherapy

- Methylphenidate
- Amphetamine/dextroamphetamine (Adderall)
- Dextroamphetamine (Dexedrine)
- Modafinil (Provigil)

Follow-Up

- Consider psychiatric evaluation if mental, emotional, or behavioral disorder is suspected
- Consider sleep lab evaluation if symptoms persist

Prognosis

- Responds poorly to treatment
- Disabling

Patient Education

- Eat three meals every day
- Exercise regularly
- Avoid use of OTC antihistamines or alcohol before bedtime
- Use bedroom for sleep or intimacy only

Narcolepsy

Background Information

Definition of Disorder
- Chronic REM sleep disorder of central origin is characterized by excessive daytime sleepiness
- Classic presenting symptoms include excessive daytime sleepiness, sleep paralysis, cataplexy, and hypnagogic hallucinations
- Nocturnal sleep disturbances are common

Etiology
- Associated with specific HLA halotypes
- Possible autoimmune etiology

Demographics
- Male to female ratio is 1.64:1
- First-degree relatives have a 10- to 40-fold higher risk than the general population
- Age of peak presentation is 15 years
- It is reported in children as young as 2 years
- Affects 0.02–0.18% of the United States and Western population
- Increases to 25–56 per 100,000 when cataplexy is not a required symptom for diagnosis

Risk Factors
- Positive family history
- Age
- At risk for motor vehicle accidents and injuries
- Pregnancy considerations
- Pediatric consideration: children rarely present with all four symptoms

Diagnosis

Differential Diagnosis
- Absence seizures
- Benign childhood epilepsy
- Brainstem glioma
- Complex partial seizures
- Periodic limb movement disorder
- REM sleep behavior disorder
- Tonic-clonic seizures
- Transient global amnesia
- Syncope and related paroxysmal spells

ICD Code
9-CM 347.00 Narcolepsy

Diagnostic Work-Up
- Symptoms
  - Nocturnal sleep disturbances
  - Short and frequent refreshing napping episodes
  - Excessive daytime sleepiness for 3 months or longer
  - Loss of muscle tone briefly
  - EOMs and respiratory function remain intact with cataplexy
  - If cataplexy event is severe and generalized, patient may fall
  - Cataplexy is often triggered by changes in emotions such as laughter or anger episodes

Initial Assessment
- Sleep hygiene
- Related medical conditions
- Snoring, sleep movements, irregular breathing patterns, length of sleep, changes in mood should be obtained from family
- Length of time with sleep disturbance
- New medications, OTC meds, or herbal supplements

Laboratory Tests
- Thyroid function studies (T3, T4, TSH)
- CMP, including glucose, calcium, albumin; total protein count; levels of sodium, potassium, CO_2 (carbon dioxide and bicarbonate), chloride, BUN, creatinine, ALP, ALT, AST, and bilirubin
- CBC with differentials: hemoglobin, hematocrit, RBC count, WBC count, WBC differential count, and platelet count
- Confirmed by MSLT as demonstrated by sleep latency of <8 minutes accompanied by REM sleep occurring within 15 minutes of sleep onset during at least 2 out of 4 nap opportunities
- Epworth sleepiness scale

- Polysomnography
- Actigraphy
- Human leukocyte antigen typing
- Cerebrospinal fluid hypocretin-1 analysis

DSM-IV-TR Diagnostic Criteria

- The individual falls asleep irresistibly, occurring daily for at least 3 months.
- The presence of one or both of the following:
  - Cataplexy (abrupt loss of muscle tone)
  - Consistent incursions of elements of REM sleep into the transitions between sleep and wakefulness
- The disturbance is not the direct physiological effect of use of a substance or of other medical conditions.

Treatment

Behavioral

- Sleep hygiene
- Scheduled naps
- Reassurance for patient and family
- Exercise programs
- Avoidance of foods high in sugar

Pharmacotherapy

- Methylphenidate
- Amphetamine/dextroamphetamine (Adderall)
- Dextroamphetamine (Dexedrine)
- Modafinil (Provigil)

Follow-Up

- Pediatric patients should be followed by a pediatrician and pediatric neurologist

Prognosis

- With medications and treatment, the patient may lead a productive life

Complications

- Adverse effects of medications
- Injury

Patient Monitoring

- Monthly follow-up is recommended to monitor response to medications

Patient Education

- Advise adult patients regarding driving responsibilities
- Educate patient regarding long-term effects of medications and need for safety precautions

Nightmare Disorder

Background Information

Definition of Disorder
- Is associated with REM sleep
- Occurs at any age
- Patient describes bizarre dream plot
- Patient is arousable from sleep
- Remembers event
- Is exacerbated by stress

Etiology
- Occurs equally in males and females
- Twenty to thirty-nine percent of children between ages 5 and 12 are affected
- Five to eight percent of adults are affected

Risk Factors
- Stress
- Sleep deprivation
- Psychiatric and neurological disorders in adults
- Medications affecting neurotransmitter levels, such as antidepressants, narcotics, or barbiturates

Diagnosis

Differential Diagnosis
- Sleep terrors
- Sleep-disordered breathing
- Restless leg syndrome

ICD Code
9-CM 304.47 Nightmare Disorder

Initial Assessment
- Sleep hygiene
- Related medical conditions
- Data on snoring, sleep movements, irregular breathing patterns, length of sleep, changes in mood should be obtained from family
- Length of time with sleep disturbance, difficulty falling asleep, repeated awakenings, or early-morning awakening history should be obtained

- New stressors
- New medications, OTC meds, or herbal supplements

Clinical Presentation
- Abrupt awakening
- Frightened and able to describe fears

DSM-IV-TR Diagnostic Criteria
- Frequent awakenings from major sleep or naps, with detailed recall of extended and ominous dreams (usually involving threats to survival, personal security, or self-esteem).
- The awakenings generally occur during the latter part of the sleep period.
- On waking, the person rapidly becomes oriented and alert.
- The disturbance that is experienced on waking causes notable distress for the individual or impairment of social functioning.
- The nightmares do not occur concurrently with and exclusively during the course of another mental disorder (e.g., delirium, posttraumatic stress disorder) and are not the direct physiological effect of substance use or another medical condition.

Treatment

Behavioral
- Comfort and reassurance are given
- Behavioral strategies or counseling, if episodes are frequent and severe

Pharmacotherapy
- None indicated

Follow-Up
- Referral to psychiatrist may be indicated if a psychiatric disturbance is suspected
- Referral to sleep lab, if history does not correlate with clinical findings to rule out sleep-disordered breathing, parasomnia, or restless leg syndrome

- Nightmares should resolve with time
- Insomnia from fear of sleeping may occur
- Daytime sleepiness may occur
- Cognitive dysfunction with protracted sleep disruption

Patient Education

- Reassure parents that the disorder should resolve with maturity
- Reinforce the need for security to parents
- Adult patients should decrease stressors

Sleep Terror Disorder

Background Information

Definition of Disorder

- Also referred to as pavor nocturnus (night terrors)
- Sleep disturbance arising from slow wave sleep nonrapid eye movement (NREM) sleep stage III or IV
- Occurs 60–90 minutes after onset of sleep in children
- Patient does not remember the event and is often confused and disoriented afterward
- Screaming, sitting upright in bed
- Frequently will have pallor, pupil dilation, tachycardia, and sweating
- Occurs most often in children age 4–12
- Typically a strong family history of parasomnias
- Exacerbated by stress and fatigue

Etiology

- It is predominant in males
- Occurs in 3% of children ages 18 months to adolescence
- Prevalence 1–4% of population

Risk Factors

- Adults are likely to have psychopathology such as substance abuse and affective disorders

Diagnosis

Differential Diagnosis

- Nocturnal panic attacks occur
- Nocturnal dissociative episodes
- Frontal lobe seizures
- Delirium is associated with medical or neurologic disorder
- Sleep-disordered breathing occurs
- Restless leg syndrome

ICD Code

9-CM 307.46 Sleep Terror Disorder

Initial Assessment

- Sleep hygiene should be examined
- Related medical conditions should be known
- Snoring, sleep movements, irregular breathing patterns, length of sleep, changes in mood should be obtained from family
- Length of time with sleep disturbance, difficulty falling asleep, repeated awakenings, or early-morning awakening history should be obtained
- New stressors should be recorded
- New medications, OTC meds, or herbal supplements should be considered

Clinical Presentation

- Patient abruptly awakens from sleep with screaming during the first one-third of major sleep
- Tachycardia, rapid breathing, pupil dilation, and sweating with each episode may occur
- Patient is unresponsive to family
- Does not recall event

Laboratory Tests

- Polysomnography
- EEG with time-synchronized video monitoring

DSM-IV-TR Diagnostic Criteria

- Abrupt awakenings from sleep, usually occurring during the first third of the sleep episode.
- A frightened scream often accompanies the awakening.
- Intense fear occurs on waking.
- Signs of autonomic stimulation: tachycardia, rapid breathing, sweating.
- Relative unresponsiveness of the individual to the efforts of others to comfort him/her.
- The episodes engender notable distress for the individual or impairment of social functioning.
- The disturbance is not the direct physiologic effect of substance use or another medical condition.

Treatment

Behavioral
- Rule out sleep-disordered breathing
- Parent reassurance should be given
- Ensure safe environment
- Timed awakening
- Suggest afternoon nap for children
- Self-hypnosis
- Short course of therapy of benzodiazepine or tricyclic in adults
- Do follow-up
- Referral to psychiatrist may be indicated if psychiatric disturbance is suspected
- Referral to sleep lab if history does not correlate with clinical findings to rule out sleep-disordered breathing, parasomnia, or restless leg syndrome

Pharmacotherapy
- Diazepam (Valium), clonazepam (Klonopin), flurazepam (Dalmane), alprazolam (Niravam), imipramine (Tofranil)

Prognosis
- Sleep terrors should resolve with maturity
- Complications may occur
- Daytime sleepiness may occur
- Cognitive dysfunction with protracted sleep disruption

Patient Monitoring
- Reassess for protracted symptomatology

Patient Education
- Family, partner reassurance should be given
- Adult patients must avoid substances that trigger events

Sleepwalking Disorder

Background Information

Definition of Disorder
- Arousal from deep NREM sleep results in sleepwalking, occurring in stage IV sleep, usually 1–2 hours into sleep
- May involve complex motor activity such as eating or driving
- May be precipitated by fever, stress, sleep deprivation, and medications
- Occurs most often in school-aged children

Etiology
- Genetic component is linked with HLA gene
- No gender predominance is shown
- Occurs typically between ages 3 and 10
- Ten to twenty percent of all children
- One to four percent in adults who had somnambulism as a child

Risk Factors
- Sleep deprivation
- Psychotropic medications may raise risk of somnambulism
- Changes in routine
- Fatigue
- Daily stress

Diagnosis

Differential Diagnosis
- Nocturnal dissociative episodes
- Frontal lobe seizures
- Delirium associated with medical or neurologic disorder
- Sleep-disordered breathing

ICD Code
9-CM 307.46 Sleepwalking Disorder

Initial Assessment
- Sleep hygiene
- Related medical conditions
- Data on snoring, sleep movements, irregular breathing patterns, length of sleep, and changes in mood should be obtained from family
- Data on length of time with sleep disturbance, difficulty falling asleep, repeated awakenings, or early-morning awakening history should be obtained
- New stressors
- New medications, OTC meds, or herbal supplements

Clinical Presentation
- Frequent episodes of rising from bed during sleep and walking about
- Usually occurs in first third of major sleep episode
- Patient has a blank face and stares straight ahead
- Is unresponsive to verbal or tactile stimuli
- May have short period of confusion, once awakened

Laboratory Tests
- None are necessary usually

DSM-IV-TR Diagnostic Criteria
- Episodes of rising from sleep and walking, usually occurring during the first third of the sleep period.
- During the sleepwalking, the individual's expression is one of vacantness.
- The individual is relatively unresponsive to the efforts of others to make contact with him/her.
- The individual can only be awakened with difficulty.
- On waking, the individual has amnesia in relation to the sleepwalking episode.
- Within several minutes of waking from the sleepwalking episode, the individual shows no impairment of mental activity (although there may be a short-lived confusion).
- Awareness of sleepwalking is likely to cause some distress for the individual and some impairment of daily and social functioning.

- The disturbance is not the direct physiological effect of substance use or other medical condition.

Treatment
- Lead patient quietly back to bed
- Scheduled awakenings before sleepwalking event normally occurs may help
- Ensure safety
- Avoid precipitating factors
- No medications are indicated for children

- In adults with a history of injurious NREM parasomnia, benzodiazepines may be helpful
- Start with clonazepam (Klonopin) at bedtime

Patient Education
- Protect patient from injury
- Bedroom should be on first floor of home
- Advise parents to avoid trying to awaken child
- Avoid stress and sleep deprivation
- Avoid medications that trigger event
- Monitor for fever and treat before bedtime

Other Resources

Evidence-Based References

American Academy of Sleep Medicine. (2005). *International classification of sleep disorders: Diagnostic and coding manual* (2nd ed.). Westchester, IL: AASM.

American Psychiatric Association. (2000). *Diagnostic and statistical manual of mental disorders (DSM-IV-TR)* (4th ed.). Washington, DC: American Psychiatric Press.

Bozorg, A. M., & Benbadis, S. R. (2008). Narcolepsy. *Medscape.* Retrieved on March 11, 2009, from http://emedicine.medscape.com/article/1188433-overview.

Burns, C. E. (2004). *Sleep and rest.* In C. E. Burns, A. M. Dunn, Brady, M. A., Starr, N. B., & Blosser, C. G. (Eds.), *Pediatric primary care* (pp. 331–343). Philadelphia, PA: Saunders.

Guilleminault, C., Palombini, L., Pelayo, R., & Chervin, R. D. (2004). Sleepwalking and sleep terrors in prepubertal children: What triggers them? *Pediatrics, 111*, 17–25.

Pagel, J. F. (2000). Nightmares and disorders of dreaming. *American Family Physician, 61*, 2037–2044.

Phillips, B. A., Colllop, N. A., Drake, C., Consens, F., Vgontzas, N., & Weaver, T. (2008). Sleep disorders and medical conditions in women. Proceedings of the women & sleep workshop, National sleep foundation, Washington, DC, March 5–6, 2007. *Journal of Women's Health, 17*, 1191–1199.

Plante, D. T., & Winkelman, J. W. (2006). Parasomnias. *Psychiatric Clinics of North America.*

Silber, M. (2001). Sleep disorders. *Neurologic Clinics, 19*, 173–186.

Thiedke, C. C. (2001). Sleep disorders and sleep problems in childhood. *American Family Physician, 63*, 277–284.

Ting, L., & Malhotra, A. (2005). Disorders of sleep. An overview. *Primary Care: Clinics in Office Practice, 32*, 305–318.

Web Resources

- Obstructive Sleep Apnea Syndrome: MediFocusHealth
  This Web site provides a comprehensive guide on obstructive sleep apnea syndrome, including an overview of symptoms, diagnosis, treatment, and current research/study results. The content of the guide is reviewed by Medical Advisory Board of top physicians and is being updated every 3 months from peer-reviewed medical journals. This is definitely a site to check out if you want to learn more about sleep apnea and the latest developments.

- SleepNet: Pro Tech Services
  Everything you wanted to know about sleep disorders but were too tired to ask. SleepNet's goal is to link all the sleep information located on the Internet. While the content isn't comprehensive, its listings of links is very large. It's very easy to get around and we really like its simplicity.

- Sleep Disorders Center, University of Maryland Medical Center: http://www
  This Web site provides information about sleep disorders in adults and children, including an overview of common conditions, treatment strategies, and methods, tips for patients, sleep study information, and more. The site also includes contact information for treatment at the center, but the majority of the site is designed to provide free information to the general public and is very thorough.

- Sleep Disorders Guide—Your Guide to All Sleep Disorders Nishanth
  This Web site provides information about all types of sleep disorders. Descriptions, symptoms, causes, and treatments of various sleep disorders, such as sleep apnea, insomnia, snoring, restless legs and narcolepsy, are explored.

- Sleep Disorders Topic Center: http://www.MentalHelp.net
  This topic center focuses on sleep disorders and includes information on symptoms, causes, treatments and ways to cope. Disorders covered include insomnia, circadian rhythm sleep disorder, sleepwalking, hypersomnia, sleep terror disorder, nightmare disorder, and narcolepsy. In addition, the topic center also includes links to valuable resources, related blog entries, questions and answers, and the opportunity to share experiences through an online support community.

III

Syndromes and Treatments in Child and Adolescent Psychiatry

18. DISORDERS PRESENTING IN INFANCY OR EARLY CHILDHOOD (0–5 YEARS OF AGE)

Asperger's Syndrome

Background Information

Definition of Disorder
- Neurodevelopmental disorder
- Characterized by significant social impairment
- Restricted interests and stereotyped movements
- Similar to autism but no significant delay in language or cognitive abilities
- Similar characteristics to nonverbal learning disability

Etiology
- Most studies are of autism in general; Asperger's syndrome (AS) is included in these studies
- Not caused by immunizations, as previously speculated
- Compelling genetic evidence
- Neuroimaging shows abnormalities in frontal and temporal lobes and amygdala
- Megalencephaly is a consistent finding
- Not fully understood

Demographics
- A total of 3 cases per 10,000 births
- Nine times more frequent in males
- Five times less common than autism

Risk Factors
- Gender: males
- No apparent socioeconomic factors
- Family history
  - Parental psychiatric history (not specifically of autism)
  - Family history of an autoimmune disease
  - Advanced paternal age, >40 years
  - Risk increases with every 10 years—maternal/paternal

Diagnosis

Comorbidities
- Attention-deficit hyperactivity disorder (ADHD)
- Anxiety disorders
- Depression
- Obsessive-compulsive disorder (OCD)
- Oppositional defiance disorder
- Schizophrenia

ICD-9 Code
299.80 Asperger's Disorder

Initial Assessment
- Developmental history
- Milestones met or delayed
- How significant is the delay?
- Onset-age/symptoms
- Symptoms/severity
- Medical history

Diagnostic Evaluation
- Interview is based on *DSM-IV-TR* (see below)
- Most interviews, testing, and scales require specialized training
- Autism diagnostic interview revised—semi-structure interview is based on *DSM*
- Neuropsychological testing
- Cognitive/IQ testing
- Childhood Asperger's syndrome test (CAST)—available online through Autistic Research Centre (ARC)
- The Asperger's syndrome diagnostic scale—Asperger/autism publishing company
- Autism spectrum screening questionnaire (ASSQ); 27-question screen must be purchased
- Gillium autism rating scale available through PRO-ED

Clinical Presentation
- Poor eye contact
- Poor social skills
- Interest in specific area that is restrictive
- Difficulty with transitions
- Sensory sensitivity
- Routine and rule driven
- Cognitively/academically on track
- Early motor clumsiness

DSM-IV-TR Diagnostic Criteria

- Notable difficulty in social interaction, as manifested by two of the following:
  - Presence of a range of restrictions in nonverbal expression/behaviors, including eye contact, facial expression, body posture, and gestures.
  - Failure to develop peer relationships commensurate with age and developmental level.
  - Absence of spontaneous activity.
  - Limited social or emotional reciprocity, limited empathy.
- Restricted and repetitive activities and interests, as manifested by at least one of the following:
  - A very narrowed range of interests, patterns of interest that are aberrant in intensity.
  - Rigid adherences to routines or rituals.
  - Persistent preoccupation with parts of objects (versus objects in their entirety).
- The overall disturbance engenders a notable impairment in social functioning.
- Linguistic development and cognitive development are relatively unaffected.
- Criteria for another pervasive developmental disorder or schizophrenia are not met.

Treatment

Behavioral

- Individual, family, and group therapies—developmentally appropriate
- Behavioral therapy
- Social skills training
- Monitor for sedation, hypotension, dystonia, akathisia, oculogyric crisis, neuroleptic malignant syndrome, elevated prolactin, galactorrhea, amenorrhea, hyperglycemia, insulin resistance, and weight gain
- Monthly, administer an AIMS (abnormal involuntary movement scale) or a DISCUS rating scale to monitor for side effects

- Educate parents about the risk/benefit profile of atypical antipsychotic
- Educate parents on how to recognize extra-pyramidal side effects and neuroleptic malignant syndrome

Pharmacotherapy

- Fluoxetine (Prozac) and fluvoxamine (Luvox) are helpful for rigid/obsessive thinking/irritability
- Fluvoxamine (Luvox) had significant side effects
- Fluoxetine (Prozac) is FDA approved for depression and OCD in children >7 years old.
- Fluoxetine (Prozac)—initiate at 10 mg, children up to 30 mg, adolescents up to 60 mg
- Risperidone (Risperdal) is FDA approved for use in children aged 5–16 for irritability, aggression, deliberate self-harm, temper tantrums, and mood fluctuations in autistic disorders
  - <20 kg (44 lb), 0.25–0.5 mg
  - ≥20 mg (44–99 lb) 0.5–1.0 mg
- An increase of risperidone (Risperdal) of 0.25–0.5 mg can be considered at 2-week intervals. Maximum daily dose is 3 mg
- Initiate risperidone (Risperdal) at 0.5 mg once daily, titrate up to 3 mg/day, divided dose
- Treat comorbid disorders as appropriate

Patient Education

- Explain diagnosis and prognosis
- Community resources
- Social skills education for patient
- Academic education with accommodations for developmental needs

Medical/Legal Pitfalls

- Depending on severity of illness, may require guardian as patient approaches adulthood.
- Informed consent for medications, most are not FDA approved for use in children; this should be part of consent.

Attention-Deficit Hyperactivity Disorder

Background Information

Definition of Disorder

A biochemically based disorder of behavior and attention that results in a persistent pattern of difficulty affecting a child's functioning at home, school, and socially. Symptoms must be outside of the range of normal behavior for developmental level.

- An inability to pay attention or to sustain attention
- Always on the move, often like driven by a motor
- Impulsivity—verbally and physically
- Symptoms interfere with multiple life domains
    - School, social, home, or work
    - Symptoms must be present before age 7

Etiology

- This is not fully understood
- It is hypothesized that inefficient neurochemical processing in the following areas accounts for the complex symptoms of ADHD
    - Dorsal anterior cingulate cortex—selective attention
    - Dorsal lateral prefrontal cortex—sustained attention and problem solving
    - Prefrontal motor cortex—hyperactivity
    - Orbital frontal cortex—impulsivity

Demographics

- About 4.7% of school-age children have ADHD
- Rates are higher among boys than girls
    - This may be secondary to boys having higher rates of disruptive behavior due to hyperactivity and impulsivity.
    - Girls are less likely to be hyperactive and if they have good social skills, they often don't come to the attention of parents, teachers, or health care providers.

Risk Factors

Gender
- Male

Family History
- Family members with ADHD
- Heritability is estimated at $\geq 75\%$

Precipitating Factors
- Infections
- Head injury
- Hypoxia
- Exposure to drugs or alcohol in utero
- Low birth weight

Comorbidity Factors
- Higher incidence of chronic health conditions than in nonaffected children
- High incidence of substance use and abuse
- Six times more likely to have psychiatric comorbidities
    - Oppositional defiant disorder and conduct disorder
    - Developmental disorders
    - Learning disorders
    - Anxiety disorders
    - Mood disorders
    - Sleep problems
        - Difficulty winding down and falling asleep

Socioeconomic Factors
- Children from single-mother families are more likely to have ADHD diagnosis
- Children with Medicaid are more likely to have ADHD diagnosis than privately insured children
- Adolescents with ADHA are more likely to drop out of school
- Higher rates of pregnancy among high school girls
- Higher incidence of legal involvement
- Higher incidence of auto accidents

Diagnosis

ICD-9 Codes

314.01 Attention-Deficit/Hyperactivity Disorder, Combined Type: if both Criteria A1 and A2 are met for the past 6 months

314.00 Attention-Deficit/Hyperactivity Disorder, Predominantly Inattentive Type: if Criterion A1 is met but Criterion A2 is not met for the past 6 months

314.01 Attention-Deficit/Hyperactivity Disorder, Predominantly Hyperactive-Impulsive Type: if Criterion A2 is met but Criterion A1 is not met for the past 6 months

Coding note: For individuals (especially adolescents and adults) who currently have symptoms that no longer meet full criteria, "In Partial Remission" should be specified.

Diagnostic Work-Up

- Vision and hearing screen may be indicated
- Complete blood count (CBC), complete metabolic panel (CMP), thyroid-stimulating hormone (TSH), free thyroxine (T4), liver function test (LFT) are all recommended
- Complete physical may be indicated
- Consider an electrocardiogram (EKG) if contemplating using a stimulant (this is not standardized practice)
- A complete psychiatric assessment is recommended
  - Overall behavior, mood, sleep, drug and alcohol use/abuse
- Rating scales for ADHD
  - Parents and teachers to complete rating scale
    - ADHD rating scale (ages 6–12)
    - Connor's parent and teacher rating scale (reliable with criterion validity)
    - SWAN rating scale (helps differentiate type of ADHD)
    - Vanderbilt (ages 6–12 with parent and teacher scales)
- School records

Initial Assessment

- Prenatal and postnatal care
- Growth and development
- Medical history
- Onset of symptoms
- Establish baseline symptoms
- Severity of symptoms
  - At home, school, work, and socially

Clinical Presentation

Symptom clusters: inattention, impulsive, and hyperactive

- Combined type has features of inattention, impulsivity, and hyperactivity
- Children often do not grasp how their behavior impacts others
  - Kids can feel demoralized by how their symptoms affect their ability to function at home, school, and at play

DSM-IV-TR Diagnostic Guidelines

Inattention Symptoms

- Six or more of the following symptoms of inattention are present for at least 6 months, to a degree that is maladaptive:
  - The individual fails to give attention to details, in schoolwork or other activities.
  - Has difficulty in sustaining attention in performance of tasks.
  - Does not seem to be listening when spoken to directly.
  - Fails to follow through on instructions, fails to complete school work or other duties (with failures not attributable to confrontational behavior or failure to understand instructions).
  - Has difficulty in organizing tasks and other activities.
  - Seeks ways to circumvent tasks that require mental effort.
  - Often loses things.
  - Individual is easily distracted by stimuli of many kinds.
  - Individual is, more often than not, forgetful in daily activities.

Hyperactivity-Impulsivity Symptoms

- Six or more of the following symptoms have persisted for at least 6 months, to a degree that is maladaptive:
  - The individual fidgets or squirms when seated.
  - Leaves seat in classroom or in other situations in which remaining seated is required.
  - Runs about in environments in which it is inappropriate to do so.
  - Has difficulty in engaging in leisure activities quietly.

- Is always on the go.
- Talks excessively.
- Gives answers to questions before questions have been fully verbalized.
- Has difficulty in waiting his or her turn.
- Interrupts the speech of others or intrudes on the activities of others.
- In adolescents and adults: the presence of feelings of extreme restlessness.
- Symptoms were present before age 7.
- Social deficits are present in two or more settings
- Clear evidence of impairment in social functioning.
- The symptoms do not occur concurrently with and exclusively during the course of a pervasive developmental disorder (PDD), schizophrenia, or other psychotic disorder, and are not more readily ascribed to another psychiatric condition.

Treatment

Behavioral
- Individual and family behavior therapy
- School
  - Individual education plans
    - Accommodations for daily work and testing

Pharmacotherapy
- Stimulants
  - Immediate release
  - Extended release
    - Medications to treat ADHD can create sleep disturbance
    - Rebound appetite
  - Twenty percent of patients do not respond to stimulants
  - For patients with substance abuse issues choose stimulants with nonabuse formulations
    - Methylphenidate (Concerta)
    - Daytrana
    - Lisdexamfetamine (Vyvanse)
- Nonstimulants
  - Atomoxetine (Strattera)
    - Black box warning.
    - Analysis of 12 studies revealed 4 out of 1000 children experienced suicidal thoughts. There were no actual suicides in the studies.

- Bupropion (Wellbutrin)
  - Contraindicated in patients with anorexia nervosa and bulimia nervosa
  - Can exacerbate tics
  - CA
  - *Caution*—lowers seizure threshold
- Guanfacine
  - Longer duration of action than with clonidine (Catapres)
  - Immediate and extended release formulation
- Clonidine (Catapres)
  - May be more helpful with hyperactive symptoms
  - Potential cardiac side effects—monitor blood pressure
    - Oral
    - Transdermal patch
- Antidepressants
  - Tricyclic antidepressants (TCA)
    - *Caution*—TCAs are lethal in overdose

Recurrence Rate
- ADHD is a lifelong condition
  - Hyperactive symptoms often dissipate with age as the brain matures and patients develop coping skills
    - Symptoms of inattention persist into adulthood
- Algorithm for treating ADHD by American Academy of Pediatrics
  - http://aappolicy.aappublications.org/cgi/reprint/pediatrics;108/4/1033.pdf

Patient Education
- Nonpharmacological intervention
  - Psychoeducation
    - Understanding of ADHD
    - Coping skills
      - Preplanning
      - Organize study time
      - Break up big tasks into smaller parts
    - Parenting strategies
      - Give one direction at a time
      - A light touch can help refocus attention

- Provide a predictable and consistent schedule
- Get kids ready for school the night before
- Keep in close contact with teachers to proactively problem solve
- Psychosocial support for child and parent
  - Higher rates of divorce are found among parents of children with ADHD
- Urge structure, structure, structure

Medical/Legal Pitfalls

- Comorbid illness: medical and psychiatric.
- Treating ADHD with stimulants can exacerbate other conditions such as bipolar mood disorder, thought disorders, and chemical dependency issues.
- Off-label prescribing.
  - Medication education includes: indications, dose, route, schedule, potential side effects, class effects, off-label use, black box warnings, and alternatives.
- Diversion of stimulants for abuse.
  - A new fad among adolescent babysitters is to go through medicine cabinets and steal prescription medications.
- Persons diagnosed with ADHD are protected under the Americans with Disabilities Act of 1990 and have recourse, should they experience discrimination at school or work.

Autism Disorders

Background Information

Definition of Disorder

Autism is a PDD, is usually evident in the initial years of life (by age 3), and is often observed with other medical abnormalities, such as chromosomal abnormalities, congenital infections, and CNS abnormalities. According to the *DSM-IV*, symptoms include:

- Markedly abnormal or impaired development of *social interaction*, including at least two of the following:
  - Impaired nonverbal behaviors (e.g., eye contact, facial expression, body postures, and gestures)
  - Failure to develop age-appropriate peer relationships
  - Lack of spontaneous activity to share enjoyment, interests, or achievements with others (e.g., play)
- Marked impairment in *communication* as indicated by at least one of the following:
  - Delay or lack of development of spoken language
  - In individuals with adequate speech, the lack of ability to initiate or sustain conversations
  - Stereotyped or repetitive use of language, or idiosyncratic language
  - Lack of spontaneous play
- Restricted repetitive or stereotyped *patterns of behavior*, as indicated by at least one of the following:
  - Narrowed range of interests
  - Inflexible adherence to specific, nonfunctional routines or rituals
  - Stereotyped and repetitive motor mannerisms
  - Persistent preoccupation with parts of objects

Etiology

There is no one known single cause of autism, but it is generally accepted that it is caused by abnormalities in the brain structure or functioning.

- A number of theories are being investigated, including the link between heredity, genetics, and medical problems. In many families there appears to be a pattern of autism or related disabilities, further supporting a genetic basis for the disorder, but no one gene has been identified as causing autism.
- It also appears that some children are born with a susceptibility to autism, but researchers have not yet identified a single "trigger" that causes autism to develop. It is possible that under certain conditions, a cluster of unstable genes may interfere with brain development.
- Other research focuses on pregnancy or delivery problems as well as environmental problems including viral infections, metabolic imbalances, and exposure to environmental chemicals.

Demographics

- A total of 1 case in 150 births, with a median rate of 5 cases per 10,000
- Among 1–1.5 million Americans, it is the fastest-growing developmental disability
- There is 10–70% annual growth in diagnosis
- Lifelong cost of care can be reduced by two-thirds with early diagnosis and intervention

  Note: It is unclear whether the higher reported rates reflect differences in methodology, increased awareness, or an increase in the frequency of autism.

Risk Factors

- Gender: rates are four to five times higher in males. Females with the disorder are more likely to exhibit more severe mental retardation (MR).
- Familial pattern: increased risk of autism among siblings (approximately 5%) and some risk for various developmental difficulties in affected siblings.
- Stressors
  - Having another mental disorder.
  - In most cases, there is an associated diagnosis of MR, ranging from mild to profound.

- Having a child with autism can be a significant stressor for families.
- Change in routine can be a major stressor for the autistic child.

Diagnosis

Differential Diagnosis
- Rett's disorder
- Childhood disintegrative disorder
- Asperger's syndrome
- Selective mutism
- Language disorders
- MR
- Stereotypic movement disorder
- Attention deficit/hyperactivity disorder
- Schizophrenia

ICD-9 Code
F84.0 Childhood Autism

Diagnostic Work-Up
- Autism tends to occur more frequently than expected among children with certain medical conditions, including Fragile X syndrome, tuberous sclerosis, congenital rubella syndrome, and untreated phenylketonuria (PKU).
- Some harmful substances ingested during pregnancy also have been associated with increased risk of autism.
- Seizures may develop, especially in adolescence, in up to 25% of cases.
- Microcephaly and macrocephaly may be observed.

Initial Assessment
- Medical history, including assessing for:
  - Maternal infections, bleeding, or other problems during gestation
  - Experiences in pre-, peri-, and neonatal periods
  - Postnatal, potentially brain-damaging events
  - Medical illnesses of infancy
  - Growth patterns normal
- Physical exam including head circumference, weight and height measurements for growth patterns, and neurological examination. Considerations include posture, gait, and what the child is grasping in his/her hand. Is child

rocking or whirling? Or catatonic? Observe for movements, such as self-biting, hands over ears, hand flapping, clasping, wringing, and clapping. Fingers or other objects in the mouth? Is there facial grimacing? Is child performing visual self-stimulation on a pattern in your office? Note and record any myoclonic jerks. If possible, observe spontaneous handedness. Record spoken language by child, if any. Observe information processing, overstimulation or distraction by visual/auditory information, tactile defensiveness, or delay in response.
- Hearing tests can determine whether hearing problems may be causing developmental delays, especially those related to social skills and language use.
- Behavioral questionnaires are commonly used, and use varies according to age and informant, and presenting symptoms. Commonly used tests are:
  - Modified checklist for autism in toddlers (M-CHAT): evaluates infants who are at least 24 months old, and is used to identify milder autistic symptoms.
  - PDD Screening: this questionnaire is completed by parents to evaluate early signs of autism.
  - Autism screening questionnaire: is used for children 4 years and older.
  - Autism behavior checklist: a screening tool that is completed by the teacher.
  - Childhood autism rating scale: rates how much a child's behavior differs from that of other children the same age (older than 24 months).
  - Autism diagnostic interview: parents provide information about their child's behaviors during this wide-ranging, structured interview.
  - Autism observation schedule: observation of the child performing activities including communication, interaction, play, and other behaviors.
- If a metabolic disorder is suspected, the DAN (Defeat Autism Now!) protocol may be used to pinpoint it; see http://www.healing-arts.org/children/assessment.htm#Metabolic for more information.

Clinical Presentation

- Symptoms of autism vary, but contain core deficiencies in social and communication skills, and behaviors, as previously described. CNS abnormalities will typically be present.
- Assess for known medical conditions, refer for specialty assessment.
- When other medical conditions are present, note on Axis III.
- Assess for sleep problems, as fatigue and attention deficits are often the result of sleep problems or exacerbate behavioral problems.
- There is an increased frequency of GERD, food allergies, and vitamin deficiencies in children with ASD.
- Assess for pain related to a wide range of physical and physiological risk factors, as pain can be a contributor to an increase in emotional and behavioral problems.

Laboratory Tests

When autism is associated with a general medical condition, lab findings consistent with the general medical condition will be tested.

- There are no medical tests for autism, but it should be diagnosed with a team of professionals.
- There are some differences with measures of serotonergic activity, but no specific pattern is clearly identified.
- Imaging studies may be abnormal.
- Electroencephalography (EEG) abnormalities are common, even in the absence of a seizure disorder.
- A laboratory and clinical assessment of malabsorption problems and nutritional deficiencies is prudent, especially if nutrition supplements are being considered.
- Test for lead poisoning, especially if a condition called pica (a craving for substances that are not food, such as dirt or flecks of paint) is present. Children with developmental delays usually continue putting items in their mouth after this stage has passed. This practice can result in lead poisoning, which should be identified and treated as soon as possible.

Treatment

Autism follows a continuous course. Language skills and intelligence are the strongest factors related to progress. In the school-age years, gains in some areas are common, however some adolescents deteriorate and some improve. In general, autistic children respond best to highly structured and specialized treatment. A program that addresses helping parents and caregivers in improving communication, social, behavioral, adaptive, and learning aspects of a child's life will be most successful. Treatments can be broken down into the following five categories.

Behavioral and Communication Approaches

- Using positive reinforcement, self-help, and social skills training to improve behavior and communication.
- Many types of treatments have been developed, including applied behavioral analysis (ABA), treatment and education of autistic and related communication-handicapped children (TEACCH), and sensory integration.

Biomedical and Dietary Approaches

- Medicines are most commonly used to treat related conditions and problem behaviors, including depression, anxiety, hyperactivity, and obsessive-compulsive behaviors.
- Some studies (most unreplicated) have found the following supplements to improve functioning: cod liver oil (with vitamins A and D), vitamins C and B, biotin, selenium, zinc, and magnesium.
- Other studies suggest avoiding copper and taking extra zinc to boost the immune system, and a need for more calcium.

Community Support and Parent Training

- Educating family members about autism and how to effectively manage the symptoms has been shown to reduce family stress and improve the functioning of the child with autism.
- Some families will need more outside assistance than others, depending on their internal functioning, established support systems, and financial situation.

Specialized Therapies

- Speech, occupational, and physical therapies are important for managing autism and should all be included in various aspects of the child's treatment program.
- Speech therapy improves language and social skills.
- Occupational and physical therapy can help improve coordination and motor skills, and help in learning to process information from the senses (sight, sound, hearing, touch, and smell) in more manageable ways.

Complementary Approaches

- Music, play, art, and animal therapy may be used.
- All can help to increase communication, develop social interaction, and provide a sense of accomplishment; and can provide a nonthreatening way to develop a positive relationship with a therapist in a safe environment. Art and music are useful in sensory integration, providing tactile, visual, and auditory stimulation. Music therapy enhances speech development and language comprehension. Songs can teach language and increase the ability to put words together.
- Art therapy can provide a nonverbal, symbolic way for expression.
- Animal therapy, including horseback riding, provides improved coordination and motor development while creating a sense of well-being and self-confidence.

  Note: With most complementary approaches, there may be little scientific research that has been conducted to support the particular therapy.

Chronic Treatment

- There is no known cure, and chronic treatment is necessary and depends on associated symptoms. There are no approved medications for autism. Targeted therapies for specific symptoms have included seratonin specific reuptake inhibitors (SSRIs) for rituals and compulsive behaviors, stimulants for attentive problems, neuroleptics for agitation and aggression, and benzodiazepines for anxiety.
- Be aware of interactions among multiple medications and assess for interactions.

- Treatment needs often change over time, as growth and development occur, and include the abovementioned treatment approaches as well as vocational training and independent living skills, when appropriate, for older youth.

Recurrence Rate

- Follow-up studies indicate that only a small percentage of individuals with autism live and work independently as adults.
- In about one-third of cases, partial independence is possible, and in the highest-functioning adults, some degree of social and communication problems exists, along with markedly restricted interests and activities.

Patient Education

It is important for families to actively seek assistance from whatever sources are available. The following measures are helpful for all families who have a member with autism:

- *Schedule breaks for caregivers.* Daily demands of caring for an autistic child can be overwhelming. Trained personnel can relieve family members from these duties as needed. Breaks can help families communicate in a less stressful context and allow parents to focus on their relationships with other children and significant others. Regular breaks may also help a family continue to care for a child at home, rather than considering out-of-home care. Government programs exist to help families with limited resources.
- *Seek assistance for a child with autism who is entering adolescence.* Community services and public programs can help families during what can be an especially difficult time for their child. An adolescent child may benefit from group home situations, special employment, and other programs designed to help the transition into adulthood.
- *Make contact with other families who have a child with autism.* Local and national groups can help connect families and provide much-needed sources of information. The Internet and targeted Web sites (e.g., www.autism-society.org) can be an important tool, and for connecting with those

with limited community resources (e.g., in rural areas).

Medical/Legal Pitfalls

- Given the complexity of medications, drug interactions, and the unpredictability of how each patient may react to a particular drug, parents should seek out and work with a provider with expertise in the area of medication management and experience with individuals with ASD.
- The U.S. Food and Drug Administration has advised that antidepressants may increase the risk of suicidal thinking in some patients, especially children and adolescents, and all young people being treated with them should be monitored closely for unusual changes in behavior.
- Individuals with ASD may be eligible for specialized education services under the IDEA Act, which mandates the creation of an individualized education program (IEP). The IEP sets goals and objectives and describes what services a child will receive as part of his or her special education program. There is a process to determine eligibility, requiring an evaluation by the child's school district. See http://www.nichcy.org/InformationResources/Documents for more information.

Childhood Disintegrative Disorder

Background Information

Definition of Disorder
- Bioneurological developmental disorder:
    - Onset is after a period of seemingly normal development until at least 2 years of age, may be up to age 10.
    - Regressions may be gradual (from weeks to months) or abrupt (days to weeks).
- After regression, the child has behaviors similar to those seen in autism with deficits in social interactions, communication, restricted range of interests.

Etiology
Etiology is unknown:
- Possibly genetic, involving multiple genes
- Possible autoimmune response
- No link is found to vaccines, infection <2 years old, bilirubin or gastrointestinal (GI) disorders
- Brain is structurally and functionally different from normal brain

Demographics
- Very rare—0.2 cases per 10,000 births
- More boys than girls are affected
- Sixty times less prevalent than autistic disorders

Risk Factors
- Gender: male
- Tuberous sclerosis—noncancerous tumors grow in the brain
- Lipid storage disease—rare group of inherited metabolic disorders
- Subacute sclerosis panencephalitis—chronic infection of brain, is a form of the measles

Diagnosis

Comorbidities
- Mood disorders
- Epilepsy
- High likelihood of MR

ICD-9 Code
299.10 Childhood Disintegrative Disorder

Diagnostic Work-Up
- Interview is based on *DSM-IV-TR* (see below)
- Psychological, neuropsychological, intellectual/cognitive testing—some testing is not valid if patient is nonverbal or has MR. These tests would be referred out
- Neurologic work-up is based on frequency of seizures associated with autism

Initial Assessment
- Parent/child early development
- Including prenatal, perinatal, and postnatal development
- Physical assessment
- Milestones
- Motor/coordination
- Medical history
- Onset of symptoms
- Severity of symptoms (communication, social, behavioral)

Clinical Presentation
- Initial normal development occurs until ages 2–10 (usually ages 3–4)
- Language impairment
- Idiosyncratic or repetitive language
- Strong reaction to sensory stimulation
- Cognitive impairment
- Difficulty with transitions, rule/routine driven
- Poor social skills/relatedness
- Do not develop peer relationships
- Difficulty with social reciprocity
- Stereotyped movements
- Delay or absence of verbal and written language
- Unusual interests or resilient focus on a chosen topic of interest

DSM-IV-TR Diagnostic Criteria
- Late onset of developmental delays, with apparently normal development (with

achievement of age-appropriate developmental milestones) for at least the first 2 years after birth.
- Clinically significant loss of previously acquired skills (before age 10) in at least 2 of the following areas:
  - Language (expressive or receptive)
  - Social skills
  - Bowel or bladder control
  - Motor skills
  - Play
- Deficits in at least 2 of the following areas:
  - Social interaction, including peer relationships.
  - Communications skills, including an inability to initiate or sustain a conversation.
  - Repetitive patterns of behavior, narrowed range of interests.
- The disturbance is not better accounted for by another pervasive developmental disorder or schizophrenia.

Treatment
- Parent education programs
- Behavior therapy
- Social skills training
- Special education in academic setting
- Music therapy is shown to be helpful with expression
- Ancillary therapies—occupational therapy, physical therapy
- Treatment of co-occurring medical conditions
- Haldol (haloperidol) has been one of the most studied medications with efficacy shown for behavioral discontrol in autism spectrum disorders but there is no FDA approval for children

- Risperdal is FDA approved for use in children ages 5–16 for irritability, aggression, deliberate self-harm, temper tantrums, and mood fluctuations in autistic disorders: $0 < 20$ kg (44 lb), 0.25–0.5 mg, $0 \geq 20$ mg (44–99 lb), 0.5–1.0 mg. An increase of risperidone (Risperdal) of 0.25–0.5 mg can be considered at 2-week intervals.
- Monitor for sedation, hypotension, dystonia, akathesia, oculogyric crisis, neuroleptic malignant syndrome, elevated prolactin, galactorrhea, amennorhea, hyperglycemia, insulin resistance, and weight gain
  - Monthly, administer an AIMS or DISCUS rating scale to monitor for side effects
  - Educate parents about the risk/benefit profile of an atypical antipsychotic
  - Educate parents on how to recognize extrapyramidal side effects and neuroleptic malignant syndrome

Patient Education
- About diagnosis, including prognosis
- Treatment options (see above)
- Available community resources
- Importance of support systems for family

Medical/Legal Pitfalls
- Most people with autism will require guardianship as they enter adulthood, 2/3 will need intensive care as adults.
- Public law 94–142 mandates provision of free appropriate education up to age 21.
- Informed consent for medications, most are not FDA approved for use in children; this should be part of consent.

Disruptive Behaviors Disorders (NOS, Not Otherwise Specified)

Background Information

Definition of Disorders

Disruptive behavior disorders comprise three disorders:

- Conduct disorder (CD)
- Oppositional-defiant disorder (ODD)
- Attention-deficit disorder (ADD)

Research indicates CD is a more severe form of ODD. Severe ODD can lead to CD. Milder ODD usually does not. The common thread that separates CD and ODD is safety. If a child has CD, there are safety concerns, either the personal safety of others in the school, family, or community, or the safety of the child with CD. These three disorders will be presented as a group to help compare and contrast the similarities and differences among the three.

Conduct Disorder

CD is a repetitive and persistent pattern of behavior in which the basic rights of others or major society rules are violated. At least three of the following criteria must be present in the last 12 months, and at least one criterion must have been present in the last 6 months:

- Aggression to people and animals
- Often bullies, threatens, or intimidates others
- Often initiates physical fights
- Has used a weapon that can cause serious physical harm to others (a bat, brick, broken bottle, knife, gun)
- Is physically cruel to animals or people
- Has stolen while confronting a victim (mugging, purse snatching, extortion, armed robbery)
- Destruction of property
- Deliberate fire setting with the intention of causing serious damage
- Deceitfulness or theft

- Has broken into someone else's house, building, or car
- Often lies to obtain goods or favors or to avoid work
- Theft is committed without confronting a victim (shoplifting, forgery)
- Seriously violates rules
- Often stays out at night despite parental prohibitions, beginning before age 13
- Running away from home overnight at least twice for a lengthy period
- Often skips school before age 13

Note: The above problems cause significant impairment in social, academic, and occupational functioning.

Oppositional-Defiant Disorder

ODD is a psychiatric disorder that is less severe than CD, and is beyond the range of simple stubbornness. The criteria for ODD are as follows. A pattern of negativistic, hostile, and defiant behavior lasting at least 6 months, during which 4 or more of the following are present:

- Often loses temper
- Often argues with adults
- Often actively defies or refuses to comply with adults' requests or rules
- Often deliberately annoys people
- Often blames others for his or her mistakes or misbehavior
- Is often touchy or easily annoyed by others
- Is often angry and resentful
- Is often spiteful and vindictive

Note: The disturbance in behavior causes clinically significant impairment in social, academic, family, or occupational functioning.

All of the criteria above include the word "often." While research indicates these behaviors occur to a varying degree in all children, for the behavior to be considered "often," apply the following criteria:

(1) Has occurred at all during the last 3 months:
   - Is spiteful and vindictive
   - Blames others for his or her mistakes or misbehavior
(2) Occurs at least twice a week:
   - Is overly touchy or easily annoyed by others
   - Loses temper
   - Argues with significant others
   - Actively defies or refuses to comply with adults' requests or rules
(3) Occurs at least four times per week:
   - Is angry and resentful
   - Deliberately annoys people

Attention-Deficit Disorder/Attention-Deficit Hyperactivity Disorder

ADHD is one of the most common disorders diagnosed in youth. The essential feature is a persistent pattern of inattention and/or hyperactivity and impulsivity that is more frequent and severe than typically observed in individuals at a comparable level of development. ADHD has been associated with impaired academic achievement, rejection, and family resentment and antagonism. The most common symptoms of ADHD are as follows:

- Impulsiveness: acting before thinking of consequences, jumping from one activity to another, disorganization, tendency to interrupt other people's conversations.
- Hyperactivity: restlessness, often characterized by an inability to sit still, fidgeting, squirminess, climbing on things, restless sleep.
- Inattention: distracted, daydreaming, not finishing work, difficulty listening.

Etiology

- Problematic behaviors are the result of both difficult temperament qualities (e.g., low frustration tolerance, demanding, inflexibility, low psychophysiological arousal) of the child and environmental influences, including poor parenting, family stress and adversity, association with deviant peers, and trauma.

- Some theorists believe ODD is the result of disruption of normal behavioral development, and that children may get stuck in the 2–4-year-old stage of development.
- Cognitions may also influence the development of CD, as these youth have been found to misinterpret or distort social cues during interactions and have deficits in social problem solving. Thus they generate fewer alternate solutions to social problems, seek less information, see problems as having a hostile basis, and anticipate fewer consequences than children without CD.
- A specific cause of ADHD and other behavior disorders is not known. There are, however, a number of factors that may contribute to ADHD, including genetics, diet, and social and physical environments.
  - *Genetic factors*: Twin studies indicate that the disorder is highly heritable and that genetics are a factor in about 75% of ADHD cases. It is believed a large majority of ADHD cases arise from a combination of various genes, many of which affect dopamine transporters. The broad selection of targets indicates that ADHD does not follow the traditional model of a "genetic disease" and should therefore be viewed as a complex interaction between genetic and environmental factors. Twin studies suggest 9–20% of the variance in ADD symptoms can be attributed to nonshared environmental or nongenetic factors.
  - *Environmental factors*: alcohol and tobacco smoke during pregnancy and environmental exposure. Premature birth may play a role. A meta-analysis found that elimination of artificial food coloring and preservatives may provide a benefit to children with ADHD. Also, children who grow up in an environment where there is poverty, alcohol or drug use, or violence are more likely to develop ODD.

Demographics

- Six percent of children in the United States may have CD. The incidence varies. For example, in a New York sample, 12% had a moderate level of

CD and 4% had severe CD. Prevalence is based primarily on referral rates, and since many youth are never referred for mental health services, the actual incidence may be higher.

- Prevalence of ODD ranges from 2 to 16%, and is strongly associated with later development of CD, and untreated; about 52% continue to exhibit problems.
- For youth with CD, the co-occurrence with ADHD is at least 50%.
- High comorbidity (32–37%) exists between behavior disorders and anxiety and depression, and learning disorders and academic failure.
- Prevalence estimates of ADHD vary according to methods of assessment, diagnostic criteria, informants, and population sampled, and prevalence in school-age children is 3–16%.

Risk Factors

- Gender: ADHD occurs twice as commonly in boys as in girls. However, there is some evidence that it is underdiagnosed in girls because they may be less likely to exhibit aggressive behaviors and so go unnoticed.
- Family history: the majority of studies performed to assess genetics in ADHD have supported a strong familial nature of this disorder. Family studies have identified a 2- to 8-fold increase in the risk for ADHD in parents and siblings of children with ADHD.
- Maternal smoking during pregnancy.
- Some theorists have proposed that a lack of empathic concern, or callous disregard for the welfare of other people, is a risk factor for CD.
- Stressors, including increased violence in media, social status competition, and decreased parental involvement, increase risk for disruptive behavior disorders.
- Having another mental disorder.
- Increased risk for CD in children with an adoptive or biological parent with antisocial personality, alcohol dependence, mood disorder, schizophrenia, ADD, or CD, or a sibling with CD.
- Increased risk for CD when there is marital conflict and child abuse/neglect, and inconsistent or harsh parenting style.

Diagnosis

Differential Diagnosis

Conduct Disorder
- Childhood mood disorder or bipolar disorder
- ADHD
- ODD

Oppositional-Defiant Disorder
- CD
- Mood disorder
- Psychotic disorder
- ADD
- MR
- Impaired language comprehension

Attention-Deficit Disorder/Attention-Deficit Hyperactivity Disorder
Problems with the diagnosis and treatment of ADD/ADHD can arise because approximately 65% of ADHD patients may have at least one of the following comorbid disorders:
- Anxiety, communication, mood, and learning disorders.
- Tourette's syndrome.
- Subnormal intelligence.
- ODD (35%) and CD (26%).
- Primary disorder of vigilance: Characterized by poor attention and concentration, as well as difficulties staying awake. These children tend to fidget, yawn, and stretch, and appear to be hyperactive in order to remain alert and active.
- Bipolar disorder: As many as 25% of children with ADHD have bipolar disorder. Children with this combination may demonstrate more aggression and behavioral problems than those with ADHD alone.
- PTSD.
- Medical conditions:
  - Medical conditions that must be excluded include *hypothyroidism*, *anemia*, *lead poisoning*, *chronic illness*, *hearing* or *vision* impairment, *substance abuse*, *medication side effects*, sleep impairment, and *child abuse*.
- Sleep conditions:
  - The relationship between ADHD and sleep is complex and includes an overlap in the central nervous system centers that regulate sleep and

those that regulate attention and arousal. Sleep disorders play a role in the clinical presentation of symptoms of inattention and behavioral dysregulation. Mechanisms that account for excessive daytime sleepiness include: chronic sleep deprivation, fragmented or disrupted sleep, sleep apnea and circadian rhythm disorders.

ICD-9 Codes
CD (F91.8), Specify Type: childhood or adolescent onset; mild, moderate, or severe
ODD (F91.3)
ADD: NOS (F90.9), Combined Type (F90.9), Predominantly Inattentive Type (F98.8), Predominantly Hyperactive/Impulsive Type (F90.0)

Diagnostic Work-Up
- Assessing a child for disruptive behavior disorders begins with complete school and family histories and a medical exam to exclude other causes. A number of medical conditions may cause signs and symptoms similar to those of ADHD, including learning disabilities, mood disturbances, hyperthyroidism, seizure disorders, fetal alcohol syndrome, vision or hearing problems, and Tourette's syndrome.
- Psychiatric interview, including substance use.
- Sleep patterns.
- Nutritional assessment.
- Check for heart conditions before treatment with stimulant medications.
- An evaluation for ADHD should also include checking for learning or language problems, depression, anxiety, and sleep disorders. These and other coexisting conditions are found in as many as one in three children with ADHD.
- Symptoms may not be obvious in an office setting, so questionnaires and interviews will be needed, including the parent, teachers and other people who know the child well, such as babysitters and coaches, may be interviewed.
- Rating scales, such as the Vanderbilt questionnaire, the Conners rating scales or the Achenbach child behavior checklist (CBCL), are helpful in diagnosing behavior disorders.

- It's important to determine not just behavior, but whether the behavior is longstanding or temporary, and when it occurs. Children with behavior disorders exhibit these behaviors over a long period of time and have particular trouble in stressful, demanding situations or in activities that require sustained attention, such as reading, doing math problems, or playing board games.
- Brain scans are not a reliable way to diagnose the disorder, nor are a child's responses to a psychostimulant medication.
- The behaviors do not occur simultaneously with a psychotic disorder.

Clinical Presentation
- Symptoms can vary greatly and are related to cognitive, emotional, and behavioral signs previously described.
- Sleep problems may be reported.
- Culture may influence how children and families communicate symptoms.

Laboratory Tests
- There are currently no laboratory tests assessing chemical status of the living brain.
- CBC with differential and platelet counts are needed periodically when using stimulants to assess for side effects such as leucopenia.
- EKG prior to, and then periodically, when stimulants are prescribed.
- Use of clonidine (Catapres) requires monitoring of blood pressure and cardiovascular parameters.
- Depending on age and assessment test for substance use.

Treatment

Conduct Disorder
- Bupropion (Wellbutrin) has been shown to improve symptoms in ADHD and CD, and SSRIs have been shown to be effective in youth with disruptive disorders and associated major depression.
- Stimulants, antidepressants, lithium, anticonvulsants, risperidone (Risperdal), and clonidine (Catapres) have all been used in the treatment of CD.

- No medications have been found consistently effective in the treatment of CD alone without other disorders such as ADHD or mood disorders.
- Initial intervention is to teach all family members clear, direct, and specific communication techniques; and how to consistently set rules, limits, and expectations. A home rules contract, setup with the help of a therapist can provide the high level of structure that is needed.
- It is helpful to set aside time each day for interacting with children or teens with CD (e.g., play, sports, shopping).
- In extreme cases, intensive behavior modification in a residential setting may be needed. The World-wide Association of Programs six-level behavior modification programs can offer hope to parents who are dealing with teens diagnosed with either CD or ODD.
- Teens with CD are poorly bonded to people and institutions, including broader social rules; and may come into contact with the juvenile justice system. Unfortunately, experiences with other deviant peers often worsen the behavior, as do group therapy programs.
- Residential programs such as military-style camps (e.g., boot camps) are popular but studies of their effectiveness indicate poorer outcomes in the young adult years, with lower employment rates and higher rates of felony arrests.

Oppositional-Defiant Disorder

- Treatments for ODD and other behavior disorders are tailored specifically to the individual child and different treatments are used for preschoolers, school-aged, children, and adolescents.
- Parent-training programs, individual and family therapy, social skills training, cognitive behavioral therapy (CBT), and social skills training are useful in combination.
- An approach developed by Russell Barkley (see Barkley, R., and Benton, C., [1998], *Your Defiant Child*, NY: Guilford Press) uses a parent-training model that focuses on positive approaches to increase compliance, only later introducing methods to extinguish negative or noncompliant behaviors.

- One study examined the use of Ritalin to treat children with both ADHD and ODD. This study found that 90% of the children treated with methylphenidate (Ritalin) no longer had the ODD by the end of the study. The study had a significant amount of dropouts, but even if these children are included as treatment failures, the study still showed a 75% success rate.
- One study showed that 80% of children with explosive behavior improved when given the mood stabilizer divalproex (Depakote).

Attention-Deficit Disorder/Attention-Deficit Hyperactivity Disorder

- Methods of treatment often involve some combination of behavior modifications, life-style changes, counseling, and medication.
- Stimulant medications (e.g., methylphenidate and amphetamine) are the most clinically and cost-effective method of treating ADHD, but are not recommended for preschool children. Stimulants improved teachers' and parents' ratings of disruptive behavior, but did not improve academic achievement. Stimulants neither increased nor decreased rates of delinquency. No significant differences between the various drugs in terms of efficacy or side effects have been found. About 70% of children improve after being treated with stimulants. Stimulants, in the short term, have been found to be safe in the appropriately selected patient and appear well tolerated over 5 years of treatment. Long-term safety has not been determined. Amphetamines such as Adderall have warnings about potential for abuse, drug dependence, and sudden death.
- It may take some time to find the best medication, dosage, and schedule. Some children respond to one type of stimulant but not another. The amount of medication needed may be adjusted over time, and scheduled upon the target outcome (e.g., performance at school, given on school days).
- Side effects occur sometimes with stimulant medication. These tend to happen early in treatment and are usually mild and short-lived. The most common side effects include the

following: decreased appetite/weight loss, sleep problems, headaches, jitteriness, social withdrawal, and stomachaches.

- Comorbid disorders or substance abuse can make the diagnosis and treatment of ADHD more difficult. Psychosocial therapy is useful in treating some comorbid conditions.
- Behavioral interventions:
  - Psychological therapies used to treat ADHD include psychoeducational input, behavior therapy, cognitive behavioral therapy, interpersonal psychotherapy, family therapy, school-based interventions, social skills training, and parent management training.
- Parent training and education have been found to have short-term benefits. Family therapy has shown to be of little use in the treatment of ADHD.
- Support groups.

Chronic Treatment

Behavior therapy, in addition to medication management, enables parents, teachers, and other caregivers to learn better ways to work with and relate to the child with ADHD. There are three basic principles to any behavior therapy approach:

- Set specific goals. Set clear goals such as staying focused on homework for a certain time or sharing toys with friends.
- Provide rewards and consequences. Give a specified reward (positive reinforcement) when she shows the desired behavior. Give a consequence (unwanted result or punishment) when she fails to meet a goal.
- Keep using the rewards and consequences. Using the rewards and consequences consistently for a long time will impact behavior in a positive way.

Recurrence Rate

- Treatment of disruptive behavior disorders is important because persistent symptoms are linked to difficulty in school, social development, and adult health.
- Children with disruptive behavior disorders who respond to initial risperidone (Risperdal) treatment continue to have decreased symptoms when continued on long-term treatment.

- ADHD diagnosed in childhood resolves in 40–90% of individuals by the time they reach adulthood. Those affected are likely to develop coping mechanisms as they mature, thus compensating for their previous ADHD. Thirty-seven percent of those with ADHD do not get a high school diploma even though many will receive special-education services. The combined outcomes of the expulsion and dropout rates indicate that almost half of all ADHD students never finish high school, and less than 5% of individuals with ADHD get a college degree as compared to 28% of the general population.
- People with ADHD tend to work better in less structured environments with fewer rules. Self-employment or jobs with greater autonomy are generally well suited for them. Hyperactive types are likely to change jobs often due to their constant need for new interests and stimulations to keep motivated.

Patient Education

Conduct Disorder

- Emphasize the seriousness of CD and the possibility of a poor prognosis if there is not significant family intervention.
- Any comorbid substance abuse should be treated first.
- Multisystemic treatment addresses serious antisocial behavior, is targeted to the home, school, and community environment; is carried out in the child's natural settings; and has been shown to reduce juvenile incarcerations and out-of-home placements.

Oppositional-Defiant Disorder

- All children with disruptive behavior disorders may be eligible for special-education services.
- The most effective way to address ODD is through parent management training and programs specific to the child's age. These programs can be quite expensive. They often cost $100/week or more and last from several months up to half a year. Insurance may not pay for such programs. However, some online and home-based programs exist that have been shown to be effective.

- Generally, the younger the child is when enrolled in such a program, the better the outcome will be.

Attention Deficit Disorder/Attention Deficit Hyperactivity Disorder

- Maintain a daily schedule. Try to keep the time that she wakes up, eats, bathes, leaves for school, and goes to sleep the same each day.
- Cut down on distractions. Loud music, computer games and television can be overstimulating. Make it a rule to keep the TV or music off during mealtime and while doing homework.
- Organize the house. If there are specific and logical places to keep schoolwork, toys, and clothes, they are less likely to be lost.
- Reward positive behavior. Offer kind words, hugs, or small prizes for reaching goals in a timely manner or for good behavior.
- Set small, reachable goals. Aim for slow progress rather than instant results. Use charts and checklists to track progress with homework or chores. Keep instructions brief. Offer frequent, friendly reminders.
- Limit choices to two or three options at a time.
- Find activities at which the young person can succeed. All children need to experience success to feel good about themselves.
- Use calm discipline. Use consequences such as time-out, removing the child from the situation, or distraction. Sometimes it is best to simply ignore the behavior. Physical punishment, such as spanking or slapping, is not helpful. Discuss the behavior when all parties are calm.

Medical/Legal Pitfalls

- There is a significantly higher risk for injury-producing automobile accidents in older adolescents and adult drivers. The major factors contributing to this higher risk were higher rates of drunken driving, street racing, and traffic violations. Those with more severe ADHD symptoms were more likely to be in danger.
- Regular checkups are needed to evaluate medication and assess for side effects.
- Due to the potential for abuse with some medications (e.g., stimulants), it is important to address this issue with the patient and family. Drug dependence with stimulants can occur and drug holidays should be considered.
- Children with disruptive behaviors are often qualified to receive specialized education services through the local school system. See http://www.nichcy.org/InformationResources/ Documents for more information.
- Early sexual activity is associated with emotional and physical health risks. Sexual activity increases risk of contracting sexually transmitted infections and pregnancy. In 2005, 18% of students in grades 9–12 who had sexual intercourse in the past 3 months reported that they used birth control pills before their prior sexual intercourse and 63% reported condom use.
- It is important to note that the U.S. Food and Drug Administration has advised that antidepressants may increase the risk of suicidal thinking in some patients, especially children and adolescents, and all people being treated with them should be monitored closely for unusual changes in behavior.
- Risperidone (Risperdal) treatment of children with disruptive behavior disorders can lead to initial weight gain, elevated prolactin levels, and somnolence.
- Youth with behavioral problems often become involved in the juvenile court system.
- Nurses are mandated reporters of suspected child abuse or neglect. See: http://www.aabs. com/PDF/childabuse.pdf for more information.

Dyslexia

Background Information

Definition of Disorder
- Language-based reading disorder
- *Dys* = difficulty, *lexia* = language
- Difficulty with written language: writing, spelling, and reading
- Combination of phonological and letter processing errors
- Persons with reading disorders have normal intellect

Etiology
- Neurobiological disorders
- Inherited genetic connections

Demographics
- Evenly distributed between sexes, cultures, and social groups
- All languages are affected
- Twenty percent of any given population is likely to have some degree of reading difficulty

Risk Factors
- Boys twice as likely as girls
- Family history of reading and learning disabilities
- Families with histories of autoimmune disease (asthma and diabetes)

Diagnosis

ICD-9 Code
315.00 Developmental Reading Disorder

Diagnostic Work-Up
- Functional hearing exam
- Functional eye exam
  Testing is standardized: refer to psychologist, education specialist, or dyslexia.

Initial Assessment
- Was there any birth trauma?
- Growth and development: Were mile stones met on time for speaking?
- Is there a family history of learning disabilities?
- History of chronic ear infections
- Has the child attended school regularly?
- Specialist

Clinical Presentation
- Delay in language acquisition—late to speak
- Does not hear sound patterns
- Difficulty with learning the names and sounds of letters
- Can read a word on one page, but not recognize it on another
- Reading comprehension is well below expected grade level
- Classic warning signs of dyslexia before age 5:
  - Speech delay
  - Slow to get words out
- Warning signs in school-age children:
  - Stuttering and articulation issues
  - Mixes up letters
  - Produces sounds out of sequence (animal = aMinal)
  - Difficulty with letters R, L, M, and N
  - Adds or eliminates words while reading
  - Difficulty with learning how to write
  - Difficulty with memorizing sequences

DSM-IV-TR Diagnostic Criteria
- An individual's ability to read is impaired.
- Reading achievement, as measured by standardized tests of reading accuracy and comprehension, is substantially below age-appropriate reading achievement levels.
- The deficit in reading achievement interferes with academic achievement and activities of daily living that require reading skills.
- If a sensory deficit is also present, the impaired reading ability is in excess of impairments associated with the sensory deficit.
- Note: If a general medical condition (e.g., a neurological condition) or sensory deficit is present, the disorder should be classified as such.

Treatment

- Individual education should plan for accommodations at school
- Small-group education
- Focus on repetition
- Therapies that integrate auditory, visual, and motor inputs

Patient Education

- Dyslexia is a lifelong condition
- Severity of disability is variable

- Treatment is important as children who have difficulty learning often believe they are incapable of learning, give up, and risk failure
- Foster the child's strengths and creativity

Medical/Legal Pitfalls

- Higher incidence of autoimmune disease in families with a history of language disorders
- Protected under the Individuals with Disabilities Education Act (IDEA)
- http://idea.ed.gov

Mental Retardation

Background Information

Definition of Disorder
- Disorder of intellectual functioning
- Limitations in adaptive skills such as communication, self care, social skills
- Mild MR is IQ 50–55 to 70
- Moderate MR is IQ 35–40 to 50–55
- Severe MR is IQ 20–25 to 35–40
- Profound MR is IQ below 20–25

Etiology
- Thirty-five percent of cases have a genetic cause
- Ten percent are caused by malformation syndrome
- Thirty-three percent are external or trauma related (prenatal, perinatal or postnatal factors)
- Causes of twenty percent of cases are unknown

Demographics
- One percent of total population is affected
- Eighty-five percent have mild MR
- Two times more likely to have medical conditions than other populations with mental issues

Risk Factors
- Parental age at birth
- Congenital heart disease
- Parental education/occupation/income
- Trauma
- Phenylketonuria
- Hydrocephalus
- Infection
- Increased lead levels
- Pre/postcerebral hemorrhage

Diagnosis

Comorbidities
- Increased level of MR severity—increased medical comorbidity
- Hypothyroidism, congenital cataracts, cardiac defects
- Fifteen to thirty percent have seizures
- Twenty to thirty percent have a motor handicap such as cerebral palsy
- Ten to twenty percent have a sensory impairment such as a vision handicap
- Five times more likely to have a diagnosable psychiatric illness
- Anxiety disorder, CD, depression, eating disorder (pica and ruminations)
- Seventy-five percent of autistic children have comorbid MR
- Seventy-five percent of people with Down syndrome may have Alzheimer's by age 60
- ADHD rates are similar to general population

ICD-9 Codes
317 Mild Mental Retardation
318.0 Moderate Mental Retardation
318.1 Severe Mental Retardation
318.2 Profound Mental Retardation

Diagnostic Work-Up
- IQ testing
- Physical exam
- Chromosomal analysis
- Brain imaging (MRI or CT)
- EEG
- Urinary amino acids, blood organic acids, lead levels
- Biochemical tests for inborn errors of metabolism

Initial Assessment
- Parent/child early development
- Including prenatal or perinatal development postnatal development
- Physical assessment
- Milestones
- Motor/coordination
- Medical history
- Onset of symptoms
- Severity of symptoms (communication, social, behavioral)

Assessment Tools
- The Aberrant Behavior Checklist—moderate to severe MR

- The Reiss Scales—8 psychopathology scales and 6 maladaptive behaviors

Clinical Presentation
- Decreased cognitive functioning
- Concrete thinking
- May have stereotypical movements
- Difficulty with change/ transitions

DSM-IV-TR Diagnostic Criteria
- Notably substandard intellectual functioning: IQ of approximately 70 or below. (For infants, a judgment of substandard intellectual functioning must be based on a clinical evaluation.)
- The individual cannot fulfill standards of adaptive functioning for his or her age group. Presence of deficits in adaptive functioning in at least 2 of the following areas: communication, care of self, home living, social and interpersonal skills, self-direction, use of community resources, academic skills, work, leisure, health, safety.
- The onset is prior to 18 years.

ICD-9 Code: Based on Degree of Severity Reflecting Level of Intellectual Impairment
- Mild Mental Retardation: IQ level, 50–55 to approximately 70
- Moderate Mental Retardation: IQ level, 35–40 to 50–55
- Severe Mental Retardation: IQ level, 20–25 to 35–40
- Profound Mental Retardation: IQ level below 20 or 25
- 319 Mental Retardation, Severity Unspecified: when there is strong presumption of Mental Retardation but the person's intelligence cannot be tested using standard IQ tests

Treatment
- Parent education programs
- Habilitation focusing on attempts to care for individuals in the community

- Behavior therapy
- Social skills training
- Special education
- Ancillary therapies—occupational therapy, physical therapy
- There are no specific meds used for MR but treat coexisting medical and psychological conditions. There are no medications FDA approved for the use in children for MR
- Neuroleptic/antipsychotics such as risperidone (Risperdal) have been used first line for behavior problems associated with MR but due to the patients limited verbal skills, monitoring side effects is difficult. Strongly weigh the risk/benefit of these meds
- People with Down's syndrome are particularly sensitive to anticholinergics
- People with MR may be disinhibited by sedative-hypnotics—paradoxical reaction
- Benzodiazepines are not used first line

Patient Education
- About diagnosis, including prognosis
- Treatment options
- Available community resources
- Importance of support systems for the family

Medical/Legal Pitfalls
- Most people with MR will require guardianship as they enter adulthood.
- Individuals with Disabilities Education Act (IDEA) guarantees children with disabilities diagnostic, educational, and support service until the age of 21.
- Public law 94–142 mandates provision of free appropriate education up to age 21.
- Informed consent for medications, most are not FDA approved for use in children; this should be part of consent.

Reactive Attachment Disorder

Background Information

Definition of Disorder
RAD is a developmental disorder that is a direct response to abuse, neglect, and disruptions in early caretaking. Attachment and social interaction are rooted in infancy and early childhood. Failures of attachment occur when a child's basic needs for emotional and physical safety, security, and predictability are not met. This failure to attach results in children being incapable of developing normal loving relationships and they exhibit maladaptive and disruptive behaviors. This disorder can be diagnosed as early as one month of age.

Etiology
- Maternal deprivation
- Birth to 36 months is a hallmark period for attachment
  - Attachment Theory—Bowlby (1969)

Demographics
Estimate of 1% of the general population. This is hard to estimate as abuse and neglect are seriously underreported in the United States.

Risk Factors
- Birth to age 5
- Emotional, physical, sexual abuse, and inconsistent care providers
- Genetic vulnerability is unclear
- Being removed from neglectfully or abusive homes
  - Children do attach to abusive care givers
  - Postpartum depression in a mother
- Unwanted pregnancy
- Living in an orphanage or institution
- Parents with abuse histories, mental illness, MR, substance abuse, and behavioral disturbance
- Long medical hospitalizations with separation from parent
- Failure to thrive
- Poverty

Diagnosis

Differential Diagnosis
- ADHD
- Autistic Disorder
- CD
- MR
- ODD
- PDD

ICD-9 Code
393.89 Reactive Attachment Disorder of Infancy or Early Childhood

Diagnostic Work-Up
- Full psychological evaluation with a multidisciplinary approach
  - Psychosocial history
  - Intellectual functioning
  - Psychometric instrument as outlined in Sherpis et al. (2003)

Initial Assessment
- Destruction of property
- Hoarding food
- Highly controlling of others and situations
- Lying about things or issues that the child doesn't need to lie about or when it would be easier to tell the truth
- Refusal to make eye contact
- Does not seek comfort from caregiver
- Failure to initiate or respond to social interactions
- Being demonstrative with strangers and refusing to be separated from new acquaintances
- Dangerous behavior with a lack of remorse
  - Assaulting others
  - Fire setting
  - Injury to self
    - Head banging
    - Hitting and biting oneself
  - Stealing
  - Sexual acting out
  - Learning problems
  - Stereotyped behaviors

- ◆ Nose picking
- ◆ Nail biting
- ◆ Rocking
- The child's negative behaviors are much easier to assess than their attachment
- Ask parents if they are afraid of their child
- Randolph Attachment Disorder Questionnaire (RADQ) is standard

Clinical Presentation

- Inhibited: inability to initiate or respond to social interactions
  - Emotionally withdrawn
  - Guarded
  - Disinterested in others
  - Does not seek comfort
  - Minimal eye contact
  - Avoidance of physical touch
- Disinherited: inability to identify an appropriate attachment figure
  - Indiscreet and superficial attachments to others
  - Knows no stranger
  - Exaggerates need for help
  - Anxious—seeks reassurance
  - Excessive childlike behaviors

DSM-IV-TR Diagnostic Criteria

- Two types
  - Inhibited type: if inhibitions predominate in the clinical presentation.
  - Disinhibited type: if indiscriminate sociability predominates in the clinical presentation.
- Disturbed and developmentally inappropriate ways of relating to others, beginning before age 5 years, as evidenced by either of the following:
  - Failure to initiate social interaction or failure to respond in a developmentally appropriate fashion to many social stimuli, as manifested by excessively inhibited or ambivalent/ contradictory responses.
  - Indiscriminate sociability, with the individual showing a marked inability to form appropriate selective attachments (e.g., excessive familiarity with strangers).
- The social deficits cannot be ascribed to developmental delay (as in mental retardation)

and do not meet criteria for a pervasive developmental disorder.
- Care of the child or infant is very likely to have included at least one of the following:
  - Persistent disregard of the child's basic emotional needs, disregard of the child's need for affection.
  - Persistent disregard of the child's physical needs.
  - Repeated changes of primary caregiver (e.g., frequent changes in foster care setting).
- There is a presumption that the unmet needs are responsible for the failures of social interaction.

Treatment

Behavioral

- There is no "gold standard" treatment for RAD
- Focus treatment effort on parents or primary caregiver
- Play therapy for patient
- Residential treatment
- Behavior management therapy
  - Provides psychoeducation and parenting strategies
- Holding therapy
  - This is not well researched and is highly controversial
- It is not mandatory that children be removed for their previously neglectful parents if those parents have changed their behavior and are now capable of providing a loving, stable relationship and environment

Pharmacotherapy

- Mood stabilizer/antiseizure medications—off label
  - Aggression
  - Mood instability
- Atypical antipsychotics—off label
  - Mood stabilization
  - Disorganized behavior
  - Behavior disturbance
  - Comorbid diagnosis
  - See specific diagnosis

Recurrence Rates

- Lifelong condition

Patient Education

- RAD children need consistent predictable relationships and environment
- Parents must be flexible
- Coach parents on how the child's behavior is not personal and rather a response to failures of empathy and protection
- Older RAD kids often have behavioral disturbances resulting in legal difficulties
- Parents are encouraged to spend time and money resources on themselves as children will get the benefit of parents who feel capable and supported
- Work closely with school and incorporate interventions into the child individual education plan

Medical/Legal Pitfalls

- It is not unusual that adopted children with RAD will be "un-adopted" by their families
- Follow mandatory reporting guidelines for abuse and neglect

Rett Disorder/Rett Syndrome

Background Information

Definition of Disorder
- Neurodevelopmental disorder
- Onset is after a period of seemingly normal development at the age of six to eight months
  - Loss of previously acquired motor and social skills
  - Severe impairment in language development
  - Poor coordination
- First stage: precocious stagnation
  - Age: 6–18 months
  - Developmental stagnation
  - Lasting a few months
- Second stage: rapidly destructive
  - Age: 1–3 years
  - Regression, irritability, crying
  - Autistic behaviors and stereotyped hand movements
  - Breathing irregularities and epilepsy may be present
- Third stage: pseudostationary
  - Ages 2–10
  - Some improvement in socialization
  - Medical difficulties present—ataxia and apraxia, spasticity, scoliosis, and tooth grinding
  - Aerophagia, forced air and saliva expulsions
- Fourth stage: later motor deterioration
  - Age: 10 years
  - Significant motor impairments: scoliosis, dystonia, choreoathetosis
  - Will usually need a wheelchair

Etiology
- Degenerative disease of the white matter
- Reductions in the frontal lobe, caudate nucleus, and mesencephalus
- Seventy-five to eighty percent have mutation of the X-linked MECP2 gene

Demographics
- About 6–7 cases per 100,000 females
- Almost exclusively seen in females
- Males with RS usually die
- Equal among race and ethnic groups

Risk Factors
- Gender: female
- Family history
  - No specific precipitating factors

Diagnosis

Comorbidities
- Epilepsy
- Scoliosis
- Cardiac-prolonged QT and bradycardia
- Breathing difficulties, i.e., apnea
- Motor difficulties, i.e., dystonia, spasticity
- Premature death may come from scoliosis, respiratory infection, or sudden death

ICD-9 Code
299.8 Rett Disorder

Diagnostic Work-Up
- Interview based on *DSM-IV-TR* criteria
- EKG—normal initially but becomes slower as illness progresses
- Molecular genetic testing—CDKL5 mutation testing is not routinely available through most diagnostic labs, go to IRSF Web site (see below) for labs
- Physical-assessing motor, seizure, cardiac respiratory, scoliosis
- Assessment of language delays
- Consult neurologist to address seizures and for help with differential diagnosis

Initial Assessment
- Growth and development including socialization
- Medical history
- Onset of symptoms
- Severity of symptoms
- Timeline of development/regression
- Compare head circumference (head circumference at birth is normal)

Clinical Presentation

- In younger children, may look like autism—often misdiagnosed early
- Significant deterioration in motor, abilities, speech, and socialization
- Few are able to speak
- Frequently present with epilepsy
- Often have stereotypic hand movement, i.e., handwashing movements
- Breathing difficulties, i.e., hyperventilation, air swallowing, breath holding
- Wide gait if able to walk (50% gain independent mobility)
- Scoliosis
- Small hands and feet, may be discolored due to poor circulation

DSM-IV-TR Diagnostic Criteria

- A neurodevelopmental syndrome characterized by all of the following:
  - Apparently normal prenatal and perinatal development.
  - Apparently normal psychomotor development for the first 5 months.
  - Normal head circumference at birth.
- The onset of all of the following after a period of normal development:
  - Deceleration of head growth between ages 5 months and 48 months.
  - Loss of previously acquired focused hand skills, between ages 5 months and 30 months, with the subsequent development of stereotyped hand movements (e.g., hand wringing).
  - Loss of social engagement early in the course of the disorder.
  - Poor gait and poorly coordinated trunk movements.
  - Markedly impaired language development and markedly poor muscle function.

Treatment

- Symptom relief
- Physical therapy for muscular difficulties
- Medications for comorbidities/complications, i.e., epilepsy
- No effective medical treatment for RS exists

Patient Education

- Educate about diagnosis
- Available community resources
- Prognosis
- Prenatal screening is available for subsequent pregnancies

Medical/Legal Pitfalls

- Most people with Rett will require guardianship as they enter adulthood
- Public law 94–142 mandates the provision of free appropriate education up to age 21
- Informed consent for medications, most are not FDA approved for use in children; this should be part of consent

Selective Mutism

Background Information

Definition of Disorder

Selective mutism is a condition where children are unable to speak in situations where talking is an expected behavior. These children are able to talk freely at home and in situations where they are comfortable. They may have articulation problems or a medical condition that affects speech, but overall, SM is an anxiety-based disorder.

Etiology

- The exact etiology is unknown.
- Children with SM are likely to have issues related to shyness, avoidance, and anxiety.

Demographics

- About 0.2–2% of population

Risk Factors

- Age: onset between ages 3 and 6
- Gender: boys and girls
- Family history
  - Parent with history of SM
  - Parents with anxiety disorders
- Precipitating factors
  - Traumatic events during the time of language development
  - Multiple moves in homes or school
  - Being threatened or bullied at school

Diagnosis

Comorbidities

- Developmental disorders
- Elimination disorders
- Learning disabilities
- ODD
- Separation anxiety disorder
- Social phobia

ICD-9 Code

312.23 Selective Mutism

Diagnostic Work-Up

- Dental exam
- Hearing evaluation
- Rule out language disorders:
  - Consultation with a speech language pathologist
- Rule out medical causes:
  - Asthma—being short of breath makes it difficult to speak
- Rating scales
  - Anxiety Disorder Interview Schedule for Children
  - Social Anxiety Scale for Children-R
  - Vineland language scale (parents and teachers)
  - Achenbach scale (parents and teachers)

Initial Assessment

- Baseline level of functioning
- Onset of symptoms
  - Difficulties may not come into focus until the child enters school
- Environments and situations where the child is mute
- How does the child communicate at home, school, and in social situations?
  - Gestures, writing, whispering
  - Will child talk on the phone?
  - Will child talk to people in one situation, but not in another?
    - Talks to a friend in the child's home, but not at school

Clinical Presentation

Refuses to speak in situations where talking is appropriate and expected.

DSM-IV-TR Diagnostic Criteria

- Consistent inability to speak in specific social situations in persons who are capable of speech in other situations.
- The disturbance interferes with educational/occupational/social functioning.
- A duration of at least 1 month (excluding the first month of school attendance).
- The failure cannot be ascribed to a lack of familiarity or comfort with the spoken language.

- The disturbance is not more easily ascribed to a communication disorder (e.g., stuttering) and does not occur concurrently with and exclusively during the course of a pervasive developmental disorder, schizophrenia, or other psychotic disorder.

Treatment
- Individual and family therapy
- Behavioral therapy
- Cognitive therapy
- Exposure therapy
- Skills training
  - Communication skills
  - Anxiety management
- Speech language pathologist

- SSRIs may be appropriate to treat anxiety symptoms
  - Case studies report benefit
    - Fluoxetine is most studied
  - Coordinate services with school

Patient Education
- SM can remit on its own without treatment
- Treatment may take several months before benefit is noted
- Reinforce positive accomplishments
- Educational pitfalls
- Hinders social development
- Interferes with reading language developmental tasks
- Hinders a child's ability to engage in regular and extracurricular activities

Separation Anxiety Disorder

Background Information

Definition of Disorder
- Anxiety disorder of childhood and early adolescence
- Characterized by unrealistic fear of separation from attachment figures
- Interferes significantly with daily life and development
- Begins before the age of 18

Etiology
- Genetic link but only in girls
- Temperamental traits
- Parental rearing styles
- Caregiver stress/support
- Life events

Demographics
- Most common anxiety disorder in childhood
- Prevalence is 2.4%
- Peak onset is 7–9 years of age

Risk Factors
- Female
- Family history of anxiety disorder or depression
- African American
- Lower-socioeconomic-status homes
- Child temperament
- Parenting styles
- Life events such as death or threat of separation

Diagnosis

Comorbidities
- Another anxiety disorder such as OCD, overanxious disorder
- Depression

ICD-9 Code
309.21 Separation Anxiety Disorder

Diagnostic Work-Up
- Clinical interview using *DSM-IV-TR* criteria (see below)
- Anxiety disorder interview schedule for *DSM-IV*—child /parent (ADIS-C/P)
- Screen for child anxiety related emotional disorders (SCARED)—parent and child versions available on line at: wpic.pitt.edu/research/ CARENET/.../PDFForms/ScaredChild-final.pdf

Initial Assessment
- Growth and development
- Current or recent life stressors for child and caregivers
- Significant losses
- Onset of symptoms
- Severity of symptoms
- Medical history
- School reports

Clinical Presentation
- Physical complaints, i.e., stomach or head, particularly on schooldays
- Distress upon separation
- Fears that something bad will happen to parent(s) or attachment figure
- School refusal
- Severe anxiety/worry
- Difficulty with sleep

DSM-IV-TR Diagnostic Criteria
- Disproportionate or extreme anxiety related to separation from the home or from persons to whom the individual is attached, as manifested by 3 or more of the following:
  - Distress for the individual, when separation from the home or "attachment figures" occurs or is anticipated.
  - Frequent worry about losing attachment figures. Worry about harm coming to attachment figures.
  - Frequent worry that an untoward event will lead to separation from attachment figures (e.g., getting lost).
  - Reluctance or refusal to go to school or elsewhere because of fear of separation.

- Reluctance or refusal to be alone or without attachment figures, at home or in other settings.
- Reluctance or refusal to go to sleep in the absence of proximity to an attachment figure, or to sleep away from home.
- Repeated nightmares that include the element of separation.
- Physical symptoms (such as headache, nausea, vomiting) when separation from attachment figures occurs or is anticipated.
- A duration of 4 weeks or more.
- Onset before age 18.
- The disturbance causes significant distress for the individual, or impairment in social functioning.
- The disturbance does not occur exclusively during the course of a pervasive developmental disorder, schizophrenia, or other psychotic disorder
- In adults and adolescents, the disturbance is not more easily ascribed to panic disorder with agoraphobia.

Treatment

- Consensus that CBT is treatment of choice
- Exposure-based CBT is preferable—refer out
- Psychopharmacology is recommended treatment for resistant SAD
- SSRI antidepressants are effective

- Sertraline (Zoloft) and fluoxetine (Prozac) are shown to be effective in RCTs
- Fluoxetine (Prozac), (>7 years old), initiate 10 mg/day; adolescents, initiate 20 mg/day, FDA approved for use in depression and OCD
- Sertraline (Zoloft), (>6 years old), initiate 25 mg/day, FDA approved for use in OCD
- Monitor antidepressants for side effects such as: nausea, agitation, sleep disturbance, suicidal thoughts, changes in appetite, and drowsiness
- SSRIs carry black box warning for increased suicidal ideation
- Results on TCA are mixed—increased risks for cardiac problems
- Benzodiazepines are effective but, due to risk/benefit considerations, are not often used in pediatric population

Patient Education

- About diagnosis
- Treatment options
- Strategies for management of symptoms such as school refusal; accommodation of symptoms makes problem worse
- Community/national resources and supports

Medical/Legal Pitfalls

- School refusal may lead to problems with truancy

Other Resources

Evidence-Based References

American Academy of Child and Adolescent Psychiatry. (2007). Practice parameters for the assessment and treatment of children and adolescents with anxiety disorders. *Journal of American Academy of Child and Adolescent Psychiatry, 46*(2), 267–283.

American Psychiatric Association. (2000). *Diagnostic and statistical manual of mental disorders* (4th ed., text revision). Washington, DC: APA.

Biederman, J. (2005). Attention-deficit/hyperactivity disorder: A selective overview. *Biological Psychiatry, 57,* 1215–1220.

Buckner, J. D., Lopez, C., Dunkle, S., & Joiner, T. E., Jr. (2008). Behavior management training for the treatment of reactive attachment disorder. *Child Maltreatment, 13*(3), 289–297. Retrieved September 1, 2009, from http://www.pubmedcentral.nih.gov/articlerender.fcgi?tool=pubmedandpubmedid=18490700.

Carr, E. G., & Herbert, M. R. *Integrating behavioral and biomedical approaches: A marriage made in heaven.*

Colman, I., Murray, J., Abbott, R. A., Maughan, B., Kuh, D., Croudace, T. J., et al. (2009). *BMJ, 8,* 338.

Cormier, E. J. (2008). Pediatr, Nurs. 2008 Oct;*23*(5):345–357. Epub 2008, June 20. Review.

DuCharme, R. W., & McGrady, R. W. (2003). What is Asperger syndrome? In R. W. DuCharme & T. P. Gullotta (Eds.), *Asperger syndrome: A guide for professionals and families* (pp. 1–20). New York: Plenum Publishers.

Farone, S. V., Perlis, R. H., Doyle, A. E., Smoller, J. W., Goralnick, J. J., Holmgren, M. A., et. al. (2005). Molecular genetics of attention-deficit/hyperactivity disorder. *Biological Psychiatry, 57,* 1313–1323.

Ferguson-Noyes, N., & Wilkinson, A. M. (2008). *Caring for individuals with ADHD throughout the lifespan: An introduction to ADHD.* Counseling Points. American Psychiatric Nurses Association and National Association of Pediatric Nurse Practitioners. Ridgewood, NJ: Delaware Media Group.

Filipek, P. (2005) Medical aspects of autism. In F. Volkmar, R. Paul, A. Klin, & C. Donald (Eds.), *Handbook of autism and pervasive developmental disorders* (pp. 534–578). Hoboken, NJ: Wiley.

Fombonne, E. (2002). Prevalence of childhood disintegrative disorder. *Autism, 6*(2), 149–157.

Fombonne, E. (2005). Epidemiological studies of pervasive developmental disorders. In F. Volkmar, R. Paul, A. Klin, C. Donald (Eds.), *Handbook of autism and pervasive developmental disorders* (pp. 42–69). Hoboken, NJ: Wiley.

Ghaziuddin, M. (2005). A family history study of Asperger syndrome. *Journal of Autism and Developmental Disorders, 35,*177–182.

Gillberg, C., Gillberg, C., Rastam, M., & Wentz, E. (2001). The Asperger syndrome (and high-functioning autism) diagnostic interview (ASDI): A preliminary study of a new structured clinical interview. *Autism, 5,* 57–66.

Hall, S. E. K., & Geher, G. (2003). Behavioral and personality characteristics of children with reactive attachment disorder. *The Journal of Psychology, 137*(2), 145–163.

Kearny, C. A., & Vecchio, J. L. (2007). When a child won't speak. *The Journal of Family Practice, 56*(11), 917–921.

Kessler, R. C., Adler, L., Barkley, R., Biederman, J., Connors, C.K., et al. (2006). The prevalence and correlates of adult ADHD in the United States: results from the National Comorbidity Survey Replication. *American Journal of Psychiatry. 163*(4). 716–723.

Kristensen, H. (2000). Selective mutism and comorbidity with developmental disorder/delay, anxiety disorder, and elimination disorder. *Journal of the American Academy of Child and Adolescent Psychiatry, 39*(2), 249–256.

Loeber, R., Burke, J. D., Pardini, D. A. (2009). *Annual Review of Clinical Psychology.*

MacDonald, H. Z., Beeghly, M., Grant-Knight, W., Augustyn, M., Woods, R. W., et al. (2008). Longitudinal association between infant disorganized attachment and childhood posttraumatic stress symptoms. *Developmental Psychopathology, 20*(2), 493–508.

Mercadante, M. T., Van der Gaag, R. J., & Schwartzman, J. S. (2006). Non-autistic pervasive developmental disorders: Rett's syndrome, childhood disintegrative disorder and pervasive developmental disorder not otherwise specified. *Revista Brasileira de Psiquiatria, 28.*

Muter, V., & Snowling, M. J. (2009). Children at familial risk of dyslexia: Practical implications for an at-risk study. *Children and Adolescent Mental Health, 14*(1), 37–41.

Sakolsky, D., & Birmaher, B. (2008). Pediatric anxiety disorders: Management in primary care. *Current Opinion in Pediatrics, 20*(5), 538–543.

Silverman, W. K., & Dick-Niederhauser, A. (2004). Separation anxiety disorder. In T. L. Morris & J. S. March (Eds.), *Anxiety disorders in children and adolescents* (2nd ed., pp. 212–240). New York: Guilford Press.

Silverman, W. K., & Ollendick, T. H. (2005). Evidence-based assessment of anxiety and its disorders in childhood. *Journal of Clinical Child and Adolescent Psychology, 34*(3), 380–411.

Scahill, L., & Martin, A. (2005). Psychopharmacology. In F. Volkmar, R. Paul, A. Klin, C. Donald (Eds.), *Handbook of autism and pervasive developmental disorders* (pp. 1102–1120). Hoboken, NJ: Wiley.

Schum, R. L. (n.d.). Selective mutism: An integrated treatment approach. The ASHS Leader Online. Retrieved December 22, 2008, from http://www.asha.org/about/publications/leader-archives/2002/q3/020924ftr.htm.

Seida, J. K., Ospina, M. B., Karkhaneh, M., Hartling, L., Smith, V., & Clark, B. (2009). *Developmental Medicine and Child Neurology, 51*(2), 95–104.

Swiezy, N., & Korzekwa, P. (2008). Bridging for success in autism: Training and collaboration across medical, educational, and community systems. *Child and Adolescent Psychiatric Clinics of North America, 17*(4), 907–922, xi, Review.

Woodbury-Smith, M. R., & Volkmar, F. R. (2008). Asperger's syndrome. *European Child and Adolescent Psychiatry, 18*(1), 1–11.

U.S. Department of Health and Human Services. (2008). *Vital and health statistics. Diagnosed attention deficit hyperactivity disorder and learning disability: United States, 2004–2006.* Series 10(237). Atlanta, GA: Centers for Disease Control and Prevention. Retrieved from http://www.cdc.gov/nchs/data/series/sr_10/Sr10_237.pdf.

Volkmar, F., Koenig, K., & State, M. (2005). Childhood disintegrative disorder. In F. R. Volkmar, R. Paul, A. Klin, & D. J. Cohen (Eds.), *Handbook of autism and pervasive developmental disorders* (pp. 70–87). Hoboken, NJ: John Wiley and Sons.

Ziegler, J. C., Castel, D., Georget-Pech, C., George, F., Alario, F. X., & Perry C. (2008). Developmental dyslexia and the dual role model of reading: Simulating individual differences and subtypes. *Cognition, 107*, 151–178.

Web Resources

- http://www.autismcenter.org/treatment_interventions.aspx.
- http://www.asatonline.org/resources/articles/evidencebasedpractice.htm.
- http://www.csha.org/protecteddirectories/magazinearticles/EvidenceBasedPracticeAutism.pdf.
- http://www.ahrq.gov/clinic/epcsums/adhdsum.htm.
- American Academy of Child and Adolescent Psychiatry: http://www.aacap.org.
- American Association on Intellectual and Developmental Disabilities (AAIDD) for professionals: http://www.aaidd.org.
- American Association on Mental Retardation: http://www.aamr.org.
- American Psychiatric Association: http://www.psych.org/.
- American Speech-Language-Hearing Association: http://www.asha.org/default.htm.
- Anxiety Disorders Association of America (ADAA): http://www.adaa.org.
- ARC of the United States: http://www.thearc.org.
- Association for the Treatment and Training in the Attachment of children: http://www.ATTACh.org.
- Autism Society of America: www.autism-society.org.
- CHADD (Children and Adults with Attention Deficit/Hyperactivity Disorder): http://www.chadd.org/.
- Dyslexia Institutes of America: http://www.diaread.com/dyslexiafacts.htm.
- International Dyslexia Association: http://www.interdys.org/.
- International Rett Syndrome Foundation (IRSF): http://www.rettsyndrome.org/.
- MAAP Services for Autism and Asperger Syndrome: http://www.asperger.org/.
- National Alliance on Mental Illness: http://www.nami.org/.
- National Autism Association: http://www.nationalautismassociation.org/.
- National Center for Health Statistics: http://www.cdc.gov/nchs/fastats/adhd.htm.
- National Guideline Clearinghouse: http://www.guideline.gov/summary/summary.aspx?doc_id=11375andnbr=005912andstring=adhd.
- National Institute of Neurological Disorders and Stroke: http://www.ninds.nih.gov/disorders.
- U.S. Autism and Asperger Association: http://www.usautism.org/.
- RAdKid.org: http://radkids.org/.
- Selective Mutism Foundation Inc.: http://www.selectivemutismfoundation.org/about.shtml.
- Selective Mutism Group: http://www.selectivemutism.org/faq/faqs?full=1.
- Southeastern Rett Syndrome Alliance (SRSA): http://www.serett.org/.

Stuttering

Background Information

Definition of Disorder
- Speech disorder characterized by disruptions in speech
- Syllable repetition
- Syllable prolongation
- Halted or interrupted flow of speech

Etiology
- Disorder is not fully understood.
- Research suggests heritability: Chromosome 12q.
- Pathology is the lack of integration between language development and the motor ability needed for a forward flow in speech production.
- Auditory processing has also been implicated as a potential factor in stuttering.
- Dysfluency can be normal in children just learning to talk and stuttering can abate on its own.
- Stuttering is not caused by an emotional disturbance.

Demographics
- One percent of the general population
- About 2.5% of preschoolers
- Male-to-female ratio is 3:1
- Some research supports higher prevalence in African American children

Risk Factors
- Age of onset is prior to ages 3–3.5
- Male
- Brain damage
- Twice as likely in families with a history of stuttering

Diagnosis

Differential Diagnosis
- Normal stuttering: dysfluency beginning before 3 years of age is likely to abate on its own.

ICD-9 Code
307.0 Stuttering

Diagnostic Work-Up
- Functional hearing evaluation
- Oral exam

Initial Assessment
- Prenatal care
- Labor and delivery
- Growth and development
- Age of onset of dysfluency
- Has stuttering lasted longer than 6–12 months?
- Symptoms of anxiety relating to speaking situations
- Does the child stutter while singing, whispering, or talking to a pet?
- Previous treatment for stuttering

Degrees of Dysfluency
This is a guideline and the actual degree of impairment is determined by a speech pathologist.

Normal stuttering (onset prior to age 3):
- Occasional repetition of sounds, syllables, or short words
- Periodic hesitation or insertion of fillers ("uh, um")
- Increases when the child is tired
- No distress to the child

Mild stuttering:
- Frequent repetition of sound, long syllables, or short words
- Physical manifestations: closing eyes, muscle strain in lips
- Occurs more of the time than not
- No distress to mild frustration noted in the child

Severe stuttering:
- Recurring long, repeated sounds: prolongations and blockages
- Pitch of utterances may increase
- Difficulty in most speaking circumstances
- Anxious, fearful, or embarrassed when speaking

Clinical Presentation

- Onset between ages 2 and 7 with a peak occurrence at 5 years
- Difficulty starting a word
- Repeating the sound of a letter or word (usually vowels)
- Repeating sounds more than once every 8–10 sentences
- Use of filler words or utterances ("um, uh")
- Change in pitch
- Rapid blinking
- Facial grimacing
- Lip pressing
- Hands about the face
- Use of physical gestures to get words out
- Looking to the side when speaking
- Emotional distress or embarrassment when speaking

DSM-IV-TR Diagnostic Criteria

- Abnormalities in the fluency, rhythms, and intonations of speech, characterized by frequent occurrences of one or more of the following:
  - Sound and/or syllable repetitions
  - Sound prolongations
  - Interjections, outbursts
  - Pauses within a word
  - Blocking (filled or unfilled pauses in speech)
  - Circumlocutions (word substitutions as a way of avoiding problematic words)
  - The individual exhibits a notable stress in the utterances of words
- The deficits in language fluency impede academic and occupational achievement.
- If a motor deficit related to speech or sensory deficit is present, the difficulties with language fluency are in excess of those usually associated with these deficits.
- *Note:* If a motor deficit related to speech, sensory deficit, or neurological condition is present, the condition should be diagnosed as such.

Treatment

- Refer to a speech/language pathologist (SLP)—first-line treatment.

- SLPs evaluates speech and language issues and establishes a hierarchy of speaking challenges.
- SLPs may recommend mechanical devices such as delayed or altered auditory feedback: patients with dysfluency can often speak fluently when talking in unison with someone else. These devices resemble a hearing aid with a pocket converter. The converter feeds back the patient's voice on a slight delay or an altered pitch and replicates the experience of speaking in unison.
- There is not a gold-standard pharmacological intervention for stuttering.
- Assess for comorbid psychiatric disorders and implement appropriate pharmacological treatments (i.e., anxiety).
- Medication studies for stuttering are with adults.
- *No* medication has been shown to consistently improve, decrease, or mediate social, emotion, or cognitive symptoms of stuttering.
- All medications prescribed for stuttering are "off label" and not FDA approved for the treatment of dysfluency—especially in children.
- Dopamine antagonist
  - Risperidone (Risperdal): 0.25–1.0 mg daily
  - Monitor for sedation, hypotension, dystonia, akathesia, oculogyric crisis, elevated prolactin, galactorrhea, amenorrhea, insulin resistance, and weight gain
  - Monthly, administer an abnormal involuntary movement scale (AIMS) or a DISCUS rating scale to monitor for side effects
  - Educate parents about the risk/benefit profile of an atypical antipsychotic
  - Educate parents on how to recognize extrapyramidal side effects

Patient Education

- Help the child to feel less anxious or self-conscious
- Wait while the child finishes a sentence
- Speak slowly to the child
- Limit questions to the child
- Practice taking talking and listening sessions with the child
- Foster acceptance

- Collaborate with schoolteachers and counselors—kids who stutter are often teased
- Support the child to practice fluency skills
- Clarify that the word "therapy" in speech therapy does not relate to counseling
- Adolescents may benefit from group speech interventions as peers are a major influence in this developmental stage

- The child's course of dysfluency often follows a family pattern in terms of whether stuttering abates on its own or requires treatment

Medical/Legal Pitfalls
- Child is protected under the Individuals with Disabilities Act and antidiscrimination laws
- http://www.stutterlaw. com/index.htm

Pervasive Developmental Disorder—Not Otherwise Specified

Background Information

Definition of Disorder
- Disorder is characterized by delayed social development, verbal, and nonverbal language delays, repetitive nonpurposeful behaviors, restricted range of interest, and unusual sensory responses.
- Clinical presentation is atypical in that there may be a later age of onset after age 3.
- Child has some but not all of the features of autism or their symptoms are a subsyndrome.

Etiology
- Not fully understood
- Multiple potential factors: genetic, neurologic, immunologic, environmental, and obstetrical
- Possible abnormal brain development in first months of life
- Serotonin, norepinephrine, and dopamine may play a role

Demographics
- A total of 1 in 150 children has autism spectrum disorder
- Three to four times more males are affected than females
- Occurs in all racial and ethnic groups

Risk Factors
- Low birth weight
- Gestational age less than 35 weeks
- Lower socioeconomic status
- Older parents (moms older than 30 and dads older than 35 years)
- Parents with psychiatric disorders
- Parents with schizoid personality traits
- Ten to fifteen percent of children with fragile X have autistic traits

Diagnosis

ICD-9 Code
299.80 Pervasive Developmental Disorder

Differential Diagnosis
- Childhood disintegrative disorder: rare, 2 cases in 100,000
- Rett syndrome: rare, 1 case in 10,000–15,000, and almost exclusively girls
- Autism disorder
- Asperger's syndrome
- Fragile X: most common form of inherited mental retardation
- Attention-deficit hyperactivity disorder
- Obsessive-compulsive disorder (OCD)
- Oppositional deviant disorder

Diagnostic Work-Up
- Well child screening hearing exam
- Lab: heavy metal—lead
- Lab: fragile X mental retardation 1 (FMR-1) DNA gene test for fragile X
- Childhood autism rating scale (ages 2 and above)
- Autism diagnosis interview—revised
- Autism diagnosis observation schedule
- Aberrant behavior checklist

Initial Assessment
- Prenatal care
- Labor and delivery
- Growth and development
- Age at onset or when parent first thought that something wasn't "quite right"
- History of self-harm behaviors during fits/tantrums
- History of seizure activity: one in four children has co-occurring seizures that begin in childhood or adolescence
- Did child seem to develop normally, but has tapered off in further language and social skill acquisition?

Clinical Presentation
- Minimal eye contact
- Limited interest in others

- Delay in language acquisition (speaking first word after 2 years of age and no phrases until after 3 years)
- Does not pick up on social cues
- Impaired social reciprocity: the give and take of a conversation or interaction
- Sensitive to sounds, lights, touch, taste, smell, and textures
- Does child know how to play with toys or use toy for intended purpose?
- The child lines up toys or objects
- Overly attached to a specific toy or item
- When overstimulated, can lose control of behavior
- Difficulty in making transitions
- Forced transitions can result in agitation or out-of-control of behavior

DSM-IV-TR Diagnostic Criteria

- A conspicuous and pervasive impairment in the development of reciprocal social skills, associated with impairment of verbal or nonverbal communication skills and/or the presence of a narrowed range of interests and behaviors.
- The criteria for a specific developmental disorder, schizophrenia, schizotypal personality disorder, or avoidant personality disorder are not met.
- *Note:* This category includes "atypical autism"—where patient histories do not meet the criteria for autistic disorder because of late age at onset, atypical symptomatology, partial symptomatology, or all of these.

Treatment

- No cure
- Less than 3 years old: early intervention (EI) programs
- Greater than or equal to 3 years old: school-based EI (individual education plan [IEP])
- Specialized according to impairment and need
- Speech therapy
- Occupational therapy
  - Risperidone (Risperdal)
  - FDA approval for ages 5–16

- For irritability, aggression, deliberate self-harm, temper tantrums, and mood fluctuations
- An increase of risperidone (Risperdal) can be considered at 2-week intervals. Monitor for sedation, hypotension, dystonia, akathesia, oculogyric crisis, neuroleptic malignant syndrome, elevated prolactin, galactorrhea, amenorrhea, hyperglycemia, insulin resistance, and weight gain
- Monthly, administer an AIMS or a DISCUS rating scale to monitor for side effects
- Educate parents about the risk/benefit profile of an atypical antipsychotic
- Educate parents on how to recognize extrapyramidal side effects and neuroleptic malignant syndrome
- SSRIs may decrease repetitive and ritualistic behavior and may improve social reciprocity, *off label, black box warning*
  - FDA approval for treating depression and OCD.
  - Monitor for nausea, agitation, sleep disturbance, suicidal thoughts, changes in appetite, and drowsiness.
- Assess for other comorbid Axis I diagnosis
- Consider referral to community mental health center for case management as child will need a multidisciplinary treatment approach

Patient Education

- Parents with a child who has autism and fragile X may want to consider genetic testing as there is a 50% likelihood that other boys will have the same constellation of autism and mental retardation.
- EI programs are mandated through the Individuals with Disabilities Education Act (IDEA), Part C (Program for Infants and Toddlers with Disabilities).
- EI programs vary from state to state.

Medical/Legal Pitfalls

- Protected under the Individuals with Disabilities Act and antidiscrimination laws.

Conduct Disorder

Background Information

Definition of Disorder

Conduct disorder (CD) is a severe form of oppositional defiant disorder (ODD). CD is characterized by a persistent pattern of behavior that ignores the rights of others with consistent violations of rules and age-appropriate behavior. A hallmark feature of CD is antisocial behavior without court involvement.

Etiology

- It is speculated that children with CDs have elevated sensory thresholds and engage in high-stimulus risk-taking behavior for optimal excitement.
- Serotonin may play a role in this excitatory process. Additionally, there is decreased communication between the amygdale and the ventromedial prefrontal context (VMPF).
- The amygdala is responsible for interpreting distress while the VMPF processes emotion and cognitions.
- Cultural factors may influence behavior where urban decay and violence shape the beliefs and behaviors of children in those communities.

Demographics

- One to four percent of children, aged 9–17 years.

Risk Factors

- Male:female (boys:girls), 5:1
- Low birth weight
- History of abuse and neglect
- Poverty
- Urban environments
- Decreased parental involvement
- Comorbidity
    - Attention-deficit hyperactivity disorder (ADHD)
    - ODD as a previous diagnosis
    - Substance abuse

Diagnosis

Differential Diagnosis

- ODD
- ADHD
- Substance use/abuse
- Depression
- Bipolar mood disorder
- Intermittent explosive disorder

ICD-9 Codes

312.81 Childhood-Onset Type
312.82 Adolescent-Onset Type
312.89 Conduct Disorder, Unspecified Onset

Diagnostic Work-Up

- Physical
- Prenatal care
- Growth and development
- School history
- Family history
- Previous psychiatric history
- Legal history

Initial Assessment

- Establish baseline behavior
    - History of ODD
- Lack of empathy and guilt

Clinical Presentation

- Consistent disregard for society norms and behavioral expectation
- Onset of symptoms in childhood and early adolescence
- Patients typically have a previous diagnosis of ODD
- Often have legal charges by adolescents

DSM-IV-TR Diagnostic Criteria

- Patterns of behavior in which the fundamental (human) rights of others are violated or in which established codes of conduct are violated, as evidenced by the presence of 3 or more of the following within the most recent 12-month period and one of the following in the most recent 6 months:

- Bullies or threatens others
- Initiates physical fights
- Has used a weapon that can bring serious physical harm to others (e.g., a broken bottle)
- Has been physically cruel to persons
- Has been physically cruel to animals
- Has stolen (e.g., has mugged someone)
- Has forced someone into sexual activity
- Has deliberately engaged in fire setting
- Has deliberately destroyed property (other than by fire setting)
- Has broken into a house, business, building, or car
- Has lied to obtain goods or favors, or to avoid obligations
- Has stolen items of some value without confronting a victim (e.g., shoplifting)
- Stays out late, despite parental or other prohibitions (starting before the age of 13 years)
- Has "run away from home," overnight, at least twice (or once without returning for a lengthy period)
- Is often truant from school (starting before the age of 13 years)

- The disturbances in behavior engender impaired social/academic/occupational functioning
- In individuals 18 years or older, the criteria for antisocial personality disorder are not met
- Type, based on age of onset:
  - Childhood-onset: onset of at least one criterion characteristic of conduct disorder prior to age 10
  - Adolescent-onset: absence of any criteria characteristic of conduct disorder prior to age 10
  - Conduct disorder—unspecified onset: when age of onset is unknown

- Severity:
  - Mild: Fewer conduct problems than are needed to make the diagnosis, and conduct problems bring only minor harm to others
  - Moderate: Number of conduct problems and effects on others are intermediate between "mild" and "severe"
  - Severe: A greater number of conduct problems than is needed to make the diagnosis, or conduct problems bring considerable harm to others

Treatment

- Medications to address aggression, inattention, hyperactivity, and impulsivity
  - Caution: avoid formulations that have abuse potential or street value
- Parent training courses
  - Intensive individual, family, and in-home therapy
- Treatment is often difficult because kids typically first interface with the juvenile justice system

Patient Education

- Several studies have found that families who participate in therapy and training courses significantly reduce the amount of time their child spends in psychiatric and legal institutions.
- Lower rates of sibling offenders in families who seek mental health services.
- Patients need education on the importance of following through with community services to reduce the risk of detention or incarceration.

Medical/Legal Pitfalls

- Patients are more likely to engage in risk taking and potentially lethal behavior than in any other psychiatric diagnosis
- Chemical use, abuse, and dependence are rampant
  - Often being under the influence of a substance is a compounding factor in illegal activity

Oppositional Defiant Disorder

Background Information

Definition of Disorder
- Disorder is a consistent pattern of negative, hostile, and disobedient behavior.
- Children with ODD are described as being "stubborn to a fault" and their disruptive behavior is exhibited at home and school.
- These children have difficulty in complying with the most simple requests or directives from adults or persons in authority.

Etiology
- Unknown

Demographics
- Five to fifteen percent in the general population
- Eight-percent lifetime prevalence.
- Up to half of all referrals for outpatient mental health services are related to ODD and conduct-related issues

Risk Factors
- Age: prior to age 8
- Gender
  - Boys more than girls
    - ODD criteria may not fully capture symptoms in girls
- Family history
  - Exposure to alcohol or in utero toxins may contribute, but this is unclear
  - Maternal depression may be a contributing factor in the development of ODD
  - Parenting style of being harsh, punitive, and inconsistent
  - Parents with alcohol abuse and legal issues
    - These children are 18% more likely to have ODD

Diagnosis

Differential Diagnosis and Comorbidities
- ADHD
  - Fifty percent comorbidity
- Mood disorders
- Substance abuse

ICD-9 Code
313.81 Oppositional Defiant Disorder

Diagnostic Work-Up
- Physical
- Establish baseline level of functioning
  - Understand that stubborn and uncooperative behavior can be normal behaviors, depending on the child's developmental stage when compared with peers
- Instruments as reported in AACAP practice parameter
  - http://www.aacap.org/galleries/PracticeParameters/JAACAP_ODD_2007.pdf
    - Conners parent rating scale (CPRS)
    - Vanderbilt ADHD diagnostic parent rating scale
    - Eyberg child behavior inventory

Initial Assessment
- Prenatal care
- Growth and development
- Medical history
- Psychiatric history
- Family history
- School history

Clinical Presentation
- Difficult temperament
- Argumentative
- Stubborn
- Refuses even the simplest request
- Explosive when told *no*
- Blames others for difficulty, failures, or negative behavior
  - "You made me do that"
- Behavioral difficulties are consistent and *not* within the context of mood symptoms

DSM-IV-TR Diagnostic Criteria
- A pattern of antagonism toward others lasting at least 6 months, during which four or more of the following are present:
  - Loses temper easily

- Is likely to be argumentative
- Refuses to comply with, or actively defies, adults' requests
- Goads others
- Is likely to blame others for his or her mistakes or misdeeds
- Is easily annoyed by others
- Is often angry or resentful
- Is often spiteful or vindictive
- *Note:* A criterion is met if the behavior occurs more frequently than is typically observed in individuals of comparable age and emotional development.
- The disturbance in behavior engenders notable impairment of social, academic, or occupational functioning.
- The antagonistic behavior does not occur concurrently with and exclusively during the course of a psychotic disorder or mood disorder.
- The criteria for conduct disorder are not met, and if the individual is 18 years or older, the criteria for antisocial personality disorder are not met.

Treatment

- ODD is not an acute presentation
- Individual therapy
  - Skills training
    - Coping skills for anger management, conflict resolution, and peer issues
- Family therapy
  - Parent skills training
    - Teaching flexibility

- Medications
  - Irritability
  - Comorbid diagnosis

Patient Education

- Start parent skills training as soon as possible
- Target and reward good behavior
- Reasonable behavioral expectations
- Logical consequences
  - Time out
    - Use a kitchen timer
    - Time starts when the children are in their room or on chairs
- Be consistent
  - The rules are the rules, are the rules
- Be flexible
  - Offer a choice
    - "I need you to take out the trash. Do you want to do it now or in 15 minutes?"
- Be very clear
  - General statements like "Straighten up" are too general
    - "I need you to stop hitting your sister"
- Make sure that the child is getting adequate sleep
- Monitor the content of video games and television
  - Aggressive content can normalize violent behavior

Medical/Legal Pitfalls

- Children may need an IEP with a behavioral component to address issues at school
- Children are more likely to interface with school and legal authorities

Learning Disorders

Background Information

Definition of Disorder

- Learning disorders (LDs) are diagnosed when achievements on standardized tests are substantially below (at least two standard deviations) than expected for age, schooling, and level of intelligence, and learning problems significantly interfere with academic achievement and activities of daily living.
- These can be categorized as reading disorder, mathematics disorder, and disorder of written expression, and learning disorders (NOS).
- Children with LDs have specific impairments in acquiring, retaining, and processing information. Standardized tests place them well below their IQ range in their area of difficulty.
- If a sensory deficit is present, the difficulties are in excess of those usually associated with it. Problematic areas may include:
  - Language development and language skills (listening, speaking, reading, writing, and spelling)
  - Social studies
  - Mathematics
  - Social skills
  - Motor skills (fine motor skills, as well as coordination)
  - Cognitive development and memory
  - Attention and organization
  - Test taking

Etiology

- There may be abnormalities in cognitive processing including deficits in visual perception, linguistic processes, attention or memory that precede or are associated with LD.
- CNS damage (prenatal or postnatal).
- LD may also be caused by such medical conditions as a traumatic brain injury or brain infections such as encephalitis or meningitis.
- LD is frequently found in association with a variety of general medical conditions (e.g., lead poisoning, fetal alcohol syndrome, or fragile X syndrome).
- Prenatal factors that may play a role in LDs include eclampsia, placental insufficiency, cord compression, malnutrition and bleeding during pregnancy.
- Ranges from 2 to 10%. Approximately, 5% of students in public schools have LDs.
- School dropout rates for children with LDs are 40% (or 1.5 times the average).
- Prevalence of specific disorders is difficult to determine because many studies focus on the prevalence of LDs in general.
- Reading disorders are the most common form of LD.
- Gender: from 60 to 80% of children with reading disorders are males, but when stringent criteria are used, the disorder has been found to occur at more equal rates in males and females. Males more often display disruptive behaviors in association with LDs.
- Family history: LD aggregates among family members and 40% of first-degree biological relatives of LD children have LDs themselves.
- Demoralization, low self-esteem, and social skill deficits are associated with LD.
- Inadequate teaching.
- Learning problems are often stressful for family members and can strain relationships.
- Children with LDs are more likely to have disruptive behavior disorders.

Diagnosis

Differential Diagnosis

- Differentiate from normal variations in academic achievement, lack of opportunity, poor teaching, and cultural factors.
- Impaired vision or hearing may affect learning, and the learning disability cannot be due to sensory impairment.
- Mental retardation.
- Pervasive developmental disorder.

- Math and written-expression disorders most commonly occur in combination with reading disorders.
- ADHD.
- Ruling out substance use as the most common feature of substance abuse is an impairment in psychosocial and academic functioning.

ICD-9 Codes

F81.0 Reading Disorder
F81.2 Mathematics Disorder
F81.8 Disorder of Written Expression
81.9 Learning Disorder NOS

Diagnostic Work-Up

- Individualized testing reflecting attention to ethnic or cultural background.
- Rule out inadequate teaching and cultural barriers to learning.
- Because standardized group testing is not accurate enough, it is important that special, psychoeducational tests be individually administered to the child to determine if he or she has an LD. In administering the test, give special attention to the child's ethnic and cultural background.
- Commonly used tests include the Wechsler intelligence scale for children (WISC-III), the Woodcock-Johnson psychoeducational battery, the Peabody individual achievement test—revised (PIAT-R), and the California verbal learning test (CVLT).
- For substance use as indicated by assessment.
- To rule out acute infection when problems occur abruptly.

Initial Assessment

- Medical history and physical examination, including hearing and vision tests.
- Psychological assessment to include self-esteem and self-confidence.
- Youth with LDs may also have CD, ADD, or depression.
- A complete medical examination to rule out an organic cause of the problem. This may include an eye exam by an ophthalmologist, a psychological exam by a psychologist, and an otolaryngology exam.

Treatment

Behavioral

- Since youth with LDs have higher rates of depression and anxiety and behavior disorders, concurrent treatment for these symptoms must be considered.
- Skill development specific to the child's limitations (e.g., social skills, problem solving, study skills, anger control, and leisure skills).
- LDs are treated with special educational methods and students with LDs frequently benefit from individualized tutoring, focusing on their specific learning problem.
- Initial strategies focus on improving a child's recognition of the sounds of letters and language through phonics training. Later strategies focus on comprehension, retention, and study skills. Students with disorders of written expression are often encouraged to keep journals and to write with a computer keyboard instead of a pencil. Instruction for students with mathematical disorders emphasizes real-world uses of arithmetic, such as balancing a checkbook or comparing prices.
- In the academic setting, short, brief assignments with time for feedback, preferential seating, reduced written tasks, support in organization and study skills, untimed tests and assignments, and colored cued materials and techniques.
- Symptoms may occur as early as kindergarten.
- Up to 40% of LD youth drop out of school, so chronic counseling, special education services, and other support are often needed.

Recurrence Rate

- LDs can continue into adulthood, but with treatment and special accommodations, symptoms can be decreased.
- Children with undiagnosed LDs or improperly treated/educated may never achieve functional literacy. They often develop serious behavior problems as a result of their frustration with school.

Patient Education

- Children with LDs are often qualified to receive specialized education services through the local school system. See http://www.nichcy.org/ InformationResources/Documents for more information.

- Parents of children with LDs should stay in close contact with educators and school administrators to ensure that their child's IEP undergoes a regular review and continues to provide the maximum educational benefit.
- School evaluations that include observations of the child in class can offer crucial information about coexisting issues.
- Mental health services may be required in addition to special academic services. Issues addressed in counseling children with LDs can include frustration, anxiety related to school performance, poor peer relationships, and depression.

Medical/Legal Issues

- Federal legislation mandates that testing be free of charge within the public school system. The IDEA guides the actions of school committees on special education in determining the eligibility for special services of students through age of 21 years.
- Parents may need legal assistance to ensure their child's needs are met by the school system.

Disorder of Written Expression

Background Information

Definition of Disorder
- Writing abilities that fall below the expected level of performance based on the child's age, education, and intellectual ability
- Difficulty with putting thoughts on paper
- Difficulty with organizing grammatically correct sentences, paragraphs, or narratives
- Poor spelling and poor handwriting

Etiology
- Genetic influences
- Deficits in writing are attributed to faulty interactions between sensory inputs and motor outputs.

Demographics
- Estimated at 4% of schoolchildren
- Equal among boys and girls

Risk Factors
- Family history of LDs: reading, writing, mathematics
- Family history of developmental disorders

Diagnosis

ICD Codes
315.2 Disorder of Written Expression
315.9 Learning Disorder, Not Otherwise Specified

Diagnostic Work-Up
- By an education or language specialist
- Evaluation of affective states (anxiety and worry) that impact writing ability
- Takes into consideration the following:
  - Legibility
  - Speed of writing
  - Spelling
  - Vocabulary
  - Punctuation and usage
  - Sentence construction
  - Organization and planning
  - Attention and concentration
- Evaluates writing ability in context of different writing components: copying, dictating, spontaneity
- Standardized testing
  - Test of written language
  - Test of early written language
  - Standardized intelligence testing

Initial Assessment
- Initial referral often made by a teacher
- Has the child attended school regularly?
- Review of child's academic record: is the child's level of performance below expected level when compared with the peers?

Clinical Presentation
- Frequent spelling errors
- Punctuation errors
- Grammatical errors
- Poor handwriting
- Letters may be reversed, backwards, or undistinguishable
- Doesn't like school because child feels inadequate
- Reluctant to participate in activities that require writing
- May have social problems

DSM-IV-TR Diagnostic Criteria
Disorder of Written Expression
- Writing skills as measured by standardized tests (or functional assessments of writing skills) are notably inferior to what would be expected on the basis of the individual's chronological age, intelligence (as measured by intelligence tests), and age-appropriate educational level.
- The presence of weak writing skills significantly interferes with academic performance and academic achievement, as well as activities of daily living that require the composition of written sentences.
- If a sensory deficit is present, the reduction in writing ability is in excess of that usually associated with that deficit.

- *Note:* If a sensory deficit or another medical condition (such as a neurological condition) is present, the condition should be diagnosed as such.

Learning Disorder—Not Otherwise Specified
- To be used for disorders in learning that do not meet the criteria for a specific learning disorder.
- Very likely to include impairment in 3 areas (reading, written expression, mathematics), which, together, significantly hinder academic achievement, even though performances on tests that measure the 3 skills individually are not substantially below what is expected on the basis of the individual's chronological age, intelligence (as measured by intelligence tests), and age-appropriate educational level.

Treatment
- No medical interventions
- Writing plan is developed by an education and writing specialist in collaboration with teachers and parents
- Family support addresses anxiety or worry related to writing performance
- IEP, which sets goals and identifies interventions for improving performance
- School accommodations: scribes, keyboards, computers, help with class notes, longer test-taking times

Patient Education
- EI is paramount in preventing the potential long-term consequences of LDs, such as poor self-esteem, decreased learning, and academic failure
- Incorporate the child's interest into writing

Medical/Legal Pitfalls
- Protected under the IDEA, http://idea.ed.gov/

Mathematics Disorder

Background Information

Definition of Disorder
- Difficulty with mathematics in a manner that is not consistent with a child's age, intellect, education, and motivation to learn.

Etiology
- Heritability genetic connection
- Cognitive deficits in visual spatial ability

Demographics
- Six to seven percent of school-age children are estimated to have MD.
- Impacts boys and girls equally.
- Two-thirds of all kids with MD have a comorbid diagnosis of language delay, dyslexia, or ADHD.

Risk Factors
- Lower social economic status
- Poor learning environment
- Family history of math disorders
- Preexisting reading disorders: kids with reading problems often have difficulty with comprehension problems, which impacts mathematics

Diagnosis

ICD-9 Code
315.1 Developmental Mathematics Disorder

Diagnostic Work-Up
- Functional eye exam
- Can the child name the number (flash cards with numbers on them)?
- Does the child understand numbering, counting?
- Does the child understand math concepts (base 10)?
- Does the child understand math procedures ($-, +, \times, \div$) or borrowing and carrying numbers?
- Does the child transpose numbers?
- Can the child retrieve math facts from memory (times tables)?

- Testing is standardized: refer to psychologist or education specialist

Initial Assessment
- Is there a family history of learning disability?
- Has the child regularly attended school?
- Is there a consistent pattern of decreased performance in math as compared to other subjects?

Clinical Presentation
- Difficulty with reading and writing numbers
- Difficulty with retaining and retrieving math facts
- Math grades are consistently lower than expected
- Child may be feel demoralized by inability to achieve in mathematics
- Difficulty may not become evident until third grade, when math reasoning is required

DSM-IV-TR Diagnostic Criteria
- Mathematical ability, as measured by standardized tests, is notably inferior to what would be expected on the basis of the individual's chronological age, intelligence (as measured by intelligence tests), and age-appropriate educational level.
- The reduced mathematical ability hinders academic performance, academic achievement, and activities of daily living that require mathematical ability.
- If a sensory deficit is present, the reduction in mathematical ability is in excess of the losses that are usually associated with the deficit.
- *Note:* If a general medical condition (such as a neurological condition) or a sensory deficit is present, the disturbance should be diagnosed as such.

Treatment
- IEP with accommodations as needed
- Teaching strategies as identified by an education specialist
- Address all areas of weakness to foster success (language processing and working memory)

- Develop the child's strengths and abilities to promote resilience
- Screen for comorbid diagnosis

Patient/Family Education

- Organize homework space at home to be free of distractions
- Allow the child to use the fingers or other items to count
- Break down assignments into manageable parts
- Check their work at each step

- Incorporate the child's interest into examples (sports statistics)
- Some children may benefit from talking math problems out or having visual learning aids
- Computer programs can be a fun, creative, and effective way of learning and practicing math skills

Medical/Legal Pitfalls

- Protected under the IDEA, http://idea.ed.gov/

Mixed Receptive-Expressive Language Disorder

Background Information

Definition of Disorder
- A mixed receptive-expressive language disorder is a language disability that causes impairment of both the understanding and the expression of language.

Etiology
- Communication disorders may be developmental or acquired.
- The cause is believed to be based on biological problems such as abnormalities of brain development, or possibly by exposure to toxins during pregnancy, such as abused substances or environmental toxins such as lead.
- A genetic factor is sometimes considered a contributing cause in some cases.
- Some causes of speech and language disorders include hearing loss, neurological disorders, brain injury, mental retardation, drug abuse, physical impairments such as a cleft lip or palate, and vocal abuse or misuse.
- Frequently, however, the cause is unknown.
- For unknown reasons, boys are diagnosed with communication disorders more often than girls.
- Children with communication disorders frequently have other developmental disorders as well.
- Most children with communication disorders are able to speak by the time they enter school; however, they continue to have problems with communication. School-aged children often have problems understanding and formulating words.
- Teens may have more difficulty with understanding or expressing abstract ideas.
- Diagnosis for receptive-expressive language disorder:
  - Most children with communication disorders are first referred for speech and language evaluations when their delays in communicating are noted.
  - A child psychiatrist is usually consulted, especially when emotional or behavioral problems are also present.
  - A comprehensive evaluation also involves psychometric testing (testing designed to assess logical reasoning abilities, reactions to different situations, and thinking performance, not tests of general knowledge) and psychological testing of cognitive abilities.
  - There are varied language disorders—for example, receptive language may be mildly delayed and expressive language may be severely delayed.
  - Knowing the type of mixed receptive-expressive language delay is important because the split may impact academics.
  - For once, the child may exhibit severely delayed receptive language skills and only mildly delayed expressive language.
  - The receptive language difficulties will most likely have a significant impact on being able to follow directions and understand classroom instruction.
  - This child will need extra help (written directions, one-on-one time) in order to be successful.
  - Many speech problems are developmental rather than physiological, and as such they respond to remedial instruction.
  - Language experiences are vital to a young child's development. In the past, children with communication disorders were routinely removed from the regular class for individual speech and language therapy.
  - This is still the case in severe instances, but the trend is toward keeping the child in the mainstream as much as possible.

- In order to accomplish this goal, teamwork among the teacher, the speech and language therapist, the audiologist, and parents is essential.
- Speech improvement and correction are blended into the regular classroom curriculum and the child's natural environment.
- It is a communication disorder in which both the receptive and expressive areas of communication may be affected in any degree, from mild to severe.
- If someone is being assessed on the Wechsler adult intelligence scale, for instance, this may show up in relatively low scores for information, vocabulary and comprehension (perhaps below the 25th percentile). If the person has difficulty with spatial concepts, such as "over," "under," "here," and "there," he or she may have arithmetic difficulties, difficulty in understanding word problems and instructions, or have difficulties using words.
- They may also have a more general problem with words or sentences, both understanding and speaking them.
- If someone is suspected to have a mixed receptive-expressive language disorder, then that person can go to a speech therapist or pathologist, and receive treatment. Most treatments are short-term, and rely on accommodations made in the person's environment, so as to be minimally interfering with work and school functioning.
- Three to five percent of all children have either a receptive or an expressive language disorder, or both.
- These children have difficulty understanding speech (language receptivity) and using language (language expression).
- The cause is unknown, but there may be genetic factors, and malnutrition may play a role.
- Problems with receptive language skills usually begin before the age of four.
- Some mixed language disorders are caused by brain injury, and these are sometimes misdiagnosed as developmental disorders.

Diagnosis

Differential Diagnosis
- Dyslexia
- Autism
- LDs
- Mental retardation

ICD Code
315.32 Mixed Receptive-Expressive Language Disorder

Clinical Presentation
The following are the most common symptoms of communication disorders. However, each child may experience symptoms differently.
- May not speak at all, or may have a limited vocabulary for their age
- Has difficulty in understanding simple directions or is unable to name objects
- Shows problems with socialization
- Inability to follow directions but show comprehension with routine, repetitive directions
- Echolalia (repeating back words or phrases either immediately or at a later time)
- Inappropriate responses to "wh" questions
- Difficulty in responding appropriately to: yes/no questions, either/or questions, who/what/where questions, when/why/how questions
- Repeats back a question first and then responds to them
- High activity level and not attending to spoken language
- Jargon (e.g., unintelligible speech) is used
- Uses "memorized" phrases and sentences
- They may have a problem with words or sentences, in both understanding and speaking them
- Learning problems and academic difficulties occur
- While many speech and language patterns can be called "baby talk" and are part of a young child's normal development, they can become problems if they are not outgrown as expected
- In this way, an initial delay in speech and language or an initial speech pattern can become a disorder, which can cause difficulties in learning. Because of the way the brain develops, it

is easier to learn language and communication skills before the age of 5

- The symptoms of communication disorders may resemble other problems or medical conditions
- Always consult your child's physician for diagnosis of:
  - Problems with language comprehension
  - Problems with language expression
  - Speech containing many articulation errors
  - Difficulty recalling early sight or sound memories

DSM-IV-TR Diagnostic Criteria

- Impairment in both receptive and expressive language development, as demonstrated by lowered scoring on standardized tests (e.g., IQ tests).
- Characterized by reductions in receptive language skills whereby a child has difficulty in extracting usable information from spoken language.
- Characterized by reductions in expressive language skills whereby a child has a diminished vocabulary, has difficulty in producing words and sentences, and uses verb tenses incorrectly.
- *Note:* Measures/tests of language development must be appropriate to and relevant to language use in the specific cultural group.
- Onset is generally before the age of 4. However, this disorder can also occur if there is physical trauma later in childhood, for example, head injury.
- With positive input, some affected children may develop normal language.
- Associated features and disorders as follows:
  - Conversational skills (e.g., waiting one's turn to speak, staying with a topic of conversation) are lacking.
  - A deficit in some aspect of sensory information processing is common (especially in auditory information processing).
  - Difficulties with the language's sound system are often present.
  - Learning disorders are often present.
  - Memory impairments.
  - May occur concurrently with attention-deficit/hyperactivity disorder,

developmental coordination disorder, or enuresis.

- The ability to process verbal output is reduced. The individual may find it difficult to absorb and recall a simple list of instructions.
- There may be high levels of competence in nonlanguage-based problem solving.
- *Note:* A school psychologist, clinical psychologist, psychiatrist, or other qualified specialist should make this diagnosis. If there is a head injury or another medical problem (e.g., encephalitis), a physician should be on the diagnostic team.

Laboratory Tests

- Standardized receptive and expressive language tests can be given to any child suspected of having this disorder.
- An audiogram should also be given to rule out the possibility of deafness, as it is one of the most common causes of language problems.
- All children diagnosed with this condition should be seen by a neurologist or a developmental pediatric specialist to determine if the cause can be reversed.
- If someone is being assessed on the Wechsler adult intelligence scale, for instance, this may show up in relatively low scores for information, vocabulary, and comprehension (perhaps below the 25th percentile). If the person has difficulty with spatial concepts, such as "over," "under," "here," and "there," he or she may have arithmetic difficulties, have difficulty understanding word problems and instructions, or have difficulties using words.

Treatment

- Speech and language therapy are the best approach to this type of language disorder.
- A coordinated effort between parents, teachers, and speech/language and mental health professionals provides the basis for individualized treatment strategies that may include individual or group remediation, special classes, or special resources.
- Special-education techniques are used to increase communication skills in the areas of the deficit.

- A second approach helps the child build on his or her strengths to overcome his or her communication deficit.
- Specific treatment for communication disorders will be determined by your child's physician, special-education teachers, and speech/language and mental health professionals on the basis of:
  - Your child's age, overall health, and medical history
  - Extent of the disorder
- Psychotherapy is also recommended because of the possibility of associated emotional or behavioral problems.
  - Type of disorder
  - Your child's tolerance for specific medications or therapies
  - Expectations for the course of the disorder
  - Your opinion or preference
- Speech-language pathologists assist children who have communication disorders in various ways.
  - They provide individual therapy for the child, consult with the child's teacher about the most effective ways to facilitate the child's communication in the class setting, and work closely with the family to develop goals and techniques for effective therapy in class and at home.
  - Early detection and intervention can address the developmental needs and academic difficulties to improve the quality of life experienced by children with communication disorders.
- The speech-language pathologist may assist vocational teachers and counselors in establishing communication goals related to the work experiences of students and suggest strategies that are effective for the important transition from school to employment and adult life.

Patient Education

- The outcome varies based on the underlying cause.
- Brain injury or other structural pathology is generally associated with a poor outcome with chronic deficiencies in language, while other, more reversible causes can be treated effectively.
- Difficulty in understanding and using language can cause problems with social interaction and in ability to function independently as an adult.
- The outcome varies based on the underlying cause.
- Brain injury or other structural pathology is generally associated with a poor outcome with chronic deficiencies in language, while other, more reversible causes can be treated effectively.
- Difficulty understanding and using language can cause problems with social interaction and ability to function independently as an adult.

Other Resources

Evidence-Based References

American Academy of Child and Adolescent Psychiatry. (1997). Practice parameter for the assessment and treatment of children and adolescents with conduct disorder. Retrieved January 2, 2009, from http://www.aacap.org/galleries/PracticeParameters/Conduct.pdf.

American Academy of Family Physicians. (2008). Oppositional defiant disorder. *American Family Physician*, 78(7), 861–868.

American Psychiatric Association. (2000). *Diagnostic and statistical manual of mental disorder* (4th ed., text revision). Washington, DC: APA.

Berninger, V. W., Abbott, R. D., Abbott, S. P., Graham, S., & Richards, T. (2002). Writing and reading: Connections between language by hand and language by eye. *Journal of Learning Disabilities*, 35(1), 39–56.

Bernstein, B. E. (2008). Learning disorder: Written expression. Retrieved February 15, 2009, from http://emedicine.medscape.com/article/918389-overview.

Bothe, A. K., Davidow, J. H., Bramlett, R. E., Franic, D. M., & Ingham, R. J. (2006). Stuttering treatment research 1970–2005: II. Systemic review incorporating trial quality assessment of pharmacological approaches. *American Journal of Speech-Language Pathology*, 15(4), 342–352.

Chandler, J. (n. d.) Oppositional defiant disorder (odd) and conduct disorder (cd) in children and adolescents: diagnosis and treatment. Retrieved January 2, 2009, from http://www.klis.com/chandler/pamphlet/oddcd/oddcdpamphlet.htm#_Toc121406159.

Department of Health and Human Services. (1999). *Mental health: A report of the Surgeon General*. Retrieved December 27, 2008, from http://www.surgeongeneral.gov/library/mentalhealth/chapter3/sec7.html.

Department of Health and Human Services. (2008). *Autism spectrum disorders: Pervasive developmental disorders*. NIH Publication No. 08-5511. Bethesda, MD: Department of Health and Human Services.

Feifer, S. G. (2007). The neuropsychology of math disorders: Diagnosis and intervention. Retrieved February 12, 2009, from http://www.ahi-online.com/schoolpsychhandouts2008/lasvegas/feiffer-mathematics.pdf.

Fitz, K. (2003). Review of theoretical and applied issues in written language expression. *Canadian Journal of School Psychology*, 18(12), 203–222.

Grigorenko, E. L. (2006). Learning disabilities in juvenile offenders. *Child and Adolescent Psychiatric Clinics of North America*, 15(2), 353–71, viii.

Hadley, P. A. (2006). Assessing the emergence of grammar in toddlers at risk for specific language impairment. *Seminars in Speech and Language*, 27(3), 173–186, Review.

Hamilton, S. S., & Glascoe, F. P. (2006). Evaluation of children with reading difficulties. American Family Physician, 74(12), 2079–2084.

Hearne, A., Packman, A., Onslow, M., & Quine, S. (2008). Stuttering and its treatment in adolescence: The perceptions of people who stutter. *Journal of Fluency Disorders*, 33, 81–98.

Howell, P., Davis, S., & Williams, S. M. (2006). Auditory abilities of speakers who persisted, or recovered, from stuttering. *Journal of Fluency Disorders*, 31, 257–270.

Jones, A. P., Laurens, K. R., Herba, C. M., Barker, G. J., & Viding, E. (2009). Amygdale hypoactivity to fearful faces in boys with conduct problems and callous-unemotional traits. *The American Journal of Psychiatry*, 166(1), 95–102.

Koenig, K., & Scahill, L. (2001). Assessment of children with pervasive developmental disorders. *Journal of Child and Adolescent Psychiatric Nursing*, 14(4), 159–166.

Lavigne, J. V., LeBailly, S. A., Gouze, K. R., Cicchetti, C., Jessup, B. W., Arend, R., et al. (2008). Predictor and moderator effects in the treatment of oppositional defiant disorder in pediatric primary care. *Journal of Pediatric Psychology*, 33(5), 462–472.

McGlaughlin, S. M., Knoop, A. J., & Holliday, G. A. (2005). Differentiating students with mathematics difficulty in college: Mathematics disabilities vs. no diagnosis. *Learning Disability Quarterly*, 28(3), 223–232.

Miller, J. L. (2000). Written expression disorder. Retrieved February 3, 2009, from http://www.athealth.com/consumer/disorders/writtenexp.html.

Rubia, K., Rozmin, H., Smith, A. B., Mohammed, M., Scott, S., Giampietro, V., et al. (2008). Dissociated functional brain abnormalities of inhibition in boys with pure conduct disorder and in boys with pure attention deficit hyperactivity disorder. *The American Journal of Psychiatry*, 165(7), 889–897.

Rubia, K., Smith, A. B., Halari, R., Matsukura, F., Mahammad, M., Taylor, E., et al. (2009). Disorder-specific dissociation of orbitofrontal dysfunction in boys with pure conduct disorder during reward and ventrolateral prefrontal dysfunction in boys with pure ADHD during sustained attention. *The American Journal of Psychiatry*, 166(1), 83–94.

Searright, H. R., Rottnek, F., & Abby, S. L. (2001). Conduct disorder: Diagnosis and treatment in primary care. *American Family Physician*, 63(8), 1579–1588.

Stigler, K. A., & McDougle, D. J. (2008). Pharmacotherapy of irritability in pervasive developmental disorders. *Child and Adolescent Psychiatric Clinics of North America*, 17(4), 739–752.

Tynan, W. D. (2008). Oppositional Defiant Disorder. eMedicine. Retrieved January 2, 2009, from http://emedicine.medscape.com/article/918095-overview.

Van Loosbroek, E., Dirkz, G., Hulstijn, W., & Janssen, F. (2009). When the mental number line involves a delay: The writing of numbers by children of different arithmetical abilities. *Journal of Experimental Child Psychology*, 102, 26–39.

Von Aster, M. G., & Shalev, R. S. (2007). Number development and developmental dyscalculia. *Developmental Medicine & Child Neurology*, 49(11), 868–873.

Woolfenden, S. R., Williams, K., & Peat, J. K. (2002). Family and parenting interventions for conduct disorder and delinquency: A meta-analysis of randomized controlled trials. *Archives of Disease in Childhood*, 86(4), 251–256.

Web Resources

- Athealth.com: http://www.athealth.com/consumer/disorders/writtenexp.html.
- Early Intervention Programs for Infants and Toddlers with Disabilities (Part C of IDEA): http://www.nectac.org/partc/partc.asp#overview.
- eMedicine, Learning Disabilities: http://emedicine.medscape.com.
- Family Self-Help Groups: http://www.nami.org.
- Family Village: http://www.familyvillage.wisc.edu/lib_stut.htm.
- The Interactive Guide to Learning Disabilities for Parents, Teachers, and Children: http://www.ldonline.org.
- Learning Disability Association of America: http://www.ldanatl.org/.
- Learning Disability Forum: Learning Disability Information and Rights: http://learningdisabilityforum.com/.
- Learning Disabilities Online Page: http://www.ldonline.org.
- National Center for Learning Disabilities (NCLD): http://www.ncld.org.
- National Education Association, IDEA/Special Education: http://www.nea.org/specialed.
- National Institute of Neurological Disorders and Stroke: http://www.ninds.nih.gov/disorders/pdd/pdd.htm.
- National Stuttering Association: http://www.nsastutter.org/content/index.php?catid = 1.
- National Youth Violence Prevention Resource Center: http://www.safeyouth.org/scripts/topics/conduct.aspnternet Support.
- Oppositional Defiant Disorder (ODD) and Conduct Disorder (CD) in Children and Adolescents: Diagnosis and Treatment: http://www.klis.com/chandler/pamphlet/oddcd/oddcdpamphlet.htm#_Toc121406159.
- Our Defiant Kids: http://ourdefiantkids.com/.
- The Stuttering Foundation: http://www.stutteringhelp.org/.

Index